Molecular Virology: Clinical Perspectives

Molecular Virology: Clinical Perspectives

Editor: Archie Harless

MURPHY & MOORE
www.murphy-moorepublishing.com

www.murphy-moorepublishing.com

MURPHY & MOORE

Cataloging-in-Publication Data

Molecular virology : clinical perspectives / edited by Archie Harless.
p. cm.
Includes bibliographical references and index.
ISBN 978-1-63987-787-4
1. Molecular virology. 2. Molecular microbiology. 3. Virology. I. Harless, Archie.
QR389 .M65 2023
579.2--dc23

Murphy & Moore Publishing
1 Rockefeller Plaza,
New York City,
NY 10020, USA

ISBN 978-1-63987-787-4

Contents

Preface

In my initial years as a student, I used to run to the library at every possible instance to grab a book and learn something new. Books were my primary source of knowledge and I would not have come such a long way without all that I learnt from them. Thus, when I was approached to edit this book; I became understandably nostalgic. It was an absolute honor to be considered worthy of guiding the current generation as well as those to come. I put all my knowledge and hard work into making this book most beneficial for its readers.

Viruses are microorganisms that replicate only inside the living cells of an organism, such as animals, plants, and microorganisms such as bacteria and archaea. Molecular virology refers to the study of viruses at the level of nucleic acids and proteins. The proliferation of one or more harmful viruses within the body of a host is called a viral infection. Molecular virology seeks to study cellular function and virus biology in order to develop techniques for inhibiting and treating viral infections. Protein-protein, protein-nucleic acid, and protein-lipid interactions control the structure of virus particles. There are several viruses that can introduce their DNA into the nucleus of the host cell. This book provides comprehensive insights into the clinical perspectives of molecular virology. The topics covered herein deal with the core subjects of this field. Researchers and students in the field of virology will be greatly assisted by this book.

I wish to thank my publisher for supporting me at every step. I would also like to thank all the authors who have contributed their researches in this book. I hope this book will be a valuable contribution to the progress of the field.

Editor

1

Impact of Chromatin on HIV Replication

Luis M. Agosto [1], Matthew Gagne [2] and Andrew J. Henderson [1,2,*]

[1] Department of Medicine, Boston University School of Medicine, Boston, MA 02118, USA; E-Mail: agosto@bu.edu

[2] Graduate Program in Microbiology, Boston University School of Medicine, Boston, MA 02118, USA; E-Mail: patsfan@bu.edu

* Author to whom correspondence should be addressed; E-Mail: andrew.henderson@bmc.org

Academic Editor: Jessica Tyler

Abstract: Chromatin influences Human Immunodeficiency Virus (HIV) integration and replication. This review highlights critical host factors that influence chromatin structure and organization and that also impact HIV integration, transcriptional regulation and latency. Furthermore, recent attempts to target chromatin associated factors to reduce the HIV proviral load are discussed.

Keywords: HIV; chromatin; integration; transcription; latency

---

1. Introduction

Retroviruses such as the Human Immunodeficiency Virus (HIV) are defined by their ability to integrate their reverse transcribed genome into the host DNA prior to proviral transcription by the cellular machinery. The role of chromatin in early HIV infection and replication has been extensively studied, revealing that chromatin influences HIV integration as well as the establishment and maintenance of a transcriptionally repressed but inducible reservoir of cells infected with HIV. These latently infected cells present a barrier to curing HIV infection since they are a persistent source of virus following the interruption of antiretroviral treatments. Recent eradication strategies have focused on developing novel compounds and testing new indications for existing drugs that target chromatin remodeling factors. This review will examine the effects of chromatin on the HIV life cycle and discuss the potential of emerging treatments that target chromatin-modifying factors.

2. Chromatin and HIV Integration

Retroviral integration is not a random event and it has been estimated that 70% of HIV provirus is integrated into introns of actively transcribed host genes [1–7]. This bias in provirus location suggests that local chromatin organization influences the site selection of integration. Integration requires a combination of viral factors including capsid, reverse transcriptase and integrase, and host factors that facilitate the HIV pre-integration complex's translocation into the nucleus and targeting the viral genome to the host DNA [8–10]. Several cellular factors have been identified as being a part of the pre-integration complex or to directly interact with HIV integrase [10,11]. These cellular factors may facilitate nuclear translocation of the preintegration complex through the nuclear pores, or influence targeting of the HIV proviral DNA by interacting with chromatin factors. However, few of these proteins have been validated as playing a role in establishing HIV provirus.

The best studied cellular factor that participates in HIV integration is LEDGF/p75 [12–15]. LEDGF/p75 is encoded by the PSIP1 gene and has been described as a transcriptional activator and a splicing factor, although, exactly how this relatively ubiquitous transcription factor functions in regulating gene expression is not clear [13,16–21]. LEDGF/p75 is part of a larger family of transcription factors, the hepatoma-derived growth factor-related proteins, which are defined by conserved N-terminal PWWP and A/T hook domains [22,23]. A/T hook domains mediate LEDGF/p75 non-specific binding [24] whereas the PWWP motif recognizes specific chromatin marks such as acetylated and methylated lysines in histone tails [25]. LEDGF also contains a C-terminal integrase binding domain (IBD) [26–28], which directly interacts with a binding pocket formed by two HIV integrase catalytic core domains (CCD) [28,29]. LEDGF/p75 involvement in HIV integration was initially suspected based on its interaction with integrase [29–31] and knockdown experiments validated the role of LEDGF/p75 in HIV infection and integration [32–36]. These studies demonstrated that although depletion of LEDGF/p75 modestly reduced HIV infection, there was an altered integration pattern with significantly reduced HIV integration into actively transcribed genes and a shift towards promoters and CpG islands being targeted by the provirus [9,14]. Structure and function studies are consistent with a model that LEDGF/p75, through its interactions with chromatin, tethers the HIV integrase dimer to the targeted DNA [24,25,29,37–40]. LEDGF/p75 may also promote integration by protecting HIV integrase from degradation and by stimulating its catalytic activity [24,30,41–43]. Recently, factors that interact with LEDGF/p75, including TOX4, NOVA1 [44], JPO2 [41,42,45] and PogZ, have been implicated in HIV integration [46]. In addition to facilitating HIV integration, LEDGF/p75 may silence HIV transcription and contribute to the establishment and maintenance of HIV latency by forming a complex with Spt6 and Iws1 that promotes the recruitment of repressive chromatin to the HIV promoter [47]. Other chromatin interacting proteins may compliment or even be functionally redundant to LEDGF/p75. For example, hepatoma-derived growth factor-related protein 2 (HRP2), which shares homology with LEDGF/p75, binds HIV integrase and rescues LEDGF/p75 activity in knockout cells [31,48,49]. Furthermore, LEDGF/p75 is not a general requirement for retroviral integration. Gammaretroviruses, such as MLV, preferentially integrate into strong transcriptional cis-elements including promoters, enhancers, and DNase hypersensitive sites and this bias is in part mediated by Bromodomain and Extra Terminal (BET) family transcription factors [8,9,50,51]. This indicates that selection of retroviral integration is specific to different retroviruses and influenced by the cellular cofactors that are usurped by the retroviruses.

Ini-1/hSNF5, a SWI/SNF ATP dependent chromatin remodeling factor, has also been suggested to influence HIV replication. The actual function of Ini-1/SNF5 in the context of HIV replication is still unclear, which may reflect the fact that Ini-1/SNF5 has multiple activities at different steps in the HIV life cycle [52–55]. Ini-1/SNF5 was originally identified as an HIV integrase-interacting partner using a yeast two-hybrid system [56] and was shown to be recruited into HIV virions and pre-integration complexes through a Gag mediated interaction [54,57]. *In vitro* assays show that Ini-1/hSNF5 facilitates integration by ATP-dependent displacement of nucleosomes to increase DNA accessibility [58]. In addition, disrupting Ini-1/SNF5-integrase interactions has been reported to alter integration [59,60]. Ini-1/SNF5 has also been suggested to have antiviral activities, inhibiting early steps of HIV replication through its interaction with HIV integrase as well as components of the Sin3a-HDAC1 repressor complex [52,54,59]. The functional relevance of Ini-1/SNF5-HIV integrase interactions warrants further investigation.

Recently, the TRIM family protein TRIM28/KAP1 has been shown to physically interact with and inhibit HIV-1 integrase [61]. TRIM28/KAP1 is a transcriptional co-repressor that interacts with KRAB zinc finger DNA proteins through its bromodomain, binding acetylated lysines to mediate gene silencing by recruiting repressor complexes to target promoters [62]. HIV integrase activity is regulated by p300 which acetylates key lysines K264, K266 and K273 within HIV integrase and TRIM28/SNF5 binds these acetylated lysines. TRIM28/KAP1 inhibits integrase activity by recruiting HDAC1 which deacetylates the lysines [61]. Therefore, Trim28/KAP1 coordinates HIV-1 integrase function with chromatin remodeling during proviral integration [61].

Using fluorescence *in situ* hybridization, immunohistochemistry and microscopy, it has been shown that the nucleus is highly organized and that genes are not randomly distributed, but are partitioned into regions that cluster expressed genes from repressed genes [63,64]. For example, transcriptionally active euchromatin is detected near nucleopore complexes, whereas transcriptionally repressed heterochromatin is enriched in areas between nucleopore complexes [65,66]. This chromatin architecture underneath the nuclear envelope is maintained by nuclear pore complex proteins including Nup153 and Tpr [67]. If expressed genes are juxtaposed to nucleopore complexes then, upon entry into the nucleus, HIV will most likely encounter actively transcribed genes with open chromatin. Furthermore, disrupting nuclear pore complexes would be predicted to compromise nuclear entry and/or integration of the HIV pre-integration complex. The pre-integration complex, HIV capsid and HIV integrase have been shown to interact with several nuclear pore proteins including transportin 3 and nucleoporins NUP153 and NUP62 [68,69]. In addition, a siRNA screen showed that targeting proteins associated with nuclear pore complexes, such as RANBP2, altered the selection of provirus integration sites [70,71]. Other nuclear pore proteins that mediate HIV infection include Nup153 and Nup98, which facilitate nuclear import of the preintegration complex and Tpr, which influences integration site selection by maintaining chromatin architecture, anchoring Nup153 and functionally associating with LEDGF/p75 [67,72–76].

Two recent reports support the possibility that HIV provirus interacts with batteries of actively expressed genes upon translocation into the nucleus. Firstly, it has been observed that HIV genomes co-localize with PML [77]. It is also interesting to note that PML functionally interacts with Ini-1/SNF5 [78]. Secondly, examination of integration sites by three-dimensional immune DNA fluorescence *in situ* hybridization suggested that integrated virus was strongly associated with chromatin regions at the outer region of the nucleus whereas integration was disfavored in lamin-associated domains located more centrally in the nucleus [79]. This bias in integration sites was dependent on Nup153 and LEDGF/p75. Most importantly, these studies demonstrate the role DNA topography plays in biasing HIV integration site selection [79].

3. Chromatin and HIV Transcription

In addition to influencing sites of integration chromatin architecture directly affects the efficiency of HIV gene expression and silencing. HIV transcription is initiated at the transcriptional start site within the R region of the 5' long terminal repeat (LTR) [80–82]. Efficient transcription of proviral DNA is tightly linked to the activation status of the cell and the availability of cellular transcription factors [83–86]. These factors recognize specific sequences within the HIV LTR and subsequently recruit the RNA polymerase II (RNAP II) transcriptional machinery. Initial transcription of the HIV provirus leads to the production of the virally encoded transcription trans-activator Tat. Tat significantly enhances the efficiency of transcription by binding a RNA stem loop at the beginning of the newly transcribed HIV RNA at the trans-activation response element or TAR. Tat recruits transcription elongation factors to the HIV promoter to facilitate provirus transcription. One critical factor recruited by Tat includes the P-TEFb complex, which phosphorylates the C-terminal domain of RNAP II as well as factors that act as negative elongation factors such as DSIF and NELF, enabling efficient processivity and elongation of the RNA transcript [87–90]. However, not all of infected cells support productive viral replication. In T cells, a subset of infected cells carries latent proviruses which are not efficiently expressed [80,91,92]. This pool of latently infected resting T cells represent an important barrier to curing HIV infection as these cells can be re-activated to produce virus at any point after the interruption of HAART and lead to the rebound of the viral load in infected individuals [93–95]. The transcriptional repression observed in latently infected cells may result from multiple mechanisms including low levels of positive transcription factors, the presence of repressive transcription factors, and epigenetic changes associated with chromatin that limit HIV transcription.

The proviral chromatin architecture includes two nucleosomes, designated as nuc-0 and nuc-1, located immediately upstream of the modulatory region within U3 and downstream of the transcription initiation site, respectively. The location of these nucleosomes were originally mapped in DNAse hyper-sensitivity studies [96]. This organization showed that the upstream cis-elements of the HIV LTR which include Sp-1, NF-κB and Ap-1 sites, are accessible and nucleosome free, whereas Nuc-1, in particular, is in a position to impede RNAP II elongation. The recruitment of histone-modifying complexes targets Histone-3 (H3) and Histone-4 (H4) of Nuc-1 to regulate HIV transcription [97–99]. A well characterized modification is acetylation of histones. Acetylation of histones by acetyltransferases (HATs) generally leads to opening of chromatin allowing accessibility of the DNA to the transcription machinery or enhanced RNAP II processivity. Cellular transcription factors including NF-AT, Sp1, NF-κB, AP-1, as well as HIV Tat recruit histone acetyltransferases such as CBP/p300, P/CAF and GCN5 to the HIV LTR (Figure 1). Acetylation of H3 and H4 of nuc-1 has been implicated in the activation of HIV transcription [100–103]. ChIP-analysis on the acetylation pattern of the nucleosomes following phorbol-ester stimulation of latently infect T cells showed increase acetylation of H3 at lysines 9 and 14 and of Histone-4 at lysines 8 and 16 [101]. Conversely, repressive transcription factors such as NF-κB p50 homodimers, YY-1, LSF, NELF and CBF-1 recruit histone de-acetylases (HDAC), leading to a closed chromatin conformation, limited access to the transcription machinery and decreased RNAP II activity [104] (Figure 1). These modifications are closely associated to the activation state of the host cell and are important for the silencing of HIV transcription and the establishment of latency. HDAC-1 [104–109], HDAC-2 [108,110,111] and HDAC-3 [88,110,112] are the main factors that mediate the de-acetylation of the nuc-1 of HIV as evidenced by ChIP analysis of repressive protein complexes, siRNA knock-downs and pharmacological inhibition. In addition to promoting opening and closing of the chromatin structure, the acetylation status of histones provides a platform for the association of additional regulatory proteins. One such protein is BRD4, which recognizes acetylated histones and transcription factors through its bromodomains. BRD4 recruits and activates P-TEFb through its P-TEFb-interacting domain (PID) [113,114]. The interaction of these proteins mediates basal transcription of the provirus in the absence of Tat. Interestingly, BRD4 competes with Tat for P-TEFb, thus acting as an antagonist for efficient proviral transcription elongation. BRD4 further antagonizes Tat transactivation by phosphorylating the CDK9 subunit of P-TEFb, thus inhibiting kinase activity within the HIV transcription initiation complex [115]. Based on these observations BRD4 has been suggested to be a critical factor for limiting HIV transcription and has been suggested to be a target for reactivating latent HIV (see below).

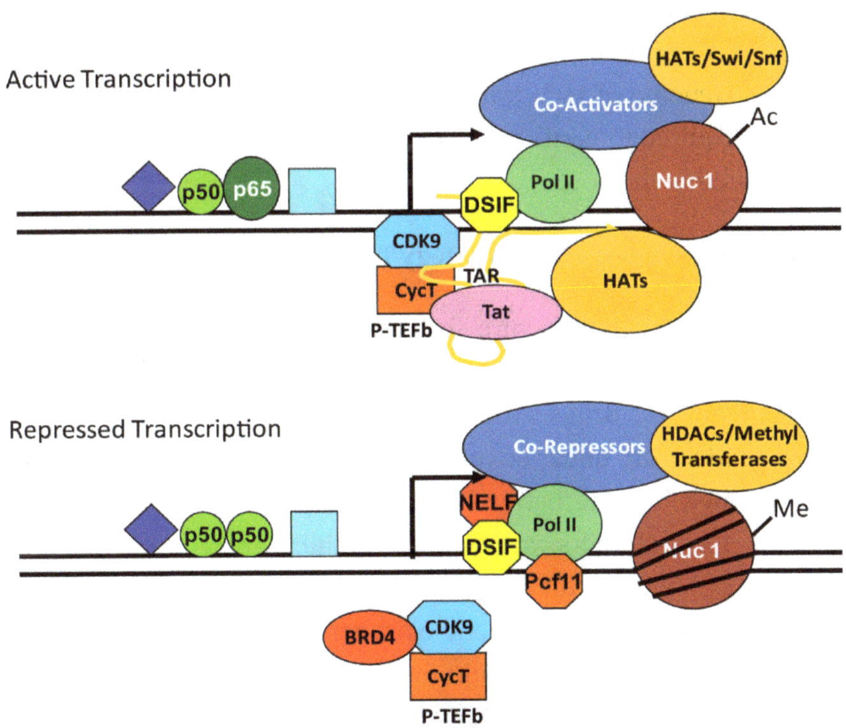

Figure 1. General regulation of HIV transcription and chromatin remodeling. Cellular transcription factors (e.g., p50/p65 NF-κB heterodimers) recognize motifs within the HIV provirus promoter region and recruit cellular co-activators, chromatin remodeling factors and transcription elongation factors. Negative transcription factors (e.g., p50/p50 NF-κB homodimers) recruit cellular co-repressors, chromatin remodeling factors and factors that hinder transcription elongation.

Histones are also modified by methylation and this modification, depending on the context and residue, either contributes to repression or to activation of transcription. Sp1 in complex with CTIP2 recruits SUV39H1 and mediates tri-methylation of H3 at lysine 9 [108]. The methyltransferase G9a also mediates repression of HIV transcription through dimethylation of H3 [116]. It remains unclear which factors mediate activation-related methylation, but it is possible that trimethylation of H3 at lysine 4 and dimethylation at lysine 36 mediated by SET1 and Smyd2 can promote proviral transcription [103,117–119]. Methyltransferases have also been shown to modify proviral DNA and HIV Tat creating additional layers of transcriptional regulation [120–123].

Another important modification to the chromatin structure is mediated by the SWI/SNF complexes. This is a large complex composed of 12 individual proteins [124]. The main function of SWI/SNF is to facilitate the mobilization of nucleosomes along the DNA in an ATP-dependent manner [124], thus facilitating access of DNA to the transcription machinery. In the context of HIV replication, SWI/SNF proteins influence integration (see above) and activate HIV transcription. Upon activation of the cell, Tat becomes acetylated. This modification of Tat allows it to bind to the catalytic subunit of the SWI/SNF complex known as Brg-1, thus recruiting the complex to the HIV promoter. The recruitment of SWI/SNF to the HIV promoter may also be facilitated by the interaction of Brg-1 with acetylated nuc-1 upon phorbol ester stimulation [125].

Chromatin re-assembly factors have also been proposed as limiting HIV transcription. Knockdown experiments of Spt6, Spt16 and Chd1, members of the facilitates chromatin transcription (FACT) complex, induced HIV transcription in latently infected cell lines [126]. These results suggest that the FACT complex promotes silencing of HIV transcription by assembling nucleosomes along the proviral DNA. Further studies are required to confirm the direct recruitment of these factors to the provirus and how their activity is regulated in the context of HIV latency.

4. Targeting Chromatin as a Therapeutic Strategy for HIV

Given the importance of DNA architecture for the efficient integration and transcription of HIV, chromatin modifying factors have been appealing targets for anti-retroviral therapies (Table 1). To block early steps in the HIV life cycle, drugs modulating the interaction between LEDGF/p75 and HIV integrase (IN), called LEDGINs, are under development. Christ *et al.* identified 2-(quinolin-3-yl) acetic acid compounds that inhibited binding between HIV integrase and LEDGF/p75 [127]. Furthermore, these LEDGINs stabilize IN multimers, allosterically inhibit integrase activity and prevent proper virion assembly [127–130]. Although the initial LEDGINs displayed IC_{50} values in the micromolar range, tert-butoxy-(4-phenyl-quinolin-3-yl) acetic acid derivatives are potent in the nanomolar range, increasing the likelihood that they will be brought to clinical trials [128].

Chromatin-targeting strategies for treating HIV also include compounds designed to work at the level of transcription such as "shock and kill" strategies to reactivate latent proviruses in conjunction with antiretroviral therapy [131]. With virus replication blocked by routine antiretroviral therapy, it is expected that the reactivated latent population will be cleared by the host immune system or by the cytopathic effects of viral replication. Many of these latency-reversing agents (LRAs) target regulators of chromatin.

Table 1. Potential HIV therapeutics that target chromatin.

Drug Class	Compounds	References
Inhibitors of Integration		
LEDGINs	2-(quinolin-3-yl) acetic acids, tert-butoxy-(4-phenyl-quinolin-3-yl) acetic acids	[127–130]
Transcriptional Activators		
Histone Deacetylase Inhibitors (HDACi)	Valproic acid, SAHA, (vorinostat), givinostat, panobinostat, entinostat, romidepsin	[132–149]
BET Bromodo main Inhibitors	JQ1	[150–154]
Histone Methyltransferase Inhibitors (HMTi)	Chaeotocin, BIX-01294, DZNep	[155–157]
DNA Methyltransferase Inhibitors (DMTi)	5-aza-2'-deoxycytidine	[121,122,157]

The most widely studied LRAs are HDAC inhibitors, which maintain an open chromatin structure by histone acetylation. The epilepsy drug, valproic acid (VPA), is a Class I/II HDAC inhibitor [132]. Phase I and II clinical trials for using VPA as a latency-reversing agent have so far shown mixed results regarding changes in the amount of integrated virus as measured by PCR. In the initial proof-of-concept study, three out of four patients obtained a mean reduction of 75% infected units per billion (IUPB) as determined by a viral outgrowth assay (VOA) [133]. A follow-up trial was only able to replicate a statistically significant decrease in IUPB for four out of 11 subjects [134]. In addition, subsequent studies indicated that valproic acid did not alter the amount of integrated latent HIV [135–137] and may increase the cognitive impairments associated with AIDS [138].

SAHA or vorinostat, a treatment for T cell lymphomas, is another promising HDAC inhibitor. It induces HIV expression in cellular models of HIV latency, such as J-LAT, JΔK, ACH-2, and U1 cells, as well as *ex vivo* experiments with patient peripheral blood mononuclear cells [139–141]. In a small clinical trial, SAHA treatment substantially increased cell-associated viral RNA levels in patients on ART, several of whom had no detectable HIV RNA before study enrollment [142]. However, a second clinical trial demonstrated that, although oral doses of vorinostat led to a significant increase in cell-associated unspliced HIV RNA for the majority of subjects, there was no change in plasma HIV RNA or the amount of integrated HIV DNA [143].

A large number of other HDAC inhibitors are under investigation, including givinostat, panobinostat, entinostat, and romidepsin [144–148]. Rasmussen *et al.* [145,149] contrasted the effects of clinically relevant concentrations of panobinostat, givinostat, vorinostat, and valproic acid on U1 and ACH2 latent cell line models as well as latently-infected resting primary cells. Panobinostat, a hydroxamic-acid pan-HDAC inhibitor, significantly increased HIV transcription as compared to the other inhibitors for all cell types [145]. A clinical trial with panobinostat demonstrated its capacity to upregulate cell-associated unspliced HIV RNA and temporarily perturb the amount of viral DNA in patients on ART [149].

Besides HDAC inhibitors, several groups have shown that the BET bromodomain inhibitor JQ1 can reactivate HIV in U1, ACH2, JΔK, and J-Lat cell models [150–154]. In addition, JQ1 induced HIV expression *ex vivo* in T cells from one out of three individuals on ART [150]. Evidence suggests that JQ1 may inhibit the BET protein BRD4, which represses transcription by sequestering PTEF-b from Tat [113,151]. However, recent studies suggest that JQ1 may function by inhibiting BRD2. Although the mechanism by which BRD2 contributes to HIV latency has not been elucidated, Boehm *et al.* postulated that BRD2 may target HDACs to the proviral LTR [154]. JQ1 has not yet been brought to clinical trials for the treatment of HIV.

Histone methyltransferases (HMTs) present another potential target for LRAs. Chaeotocin, a fungal toxin and SUV39H1 HMT inhibitor (HMTi), reactivates HIV in latently infected cell models [155,156]. Furthermore, chaeotocin and BIX-01294, a G9a HMTi, can stimulate HIV transcription *ex vivo* in PBMCs from ART-suppressed HIV^+ patients. In contrast, other evidence indicates that DZNep, which inhibits several HMTs including EZH2, is a more potent inducer of HIV transcription than either chaeotocin or BIX-01294 in latently infected Jurkats [157]. These HMTis, however, are too toxic to be used as single agents in clinical trials. DNA methyltransferase inhibitors, while also appealing, have not yet demonstrated the same potential to induce latent HIV expression as HMTi's. 5-aza-2'-deoxycytidine, which inhibits the cytosine methylation associated with CpG islands, weakly reactivates HIV but can synergize with other LRAs such as the protein kinase C modulator prostratin [121,122,157].

In spite of promising results obtained with cellular models of latency and *ex vivo* activation of $CD4^+$ T cells from HIV patients, LRAs have had little success in clinical settings. Other than early trials of valproic acid in combination with ART [133], none have successfully reduced the viral reservoir *in vivo*. However, the potential for global T cell activation, specifically for HDAC inhibitors, may have had significant negative repercussions within these trials and would have limited the dosages, perhaps below the therapeutic threshold. This has led to the search for non-T cell stimulating agents that reactivate latent HIV, like protein kinase C activators. These compounds, which use mechanisms of action unrelated to chromatin dynamics, may have increased efficacy after other LRAs have reorganized the DNA architecture. Indeed, several studies have identified that combinatorial approaches maximally induce HIV expression in latently infected primary cells and cell models [43,140,152,153,157–159]. For example, it was demonstrated that several minimally effective small molecules synergize with known activators such as prostratin to induce HIV expression in J-Lat cells [160].

Multifaceted strategies to induce HIV expression will be essential to significantly perturb the HIV reservoir. New evidence indicates that we may be substantially underestimating the size of the viral reservoir. With VOA-based measurements, about one in 10^6 resting $CD4^+$ T cells are estimated to be inducible [161,162]. In contrast, genomic PCR indicates that nearly 200 in 10^6 resting $CD4^+$ T cells contain integrated provirus [163] and this proviral load may be dynamic and vary between patients. It has been assumed that the majority of these integrated proviruses are replication-incompetent. However, the Siliciano lab sequenced 213 proviruses from eight patients on ART that were incapable of being activated by the standard LRA phytohemagglutinin and showed that approximately 10% of proviruses deemed non-inducible by VOA were actually capable of infection and replication [164]. Therefore, with this uncertainty surrounding the size and location of the latent reservoir, the potential of LRAs may need to be further evaluated.

Future design of HIV/AIDS therapeutics must incorporate drugs designed to work at the level of chromatin. Host and proviral genomic architecture have profound repercussions for the fate of infected cells. Specific manipulation of chromatin would allow us to modify the balance between the maintenance of latently infected cells and cells containing transcriptionally active proviruses that can then be targeted and finally cleared.

5. Conclusions

Chromatin influences HIV integration and transcription which has implications for efficient HIV replication and latency. Therapeutically targeting chromatin and associated factors provides promising strategies for preventing HIV infection and reducing the size of the latent reservoir.

Acknowledgments

This work was in part supported by NIH grants A1AI097117, DE 023950 and AI108447 awarded to Andrew J. Henderson. Luis M. Agosto and Matthew Gagne were supported by the Immunology Training Grant T32-AI007309.

Author Contributions

All authors contributed equally to scholarship and writing of the manuscript.

References

1. Lewinski, M.K.; Bisgrove, D.; Shinn, P.; Chen, H.; Hoffmann, C.; Hannenhalli, S.; Verdin, E.; Berry, C.C.; Ecker, J.R.; Bushman, F.D. Genome-wide analysis of chromosomal features repressing human immunodeficiency virus transcription. *J. Virol.* **2005**, *79*, 6610–6619.
2. Shan, L.; Yang, H.C.; Rabi, S.A.; Bravo, H.C.; Shroff, N.S.; Irizarry, R.A.; Zhang, H.; Margolick, J.B.; Siliciano, J.D.; Siliciano, R.F. Influence of host gene transcription level and orientation on HIV-1 latency in a primary-cell model. *J. Virol.* **2011**, *85*, 5384–5393.
3. Sherrill-Mix, S.; Lewinski, M.K.; Famiglietti, M.; Bosque, A.; Malani, N.; Ocwieja, K.E.; Berry, C.C.; Looney, D.; Shan, L.; Agosto, L.M.; *et al.* HIV latency and integration site placement in five cell-based models. *Retrovirology* **2013**, doi:10.1186/1742-4690-10-90.
4. Lenasi, T.; Contreras, X.; Peterlin, B.M. Transcriptional interference antagonizes proviral gene expression to promote HIV latency. *Cell Host Microbe* **2008**, *4*, 123–133.
5. Ding, D.; Qu, X.; Li, L.; Zhou, X.; Liu, S.; Lin, S.; Wang, P.; Kong, C.; Wang, X.; Liu, L.; *et al.* Involvement of histone methyltransferase GLP in HIV-1 latency through catalysis of H3K9 dimethylation. *Virology* **2013**, *440*, 182–189.
6. Han, Y.; Lassen, K.; Monie, D.; Sedaghat, A.R.; Shimoji, S.; Liu, X.; Pierson, T.C.; Margolick, J.B.; Siliciano, R.F.; Siliciano, J.D. Resting $CD4^+$ T cells from HIV-1 infected individuals carry integrated HIV-1 genomes within actively transcribed host genes. *J. Virol.* **2004**, *78*, 6122–6133.
7. Rezaei, S.D.; Cameron, P.U. Human immunodeficiency virus (HIV)-1 integration sites in viral latency. *Curr. HIV/AIDS Rep.* **2015**, *12*, 88–96.
8. Krishnan, L.; Engelman, A. Retroviral integrase proteins and HIV-1 DNA integration. *J. Biol. Chem.* **2012**, *287*, 40858–40866.

9. Craigie, R.; Bushman, F.D. HIV DNA integration. *Cold Spring Harb. Perspect. Med.* **2012**, doi:10.1101/cshperspect.a006890.

10. Van Maele, B.; Busschots, K.; Vandekerckhove, L.; Christ, F.; Debyser, Z. Cellular co-factors of HIV-1 integration. *Trends Biochem. Sci.* **2006**, *31*, 98–105.

11. Vandegraaff, N.; Engelman, A. Molecular mechanisms of HIV integration and therapeutic intervention. *Expert Rev. Mol. Med.* **2007**, *9*, 1–19.

12. Ciuffi, A.; Bushman, F.D. Retroviral DNA integration: HIV and the role of LEDGF/p75. *Trends Genet.* **2006**, *22*, 388–395.

13. Llano, M.; Morrison, J.; Poeschla, E.M. Virological and cellular roles of the transcriptional coactivator LEDGF/p75. *Curr. Top. Microbiol. Immunol.* **2009**, *339*, 125–146.

14. Engelman, A.; Cherepanov, P. The lentiviral integrase binding protein LEDGF/p75 and HIV-1 replication. *PLoS Pathog.* **2008**, *4*, e1000046.

15. Christ, F.; Debyser, Z. The LEDGF/p75 integrase interaction, a novel target for anti-HIV therapy. *Virology* **2013**, *435*, 102–109.

16. Ge, H.; Si, Y.; Roeder, R.G. Isolation of cDNAs encoding novel transcription coactivators p52 and p75 reveals an alternate regulatory mechanism of transcriptional activation. *EMBO J.* **1998**, *17*, 6723–6729.

17. Shinohara, T.; Singh, D.P.; Fatma, N. LEDGF, a survival factor, activates stress-related genes. *Prog. Retin. Eye Res.* **2002**, *21*, 341–358.

18. Sutherland, H.G.; Newton, K.; Brownstein, D.G.; Holmes, M.C.; Kress, C.; Semple, C.A.; Bickmore, W.A. Disruption of LEDGF/PSIP1 results in perinatal mortality and homeotic skeletal transformations. *Mol. Cell. Biol.* **2006**, *26*, 7201–7210.

19. Pradeepa, M.M.; Sutherland, H.G.; Ule, J.; Grimes, G.R.; Bickmore, W.A. PSIP1/LEDGF p52 binds methylated histone H3K36 and splicing factors and contributes to the regulation of alternative splicing. *PLoS Genet.* **2012**, *8*, e1002717.

20. Singh, D.P.; Fatma, N.; Kimura, A.; Chylack, L.T., Jr.; Shinohara, T. LEDGF binds to heat shock and stress-related element to activate the expression of stress-related genes. *Biochem. Biophys. Res. Commun.* **2001**, *283*, 943–955.

21. Singh, D.P.; Ohguro, N.; Kikuchi, T.; Sueno, T.; Reddy, V.N.; Yuge, K.; Chylack, L.T., Jr.; Shinohara, T. Lens epithelium-derived growth factor: Effects on growth and survival of lens epithelial cells, keratinocytes, and fibroblasts. *Biochem. Biophys. Res. Commun.* **2000**, *267*, 373–381.

22. Dietz, F.; Franken, S.; Yoshida, K.; Nakamura, H.; Kappler, J.; Gieselmann, V. The family of hepatoma-derived growth factor proteins: Characterization of a new member HRP-4 and classification of its subfamilies. *Biochem. J.* **2002**, *366*, 491–500.

23. Nameki, N.; Tochio, N.; Koshiba, S.; Inoue, M.; Yabuki, T.; Aoki, M.; Seki, E.; Matsuda, T.; Fujikura, Y.; Saito, M.; *et al.* Solution structure of the PWWP domain of the hepatoma-derived growth factor family. *Protein Sci.* **2005**, *14*, 756–764.

24. Turlure, F.; Maertens, G.; Rahman, S.; Cherepanov, P.; Engelman, A. A tripartite DNA-binding element, comprised of the nuclear localization signal and two AT-hook motifs, mediates the association of LEDGF/p75 with chromatin *in vivo*. *Nucleic Acids Res.* **2006**, *34*, 1653–1665.

25. Gijsbers, R.; Vets, S.; de Rijck, J.; Ocwieja, K.E.; Ronen, K.; Malani, N.; Bushman, F.D.; Debyser, Z. Role of the PWWP domain of lens epithelium-derived growth factor (LEDGF)/p75 cofactor in lentiviral integration targeting. *J. Biol. Chem.* **2011**, *286*, 41812–41825.
26. Vanegas, M.; Llano, M.; Delgado, S.; Thompson, D.; Peretz, M.; Poeschla, E. Identification of the LEDGF/p75 HIV-1 integrase-interaction domain and NLS reveals NLS-independent chromatin tethering. *J. Cell Sci.* **2005**, *118*, 1733–1743.
27. De Rijck, J.; Vandekerckhove, L.; Gijsbers, R.; Hombrouck, A.; Hendrix, J.; Vercammen, J.; Engelborghs, Y.; Christ, F.; Debyser, Z. Overexpression of the lens epithelium-derived growth factor/p75 integrase binding domain inhibits human immunodeficiency virus replication. *J. Virol.* **2006**, *80*, 11498–11509.
28. Cherepanov, P.; Ambrosio, A.L.; Rahman, S.; Ellenberger, T.; Engelman, A. Structural basis for the recognition between HIV-1 integrase and transcriptional coactivator p75. *Proc. Natl. Acad. Sci. USA* **2005**, *102*, 17308–17313.
29. Cherepanov, P.; Sun, Z.Y.; Rahman, S.; Maertens, G.; Wagner, G.; Engelman, A. Solution structure of the HIV-1 integrase-binding domain in LEDGF/p75. *Nat. Struct. Mol. Biol.* **2005**, *12*, 526–532.
30. Cherepanov, P.; Maertens, G.; Proost, P.; Devreese, B.; van Beeumen, J.; Engelborghs, Y.; de Clercq, E.; Debyser, Z. HIV-1 integrase forms stable tetramers and associates with LEDGF/p75 protein in human cells. *J. Biol. Chem.* **2003**, *278*, 372–381.
31. Cherepanov, P.; Devroe, E.; Silver, P.A.; Engelman, A. Identification of an evolutionarily conserved domain in human lens epithelium-derived growth factor/transcriptional co-activator p75 (LEDGF/p75) that binds HIV-1 integrase. *J. Biol. Chem.* **2004**, *279*, 48883–48892.
32. Llano, M.; Saenz, D.T.; Meehan, A.; Wongthida, P.; Peretz, M.; Walker, W.H.; Teo, W.; Poeschla, E.M. An essential role for LEDGF/p75 in HIV integration. *Science* **2006**, *314*, 461–464.
33. Ciuffi, A.; Llano, M.; Poeschla, E.; Hoffmann, C.; Leipzig, J.; Shinn, P.; Ecker, J.R.; Bushman, F. A role for LEDGF/p75 in targeting HIV DNA integration. *Nat. Med.* **2005**, *11*, 1287–1289.
34. Fadel, H.J.; Morrison, J.H.; Saenz, D.T.; Fuchs, J.R.; Kvaratskhelia, M.; Ekker, S.C.; Poeschla, E.M. TALEN knockout of the PSIP1 gene in human cells: Analyses of HIV-1 replication and allosteric integrase inhibitor mechanism. *J. Virol.* **2014**, *88*, 9704–9717.
35. Badia, R.; Pauls, E.; Riveira-Munoz, E.; Clotet, B.; Este, J.A.; Ballana, E. Zinc finger endonuclease targeting PSIP1 inhibits HIV-1 integration. *Antimicrob. Agents Chemother.* **2014**, *58*, 4318–4327.
36. Shun, M.C.; Raghavendra, N.K.; Vandegraaff, N.; Daigle, J.E.; Hughes, S.; Kellam, P.; Cherepanov, P.; Engelman, A. LEDGF/p75 functions downstream from preintegration complex formation to effect gene-specific HIV-1 integration. *Genes Dev.* **2007**, *21*, 1767–1778.
37. Hare, S.; Shun, M.C.; Gupta, S.S.; Valkov, E.; Engelman, A.; Cherepanov, P. A novel co-crystal structure affords the design of gain-of-function lentiviral integrase mutants in the presence of modified PSIP1/LEDGF/p75. *PLoS Pathog.* **2009**, *5*, e1000259.
38. Botbol, Y.; Raghavendra, N.K.; Rahman, S.; Engelman, A.; Lavigne, M. Chromatinized templates reveal the requirement for the LEDGF/p75 PWWP domain during HIV-1 integration *in vitro*. *Nucleic Acids Res.* **2008**, *36*, 1237–1246.

39. Rahman, S.; Lu, R.; Vandegraaff, N.; Cherepanov, P.; Engelman, A. Structure-based mutagenesis of the integrase-LEDGF/p75 interface uncouples a strict correlation between *in vitro* protein binding and HIV-1 fitness. *Virology* **2007**, *357*, 79–90.
40. Llano, M.; Vanegas, M.; Hutchins, N.; Thompson, D.; Delgado, S.; Poeschla, E.M. Identification and characterization of the chromatin-binding domains of the HIV-1 integrase interactor LEDGF/p75. *J. Mol. Biol.* **2006**, *360*, 760–773.
41. Hendrix, J.; van Heertum, B.; Vanstreels, E.; Daelemans, D.; de Rijck, J. Dynamics of the ternary complex formed by c-Myc interactor JPO2, transcriptional co-activator LEDGF/p75, and chromatin. *J. Biol. Chem.* **2014**, *289*, 12494–12506.
42. Maertens, G.N.; Cherepanov, P.; Engelman, A. Transcriptional co-activator p75 binds and tethers the Myc-interacting protein JPO2 to chromatin. *J. Cell Sci.* **2006**, *119*, 2563–2571.
43. Llano, M.; Delgado, S.; Vanegas, M.; Poeschla, E.M. Lens epithelium-derived growth factor/p75 prevents proteasomal degradation of HIV-1 integrase. *J. Biol. Chem.* **2004**, *279*, 55570–55577.
44. Morchikh, M.; Naughtin, M.; di Nunzio, F.; Xavier, J.; Charneau, P.; Jacob, Y.; Lavigne, M. TOX4 and NOVA1 proteins are partners of the LEDGF PWWP domain and affect HIV-1 replication. *PLoS ONE* **2013**, *8*, e81217.
45. Bartholomeeusen, K.; de Rijck, J.; Busschots, K.; Desender, L.; Gijsbers, R.; Emiliani, S.; Benarous, R.; Debyser, Z.; Christ, F. Differential interaction of HIV-1 integrase and JPO2 with the C terminus of LEDGF/p75. *J. Mol. Biol.* **2007**, *372*, 407–421.
46. Bartholomeeusen, K.; Christ, F.; Hendrix, J.; Rain, J.C.; Emiliani, S.; Benarous, R.; Debyser, Z.; Gijsbers, R.; de Rijck, J. Lens epithelium-derived growth factor/p75 interacts with the transposase-derived DDE domain of PogZ. *J. Biol. Chem.* **2009**, *284*, 11467–11477.
47. Gerard, A.; Segeral, E.; Naughtin, M.; Abdouni, A.; Charmeteau, B.; Cheynier, R.; Rain, J.C.; Emiliani, S. The integrase cofactor LEDGF/p75 associates with Iws1 and Spt6 for postintegration silencing of HIV-1 gene expression in latently infected cells. *Cell Host Microbe* **2015**, *17*, 107–117.
48. Wang, H.; Jurado, K.A.; Wu, X.; Shun, M.C.; Li, X.; Ferris, A.L.; Smith, S.J.; Patel, P.A.; Fuchs, J.R.; Cherepanov, P.; *et al.* HRP2 determines the efficiency and specificity of HIV-1 integration in LEDGF/p75 knockout cells but does not contribute to the antiviral activity of a potent LEDGF/p75-binding site integrase inhibitor. *Nucleic Acids Res.* **2012**, *40*, 11518–11530.
49. Vandegraaff, N.; Devroe, E.; Turlure, F.; Silver, P.A.; Engelman, A. Biochemical and genetic analyses of integrase-interacting proteins lens epithelium-derived growth factor (LEDGF)/p75 and hepatoma-derived growth factor related protein 2 (HRP2) in preintegration complex function and HIV-1 replication. *Virology* **2006**, *346*, 415–426.
50. Gupta, S.S.; Maetzig, T.; Maertens, G.N.; Sharif, A.; Rothe, M.; Weidner-Glunde, M.; Galla, M.; Schambach, A.; Cherepanov, P.; Schulz, T.F. Bromo- and extraterminal domain chromatin regulators serve as cofactors for murine leukemia virus integration. *J. Virol.* **2013**, *87*, 12721–12736.
51. Sharma, A.; Larue, R.C.; Plumb, M.R.; Malani, N.; Male, F.; Slaughter, A.; Kessl, J.J.; Shkriabai, N.; Coward, E.; Aiyer, S.S.; *et al.* BET proteins promote efficient murine leukemia virus integration at transcription start sites. *Proc. Natl. Acad. Sci. USA* **2013**, *110*, 12036–12041.
52. Sorin, M.; Yung, E.; Wu, X.; Kalpana, G.V. HIV-1 replication in cell lines harboring INI1/hSNF5 mutations. *Retrovirology* **2006**, doi:10.1186/1742-4690-3-56.

53. Ariumi, Y.; Serhan, F.; Turelli, P.; Telenti, A.; Trono, D. The integrase interactor 1 (INI1) proteins facilitate Tat-mediated human immunodeficiency virus type 1 transcription. *Retrovirology* **2006**, doi:10.1186/1742-4690-3-47.
54. Cano, J.; Kalpana, G.V. Inhibition of early stages of HIV-1 assembly by INI1/hSNF5 transdominant negative mutant S6. *J. Virol.* **2011**, *85*, 2254–2265.
55. Boese, A.; Sommer, P.; Holzer, D.; Maier, R.; Nehrbass, U. Integrase interactor 1 (Ini1/hSNF5) is a repressor of basal human immunodeficiency virus type 1 promoter activity. *J. Gen. Virol.* **2009**, *90*, 2503–2512.
56. Kalpana, G.V.; Marmon, S.; Wang, W.; Crabtree, G.R.; Goff, S.P. Binding and stimulation of HIV-1 integrase by a human homolog of yeast transcription factor SNF5. *Science* **1994**, *266*, 2002–2006.
57. Yung, E.; Sorin, M.; Pal, A.; Craig, E.; Morozov, A.; Delattre, O.; Kappes, J.; Ott, D.; Kalpana, G.V. Inhibition of HIV-1 virion production by a transdominant mutant of integrase interactor 1. *Nat. Med.* **2001**, *7*, 920–926.
58. Lesbats, P.; Botbol, Y.; Chevereau, G.; Vaillant, C.; Calmels, C.; Arneodo, A.; Andreola, M.L.; Lavigne, M.; Parissi, V. Functional coupling between HIV-1 integrase and the SWI/SNF chromatin remodeling complex for efficient *in vitro* integration into stable nucleosomes. *PLoS Pathog.* **2011**, *7*, e1001280.
59. Mathew, S.; Nguyen, M.; Wu, X.; Pal, A.; Shah, V.B.; Prasad, V.R.; Aiken, C.; Kalpana, G.V. INI1/hSNF5-interaction defective HIV-1 IN mutants exhibit impaired particle morphology, reverse transcription and integration *in vivo*. *Retrovirology* **2013**, doi:10.1186/1742-4690-10-66.
60. Maillot, B.; Levy, N.; Eiler, S.; Crucifix, C.; Granger, F.; Richert, L.; Didier, P.; Godet, J.; Pradeau-Aubreton, K.; Emiliani, S.; *et al.* Structural and functional role of INI1 and LEDGF in the HIV-1 preintegration complex. *PLoS ONE* **2013**, *8*, e60734.
61. Allouch, A.; di Primio, C.; Alpi, E.; Lusic, M.; Arosio, D.; Giacca, M.; Cereseto, A. The TRIM family protein KAP1 inhibits HIV-1 integration. *Cell Host Microbe* **2011**, *9*, 484–495.
62. Iyengar, S.; Farnham, P.J. KAP1 protein: An enigmatic master regulator of the genome. *J. Biol. Chem.* **2011**, *286*, 26267–26276.
63. Burns, L.T.; Wente, S.R. From hypothesis to mechanism: Uncovering nuclear pore complex links to gene expression. *Mol. Cell. Biol.* **2014**, *34*, 2114–2120.
64. Ibarra, A.; Hetzer, M.W. Nuclear pore proteins and the control of genome functions. *Genes Dev.* **2015**, *29*, 337–349.
65. Torok, D.; Ching, R.W.; Bazett-Jones, D.P. PML nuclear bodies as sites of epigenetic regulation. *Front. Biosci.* **2009**, *14*, 1325–1336.
66. Krull, S.; Dorries, J.; Boysen, B.; Reidenbach, S.; Magnius, L.; Norder, H.; Thyberg, J.; Cordes, V.C. Protein Tpr is required for establishing nuclear pore-associated zones of heterochromatin exclusion. *EMBO J.* **2010**, *29*, 1659–1673.
67. Krull, S.; Thyberg, J.; Bjorkroth, B.; Rackwitz, H.R.; Cordes, V.C. Nucleoporins as components of the nuclear pore complex core structure and Tpr as the architectural element of the nuclear basket. *Mol. Biol. Cell* **2004**, *15*, 4261–4277.
68. Krishnan, L.; Matreyek, K.A.; Oztop, I.; Lee, K.; Tipper, C.H.; Li, X.; Dar, M.J.; Kewalramani, V.N.; Engelman, A. The requirement for cellular transportin 3 (TNPO3 or TRN-SR2) during infection maps to human immunodeficiency virus type 1 capsid and not integrase. *J. Virol.* **2010**, *84*, 397–406.

69. Ao, Z.; Jayappa, K.D.; Wang, B.; Zheng, Y.; Wang, X.; Peng, J.; Yao, X. Contribution of host nucleoporin 62 in HIV-1 integrase chromatin association and viral DNA integration. *J. Biol. Chem.* **2012**, *287*, 10544–10555.

70. Ocwieja, K.E.; Brady, T.L.; Ronen, K.; Huegel, A.; Roth, S.L.; Schaller, T.; James, L.C.; Towers, G.J.; Young, J.A.; Chanda, S.K.; *et al.* HIV integration targeting: A pathway involving Transportin-3 and the nuclear pore protein RanBP2. *PLoS Pathog.* **2011**, *7*, e1001313.

71. Schaller, T.; Ocwieja, K.E.; Rasaiyaah, J.; Price, A.J.; Brady, T.L.; Roth, S.L.; Hue, S.; Fletcher, A.J.; Lee, K.; KewalRamani, V.N.; *et al.* HIV-1 capsid-cyclophilin interactions determine nuclear import pathway, integration targeting and replication efficiency. *PLoS Pathog.* **2011**, *7*, e1002439.

72. Price, A.J.; Jacques, D.A.; McEwan, W.A.; Fletcher, A.J.; Essig, S.; Chin, J.W.; Halambage, U.D.; Aiken, C.; James, L.C. Host cofactors and pharmacologic ligands share an essential interface in HIV-1 capsid that is lost upon disassembly. *PLoS Pathog.* **2014**, *10*, e1004459.

73. Matreyek, K.A.; Yucel, S.S.; Li, X.; Engelman, A. Nucleoporin NUP153 phenylalanine-glycine motifs engage a common binding pocket within the HIV-1 capsid protein to mediate lentiviral infectivity. *PLoS Pathog.* **2013**, *9*, e1003693.

74. Di Nunzio, F.; Fricke, T.; Miccio, A.; Valle-Casuso, J.C.; Perez, P.; Souque, P.; Rizzi, E.; Severgnini, M.; Mavilio, F.; Charneau, P.; *et al.* Nup153 and Nup98 bind the HIV-1 core and contribute to the early steps of HIV-1 replication. *Virology* **2013**, *440*, 8–18.

75. Lelek, M.; Casartelli, N.; Pellin, D.; Rizzi, E.; Souque, P.; Severgnini, M.; di Serio, C.; Fricke, T.; Diaz-Griffero, F.; Zimmer, C.; *et al.* Chromatin organization at the nuclear pore favours HIV replication. *Nat. Commun.* **2015**, doi:10.1038/ncomms7483.

76. Ebina, H.; Aoki, J.; Hatta, S.; Yoshida, T.; Koyanagi, Y. Role of Nup98 in nuclear entry of human immunodeficiency virus type 1 cDNA. *Microbes Infect.* **2004**, *6*, 715–724.

77. Lusic, M.; Marini, B.; Ali, H.; Lucic, B.; Luzzati, R.; Giacca, M. Proximity to PML nuclear bodies regulates HIV-1 latency in $CD4^+$ T cells. *Cell Host Microbe* **2013**, *13*, 665–677.

78. Turelli, P.; Doucas, V.; Craig, E.; Mangeat, B.; Klages, N.; Evans, R.; Kalpana, G.; Trono, D. Cytoplasmic recruitment of INI1 and PML on incoming HIV preintegration complexes: Interference with early steps of viral replication. *Mol. Cell* **2001**, *7*, 1245–1254.

79. Marini, B.; Kertesz-Farkas, A.; Ali, H.; Lucic, B.; Lisek, K.; Manganaro, L.; Pongor, S.; Luzzati, R.; Recchia, A.; Mavilio, F.; *et al.* Nuclear architecture dictates HIV-1 integration site selection. *Nature* **2015**, *521*, 227–231.

80. Karn, J.; Stoltzfus, C.M. Transcriptional and posttranscriptional regulation of HIV-1 gene expression. *Cold Spring Harb. Perspect. Med.* **2012**, doi:10.1101/cshperspect.a006916.

81. Schiralli Lester, G.M.; Henderson, A.J. Mechanisms of HIV Transcriptional Regulation and Their Contribution to Latency. *Mol. Biol. Int.* **2012**, doi:10.1155/2012/614120.

82. Van Lint, C.; Bouchat, S.; Marcello, A. HIV-1 transcription and latency: An update. *Retrovirology* **2013**, doi:10.1186/1742-4690-10-67.

83. Griffin, G.E.; Leung, K.; Folks, T.M.; Kunkel, S.; Nabel, G.J. Activation of HIV gene expression during monocyte differentiation by induction of NF-kB. *Nature* **1989**, *339*, 70–73.

84. Moses, A.V.; Ibanez, C.; Gaynor, R.; Ghazal, P.; Nelson, J.A. Differential role of long terminal repeat control elements for the regulation of basal and Tat-mediated transcription of the human immunodeficiency virus in stimulated and unstimulated primary human macrophages. *J. Virol.* **1994**, *68*, 298–307.
85. Nabel, G.; Baltimore, D. An inducible transcription factor activates expression of human immunodeficiency virus in T cells. *Nature* **1987**, *326*, 711–713.
86. Perkins, N.D.; Edwards, N.L.; Duckett, C.S.; Agranoff, A.B.; Schmid, R.M.; Nabel, G.J. A cooperative interaction between NF-kappa B and Sp1 is required for HIV-1 enhancer activation. *EMBO J.* **1993**, *12*, 3551–3558.
87. Ping, Y.H.; Rana, T.M. DSIF and NELF interact with RNA polymerase II elongation complex and HIV-1 Tat stimulates P-TEFb-mediated phosphorylation of RNA polymerase II and DSIF during transcription elongation. *J. Biol. Chem.* **2001**, *276*, 12951–12958.
88. Natarajan, M.; Schiralli Lester, G.M.; Lee, C.; Missra, A.; Wasserman, G.A.; Steffen, M.; Gilmour, D.S.; Henderson, A.J. Negative elongation factor (NELF) coordinates RNA polymerase II pausing, premature termination, and chromatin remodeling to regulate HIV transcription. *J. Biol. Chem.* **2013**, *288*, 25995–26003.
89. Zhang, Z.; Klatt, A.; Henderson, A.J.; Gilmour, D.S. Transcription termination factor Pcf11 limits the processivity of Pol II on an HIV provirus to repress gene expression. *Genes Dev.* **2007**, *21*, 1609–1614.
90. Wei, P.; Garber, M.E.; Fang, S.-M.; Fischer, W.H.; Jones, K.A. A novel CDK9-associated C-type cyclin interacts directly with HIV-1 Tat and mediates its high-affinity, loop-specific binding to TAR RNA. *Cell* **1998**, *92*, 451–462.
91. Kaczmarek, K.; Morales, A.; Henderson, A.J. T Cell Transcription Factors and Their Impact on HIV Expression. *Virol. Res. Treat.* **2013**, *2013*, 41–47.
92. Siliciano, R.F.; Greene, W.C. HIV latency. *Cold Spring Harb. Perspect. Med.* **2011**, doi:10.1101/cshperspect.a007096.
93. Davey, R.T.; Bhat, N.; Yoder, C.; Chun, T.-W.; Metcalf, J.A.; Dewar, R.; Natarajan, V.; Lempicki, R.A.; Adelsberger, J.W.; Miller, K.D.; *et al.* HIV-1 and T cell dynamics after interruption of highly active antiretroviral therapy (HAART) in patients with a history of sustained viral suppression. *Proc. Natl. Acad. Sci. USA* **1999**, *96*, 15109–15114.
94. Chun, T.W.; Stuyver, L.; Mizell, S.B.; Ehler, L.A.; Mican, J.A.; Baseler, M.; Lloyd, A.L.; Nowak, M.A.; Fauci, A.S. Presence of an inducible HIV-1 latent reservoir during highly active antiretroviral therapy. *Proc. Natl. Acad. Sci. USA* **1997**, *94*, 13193–13197.
95. Wong, J.K.; Hezareh, M.; Günthard, H.F.; Havlir, D.V.; Ignacio, C.C.; Spina, C.A.; Richman, D.D. Recovery of replication-competent HIV despite prolonged suppression of plasma viremia. *Science* **1997**, *278*, 1291–1295.
96. Verdin, E.; Paras, P., Jr.; van Lint, C. Chromatin disruption in the promoter of human immunodeficiency virus type 1 during transcriptional activation. *EMBO J.* **1993**, *12*, 3249–3259.
97. Van Lint, C.; Emiliani, S.; Ott, M.; Verdin, E. Transcriptional activation and chromatin remodeling of the HIV-1 promoter in response to histone acetylation. *EMBO J.* **1996**, *15*, 1112–1120.
98. Van Lint, C.; Emiliani, S.; Verdin, E. The expression of a small fraction of cellular genes is changed in response to histone hyperacetylation. *Gene Expr.* **1996**, *5*, 245–253.

99. Quivy, V.; de Walque, S.; van Lint, C. Chromatin-associated regulation of HIV-1 transcription: Implications for the development of therapeutic strategies. *Subcell. Biochem.* **2007**, *41*, 371–396.
100. He, G.; Margolis, D.M. Counterregulation of chromatin deacetylation and histone deacetylase occupancy at the integrated promoter of human immunodeficiency virus type 1 (HIV-1) by the HIV-1 repressor YY1 and HIV-1 activator Tat. *Mol. Cell. Biol.* **2002**, *22*, 2965–2973.
101. Lusic, M.; Marcello, A.; Cereseto, A.; Giacca, M. Regulation of HIV-1 gene expression by histone acetylation and factor recruitment at the LTR promoter. *EMBO J.* **2003**, *22*, 6550–6561.
102. Thierry, S.; Marechal, V.; Rosenzwajg, M.; Sabbah, M.; Redeuilh, G.; Nicolas, J.C.; Gozlan, J. Cell cycle arrest in G2 induces human immunodeficiency virus type 1 transcriptional activation through histone acetylation and recruitment of CBP, NF-κB, and c-Jun to the long terminal repeat promoter. *J. Virol.* **2004**, *78*, 12198–12206.
103. Hakre, S.; Chavez, L.; Shirakawa, K.; Verdin, E. Epigenetic regulation of HIV latency. *Curr. Opin. HIV AIDS* **2011**, *6*, 19–24.
104. Tyagi, M.; Karn, J. CBF-1 promotes transcriptional silencing during the establishment of HIV-1 latency. *EMBO J.* **2007**, *26*, 4985–4995.
105. Coull, J.J.; Romerio, F.; Sun, J.M.; Volker, J.L.; Galvin, K.M.; Davie, J.R.; Shi, Y.; Hansen, U.; Margolis, D.M. The human factors YY1 and LSF repress the human immunodeficiency virus type 1 long terminal repeat via recruitment of histone deacetylase 1. *J. Virol.* **2000**, *74*, 6790–6799.
106. Williams, S.A.; Chen, L.F.; Kwon, H.; Ruiz-Jarabo, C.M.; Verdin, E.; Greene, W.C. NF-κB p50 promotes HIV latency through HDAC recruitment and repression of transcriptional initiation. *EMBO J.* **2006**, *25*, 139–149.
107. Imai, K.; Okamoto, T. Transcriptional repression of human immunodeficiency virus type 1 by AP-4. *J. Biol. Chem.* **2006**, *281*, 12495–12505.
108. Marban, C.; Suzanne, S.; Dequiedt, F.; de Walque, S.; Redel, L.; van Lint, C.; Aunis, D.; Rohr, O. Recruitment of chromatin-modifying enzymes by CTIP2 promotes HIV-1 transcriptional silencing. *EMBO J.* **2007**, *26*, 412–423.
109. Jiang, G.; Espeseth, A.; Hazuda, D.J.; Margolis, D.M. c-Myc and Sp1 contribute to proviral latency by recruiting histone deacetylase 1 to the human immunodeficiency virus type 1 promoter. *J. Virol.* **2007**, *81*, 10914–10923.
110. Keedy, K.S.; Archin, N.M.; Gates, A.T.; Espeseth, A.; Hazuda, D.J.; Margolis, D.M. A limited group of class I histone deacetylases acts to repress human immunodeficiency virus type 1 expression. *J. Virol.* **2009**, *83*, 4749–4756.
111. Malcolm, T.; Chen, J.; Chang, C.; Sadowski, I. Induction of chromosomally integrated HIV-1 LTR requires RBF-2 (USF/TFII-I) and Ras/MAPK signaling. *Virus Genes* **2007**, *35*, 215–223.
112. Huber, K.; Doyon, G.; Plaks, J.; Fyne, E.; Mellors, J.W.; Sluis-Cremer, N. Inhibitors of histone deacetylases: Correlation between isoform specificity and reactivation of HIV type 1 (HIV-1) from latently infected cells. *J. Biol. Chem.* **2011**, *286*, 22211–22218.
113. Bisgrove, D.A.; Mahmoudi, T.; Henklein, P.; Verdin, E. Conserved P-TEFb-interacting domain of BRD4 inhibits HIV transcription. *Proc. Natl. Acad. Sci. USA* **2007**, *104*, 13690–13695.
114. Yang, Z.; Yik, J.H.; Chen, R.; He, N.; Jang, M.K.; Ozato, K.; Zhou, Q. Recruitment of P-TEFb for stimulation of transcriptional elongation by the bromodomain protein Brd4. *Mol. Cell* **2005**, *19*, 535–545.

115. Zhou, M.; Huang, K.; Jung, K.J.; Cho, W.K.; Klase, Z.; Kashanchi, F.; Pise-Masison, C.A.; Brady, J.N. Bromodomain protein Brd4 regulates human immunodeficiency virus transcription through phosphorylation of CDK9 at threonine 29. *J. Virol.* **2009**, *83*, 1036–1044.
116. Imai, K.; Togami, H.; Okamoto, T. Involvement of histone H3 lysine 9 (H3K9) methyltransferase G9a in the maintenance of HIV-1 latency and its reactivation by BIX01294. *J. Biol. Chem.* **2010**, *285*, 16538–16545.
117. Zhou, M.; Deng, L.; Lacoste, V.; Park, H.U.; Pumfery, A.; Kashanchi, F.; Brady, J.N.; Kumar, A. Coordination of transcription factor phosphorylation and histone methylation by the P-TEFb kinase during human immunodeficiency virus type 1 transcription. *J. Virol.* **2004**, *78*, 13522–13533.
118. Guccione, E.; Bassi, C.; Casadio, F.; Martinato, F.; Cesaroni, M.; Schuchlautz, H.; Luscher, B.; Amati, B. Methylation of histone H3R2 by PRMT6 and H3K4 by an MLL complex are mutually exclusive. *Nature* **2007**, *449*, 933–937.
119. Brown, M.A.; Sims, R.J., 3rd; Gottlieb, P.D.; Tucker, P.W. Identification and characterization of Smyd2: A split SET/MYND domain-containing histone H3 lysine 36-specific methyltransferase that interacts with the Sin3 histone deacetylase complex. *Mol. Cancer* **2006**, doi:10.1186/1476-4598-5-26.
120. Sakane, N.; Kwon, H.S.; Pagans, S.; Kaehlcke, K.; Mizusawa, Y.; Kamada, M.; Lassen, K.G.; Chan, J.; Greene, W.C.; Schnoelzer, M.; *et al.* Activation of HIV transcription by the viral Tat protein requires a demethylation step mediated by lysine-specific demethylase 1 (LSD1/KDM1). *PLoS Pathog.* **2011**, *7*, e1002184.
121. Kauder, S.E.; Bosque, A.; Lindqvist, A.; Planelles, V.; Verdin, E. Epigenetic regulation of HIV-1 latency by cytosine methylation. *PLoS Pathog.* **2009**, *5*, e1000495.
122. Blazkova, J.; Trejbalova, K.; Gondois-Rey, F.; Halfon, P.; Philibert, P.; Guiguen, A.; Verdin, E.; Olive, D.; van Lint, C.; Hejnar, J.; *et al.* CpG methylation controls reactivation of HIV from latency. *PLoS Pathog.* **2009**, *5*, e1000554.
123. Blazkova, J.; Murray, D.; Justement, J.S.; Funk, E.K.; Nelson, A.K.; Moir, S.; Chun, T.W.; Fauci, A.S. Paucity of HIV DNA methylation in latently infected, resting $CD4^+$ T cells from infected individuals receiving antiretroviral therapy. *J. Virol.* **2012**, *86*, 5390–5392.
124. Bowman, G.D. Mechanisms of ATP-dependent nucleosome sliding. *Curr. Opin. Struct. Biol.* **2010**, *20*, 73–81.
125. Henderson, A.; Holloway, A.; Reeves, R.; Tremethick, D.J. Recruitment of SWI/SNF to the human immunodeficiency virus type 1 promoter. *Mol. Cell. Biol.* **2004**, *24*, 389–397.
126. Gallastegui, E.; Millan-Zambrano, G.; Terme, J.M.; Chavez, S.; Jordan, A. Chromatin reassembly factors are involved in transcriptional interference promoting HIV latency. *J. Virol.* **2011**, *85*, 3187–3202.
127. Christ, F.; Voet, A.; Marchand, A.; Nicolet, S.; Desimmie, B.A.; Marchand, D.; Bardiot, D.; van der Veken, N.J.; van Remoortel, B.; Strelkov, S.V.; *et al.* Rational design of small-molecule inhibitors of the LEDGF/p75-integrase interaction and HIV replication. *Nat. Chem. Biol.* **2010**, *6*, 442–448.
128. Tsiang, M.; Jones, G.S.; Niedziela-Majka, A.; Kan, E.; Lansdon, E.B.; Huang, W.; Hung, M.; Samuel, D.; Novikov, N.; Xu, Y.; *et al.* New class of HIV-1 integrase (IN) inhibitors with a dual mode of action. *J. Biol. Chem.* **2012**, *287*, 21189–21203.

129. Desimmie, B.A.; Schrijvers, R.; Demeulemeester, J.; Borrenberghs, D.; Weydert, C.; Thys, W.; Vets, S.; van Remoortel, B.; Hofkens, J.; de Rijck, J.; *et al.* LEDGINs inhibit late stage HIV-1 replication by modulating integrase multimerization in the virions. *Retrovirology* **2013**, doi:10.1186/1742-4690-10-57.
130. Jurado, K.A.; Wang, H.; Slaughter, A.; Feng, L.; Kessl, J.J.; Koh, Y.; Wang, W.; Ballandras-Colas, A.; Patel, P.A.; Fuchs, J.R.; *et al.* Allosteric integrase inhibitor potency is determined through the inhibition of HIV-1 particle maturation. *Proc. Natl. Acad. Sci. USA* **2013**, *110*, 8690–8695.
131. Hamer, D.H. Can HIV be Cured? Mechanisms of HIV persistence and strategies to combat it. *Curr. HIV Res.* **2004**, *2*, 99–111.
132. Gottlicher, M.; Minucci, S.; Zhu, P.; Kramer, O.H.; Schimpf, A.; Giavara, S.; Sleeman, J.P.; Lo Coco, F.; Nervi, C.; Pelicci, P.G.; *et al.* Valproic acid defines a novel class of HDAC inhibitors inducing differentiation of transformed cells. *EMBO J.* **2001**, *20*, 6969–6978.
133. Lehrman, G.; Hogue, I.B.; Palmer, S.; Jennings, C.; Spina, C.A.; Wiegand, A.; Landay, A.L.; Coombs, R.W.; Richman, D.D.; Mellors, J.W.; *et al.* Depletion of latent HIV-1 infection *in vivo*: A proof-of-concept study. *Lancet* **2005**, *366*, 549–555.
134. Archin, N.M.; Eron, J.J.; Palmer, S.; Hartmann-Duff, A.; Martinson, J.A.; Wiegand, A.; Bandarenko, N.; Schmitz, J.L.; Bosch, R.J.; Landay, A.L.; *et al.* Valproic acid without intensified antiviral therapy has limited impact on persistent HIV infection of resting $CD4^+$ T cells. *AIDS* **2008**, *22*, 1131–1135.
135. Sagot-Lerolle, N.; Lamine, A.; Chaix, M.L.; Boufassa, F.; Aboulker, J.P.; Costagliola, D.; Goujard, C.; Pallier, C.; Delfraissy, J.F.; Lambotte, O. Prolonged valproic acid treatment does not reduce the size of latent HIV reservoir. *AIDS* **2008**, *22*, 1125–1129.
136. Archin, N.M.; Cheema, M.; Parker, D.; Wiegand, A.; Bosch, R.J.; Coffin, J.M.; Eron, J.; Cohen, M.; Margolis, D.M. Antiretroviral intensification and valproic acid lack sustained effect on residual HIV-1 viremia or resting $CD4^+$ cell infection. *PLoS ONE* **2010**, *5*, e9390.
137. Routy, J.P.; Tremblay, C.L.; Angel, J.B.; Trottier, B.; Rouleau, D.; Baril, J.G.; Harris, M.; Trottier, S.; Singer, J.; Chomont, N.; *et al.* Valproic acid in association with highly active antiretroviral therapy for reducing systemic HIV-1 reservoirs: Results from a multicentre randomized clinical study. *HIV Med.* **2012**, *13*, 291–296.
138. Cysique, L.A.; Maruff, P.; Brew, B.J. Valproic acid is associated with cognitive decline in HIV^-infected individuals: A clinical observational study. *BMC Neurol.* **2006**, doi:10.1186/1471-2377-6-42.
139. Contreras, X.; Schweneker, M.; Chen, C.S.; McCune, J.M.; Deeks, S.G.; Martin, J.; Peterlin, B.M. Suberoylanilide hydroxamic acid reactivates HIV from latently infected cells. *J. Biol. Chem.* **2009**, *284*, 6782–6789.
140. Reuse, S.; Calao, M.; Kabeya, K.; Guiguen, A.; Gatot, J.S.; Quivy, V.; Vanhulle, C.; Lamine, A.; Vaira, D.; Demonte, D.; *et al.* Synergistic activation of HIV-1 expression by deacetylase inhibitors and prostratin: Implications for treatment of latent infection. *PLoS ONE* **2009**, *4*, e6093.
141. Archin, N.M.; Espeseth, A.; Parker, D.; Cheema, M.; Hazuda, D.; Margolis, D.M. Expression of latent HIV induced by the potent HDAC inhibitor suberoylanilide hydroxamic acid. *AIDS Res. Hum. Retrovir.* **2009**, *25*, 207–212.

142. Archin, N.M.; Liberty, A.L.; Kashuba, A.D.; Choudhary, S.K.; Kuruc, J.D.; Crooks, A.M.; Parker, D.C.; Anderson, E.M.; Kearney, M.F.; Strain, M.C.; *et al.* Administration of vorinostat disrupts HIV-1 latency in patients on antiretroviral therapy. *Nature* **2012**, *487*, 482–485.
143. Elliott, J.H.; Wightman, F.; Solomon, A.; Ghneim, K.; Ahlers, J.; Cameron, M.J.; Smith, M.Z.; Spelman, T.; McMahon, J.; Velayudham, P.; *et al.* Activation of HIV transcription with short-course vorinostat in HIV-infected patients on suppressive antiretroviral therapy. *PLoS Pathog.* **2014**, *10*, e1004473.
144. Matalon, S.; Palmer, B.E.; Nold, M.F.; Furlan, A.; Kassu, A.; Fossati, G.; Mascagni, P.; Dinarello, C.A. The histone deacetylase inhibitor ITF2357 decreases surface CXCR4 and CCR5 expression on $CD4^+$ T-cells and monocytes and is superior to valproic acid for latent HIV-1 expression *in vitro*. *J Acquir. Immune Defic. Syndr.* **2010**, *54*, 1–9.
145. Rasmussen, T.A.; Schmeltz Sogaard, O.; Brinkmann, C.; Wightman, F.; Lewin, S.R.; Melchjorsen, J.; Dinarello, C.; Ostergaard, L.; Tolstrup, M. Comparison of HDAC inhibitors in clinical development: Effect on HIV production in latently infected cells and T-cell activation. *Hum. Vaccines Immunother.* **2013**, *9*, 993–1001.
146. Lu, H.K.; Gray, L.R.; Wightman, F.; Ellenberg, P.; Khoury, G.; Cheng, W.J.; Mota, T.M.; Wesselingh, S.; Gorry, P.R.; Cameron, P.U.; *et al. Ex vivo* response to histone deacetylase (HDAC) inhibitors of the HIV long terminal repeat (LTR) derived from HIV-infected patients on antiretroviral therapy. *PLoS ONE* **2014**, *9*, e113341.
147. Wightman, F.; Lu, H.K.; Solomon, A.E.; Saleh, S.; Harman, A.N.; Cunningham, A.L.; Gray, L.; Churchill, M.; Cameron, P.U.; Dear, A.E.; *et al.* Entinostat is a histone deacetylase inhibitor selective for class 1 histone deacetylases and activates HIV production from latently infected primary T cells. *AIDS* **2013**, *27*, 2853–2862.
148. Wei, D.G.; Chiang, V.; Fyne, E.; Balakrishnan, M.; Barnes, T.; Graupe, M.; Hesselgesser, J.; Irrinki, A.; Murry, J.P.; Stepan, G.; *et al.* Histone deacetylase inhibitor romidepsin induces HIV expression in CD4 T cells from patients on suppressive antiretroviral therapy at concentrations achieved by clinical dosing. *PLoS Pathog.* **2014**, *10*, e1004071.
149. Rasmussen, T.A.; Tolstrup, M.; Brinkmann, C.R.; Olesen, R.; Erikstrup, C.; Solomon, A.; Winckelmann, A.; Palmer, S.; Dinarello, C.; Buzon, M.; *et al.* Panobinostat, a histone deacetylase inhibitor, for latent-virus reactivation in HIV-infected patients on suppressive antiretroviral therapy: A phase 1/2, single group, clinical trial. *Lancet HIV* **2014**, *1*, e13–e21.
150. Banerjee, C.; Archin, N.; Michaels, D.; Belkina, A.C.; Denis, G.V.; Bradner, J.; Sebastiani, P.; Margolis, D.M.; Montano, M. BET bromodomain inhibition as a novel strategy for reactivation of HIV-1. *J. Leukoc. Biol.* **2012**, *92*, 1147–1154.
151. Bartholomeeusen, K.; Xiang, Y.; Fujinaga, K.; Peterlin, B.M. Bromodomain and extra-terminal (BET) bromodomain inhibition activate transcription via transient release of positive transcription elongation factor b (P-TEFb) from 7SK small nuclear ribonucleoprotein. *J. Biol. Chem.* **2012**, *287*, 36609–36616.
152. Zhu, J.; Gaiha, G.D.; John, S.P.; Pertel, T.; Chin, C.R.; Gao, G.; Qu, H.; Walker, B.D.; Elledge, S.J.; Brass, A.L. Reactivation of latent HIV-1 by inhibition of BRD4. *Cell Rep.* **2012**, *2*, 807–816.
153. Li, Z.; Guo, J.; Wu, Y.; Zhou, Q. The BET bromodomain inhibitor JQ1 activates HIV latency through antagonizing Brd4 inhibition of Tat-transactivation. *Nucleic Acids Res.* **2013**, *41*, 277–287.

154. Boehm, D.; Calvanese, V.; Dar, R.D.; Xing, S.; Schroeder, S.; Martins, L.; Aull, K.; Li, P.C.; Planelles, V.; Bradner, J.E.; *et al.* BET bromodomain-targeting compounds reactivate HIV from latency via a Tat-independent mechanism. *Cell Cycle* **2013**, *12*, 452–462.
155. Bernhard, W.; Barreto, K.; Saunders, A.; Dahabieh, M.S.; Johnson, P.; Sadowski, I. The Suv39H1 methyltransferase inhibitor chaetocin causes induction of integrated HIV-1 without producing a T cell response. *FEBS Lett.* **2011**, *585*, 3549–3554.
156. Bouchat, S.; Gatot, J.S.; Kabeya, K.; Cardona, C.; Colin, L.; Herbein, G.; de Wit, S.; Clumeck, N.; Lambotte, O.; Rouzioux, C.; *et al.* Histone methyltransferase inhibitors induce HIV-1 recovery in resting $CD4^+$ T cells from HIV-1-infected HAART-treated patients. *AIDS* **2012**, *26*, 1473–1482.
157. Friedman, J.; Cho, W.K.; Chu, C.K.; Keedy, K.S.; Archin, N.M.; Margolis, D.M.; Karn, J. Epigenetic silencing of HIV-1 by the histone H3 lysine 27 methyltransferase enhancer of Zeste 2. *J. Virol.* **2011**, *85*, 9078–9089.
158. Burnett, J.C.; Lim, K.I.; Calafi, A.; Rossi, J.J.; Schaffer, D.V.; Arkin, A.P. Combinatorial latency reactivation for HIV-1 subtypes and variants. *J. Virol.* **2010**, *84*, 5958–5974.
159. Laird, G.M.; Bullen, C.K.; Rosenbloom, D.I.; Martin, A.R.; Hill, A.L.; Durand, C.M.; Siliciano, J.D.; Siliciano, R.F. *Ex vivo* analysis identifies effective HIV-1 latency-reversing drug combinations. *J. Clin. Investig.* **2015**, *125*, 1901–1912.
160. Dar, R.D.; Hosmane, N.N.; Arkin, M.R.; Siliciano, R.F.; Weinberger, L.S. Screening for noise in gene expression identifies drug synergies. *Science* **2014**, *344*, 1392–1396.
161. Finzi, D.; Hermankova, M.; Pierson, T.; Carruth, L.M.; Buck, C.; Chaisson, R.E.; Quinn, T.C.; Chadwick, K.; Margolick, J.; Brookmeyer, R.; *et al.* Identification of a reservoir for HIV-1 in patients on highly active antiretroviral therapy. *Science* **1997**, *278*, 1295–1300.
162. Siliciano, J.D.; Kajdas, J.; Finzi, D.; Quinn, T.C.; Chadwick, K.; Margolick, J.B.; Kovacs, C.; Gange, S.J.; Siliciano, R.F. Long-term follow-up studies confirm the stability of the latent reservoir for HIV-1 in resting $CD4^+$ T cells. *Nat. Med.* **2003**, *9*, 727–728.
163. Eriksson, S.; Graf, E.H.; Dahl, V.; Strain, M.C.; Yukl, S.A.; Lysenko, E.S.; Bosch, R.J.; Lai, J.; Chioma, S.; Emad, F.; *et al.* Comparative analysis of measures of viral reservoirs in HIV-1 eradication studies. *PLoS Pathog.* **2013**, *9*, e1003174.
164. Ho, Y.C.; Shan, L.; Hosmane, N.N.; Wang, J.; Laskey, S.B.; Rosenbloom, D.I.; Lai, J.; Blankson, J.N.; Siliciano, J.D.; Siliciano, R.F. Replication-competent noninduced proviruses in the latent reservoir increase barrier to HIV-1 cure. *Cell* **2013**, *155*, 540–551.

2

Chromatinization of the KSHV Genome During the KSHV Life Cycle

Timsy Uppal [1], Hem C. Jha [2], Subhash C. Verma [1] and Erle S. Robertson [2,*]

[1] Department of Microbiology and Immunology, School of Medicine, University of Nevada, 1664 N Virginia Street, MS 320, Reno, NV 89557, USA; E-Mails: tuppal@medicine.nevada.edu (T.U.); scverma@medicine.nevada.edu (S.C.V.)

[2] Department of Microbiology and the Tumor Virology Program of the Abramson Cancer Center, Perelman School of Medicine at the University of Pennsylvania, 201E Johnson Pavilion, 3610 Hamilton Walk, Philadelphia, PA 19104, USA; E-Mail: hemjha@mail.med.upenn.edu

* Author to whom correspondence should be addressed; E-Mail: erle@mail.med.upenn.edu

Academic Editor: Elena Kashuba

Abstract: Kaposi's sarcoma-associated herpesvirus (KSHV) belongs to the gamma herpesvirus family and is the causative agent of various lymphoproliferative diseases in humans. KSHV, like other herpesviruses, establishes life-long latent infection with the expression of a limited number of viral genes. Expression of these genes is tightly regulated by both the viral and cellular factors. Recent advancements in identifying the expression profiles of viral transcripts, using tilling arrays and next generation sequencing have identified additional coding and non-coding transcripts in the KSHV genome. Determining the functions of these transcripts will provide a better understanding of the mechanisms utilized by KSHV in altering cellular pathways involved in promoting cell growth and tumorigenesis. Replication of the viral genome is critical in maintaining the existing copies of the viral episomes during both latent and lytic phases of the viral life cycle. The replication of the viral episome is facilitated by viral components responsible for recruiting chromatin modifying enzymes and replication factors for altering the chromatin complexity and replication initiation functions, respectively. Importantly, chromatin modification of the viral genome plays a crucial role in determining whether the viral genome will persist as latent episome or undergo lytic reactivation. Additionally, chromatinization of the incoming virion DNA, which lacks chromatin structure, in the target cells during primary infection, helps in establishing latent infection. Here, we discuss the recent advancements on our understating of KSHV genome chromatinization and the consequences of chromatin modifications on viral life cycle.

Keywords: KSHV; oncogenic virus; LANA; RTA; epigenetics; viral chromatin; histone modifications; DNA methylation; PAN RNA; *de novo* infection

---

1. Introduction

Kaposi's Sarcoma (KS), first described in 1872 by the Hungarian dermatologist Moritz Kaposi, is defined as a multiple idiopathic sarcoma of the skin. The causative agent of Kaposi's sarcoma was identified as the human herpesvirus 8 (HHV8), or Kaposi's sarcoma-associated herpesvirus (KSHV) from the tissue biopsies of AIDS-associated KS by Chang and Moore in 1994, using the representational difference analysis approach [1]. KSHV is an oncogenic γ-herpesvirus that establishes life-long persistent infection and causes tumors in immunosuppressed individuals; particularly, in transplant recipients and patients infected with HIV. Since its initial discovery in KS lesions, KSHV has been tightly linked with endothelial tumors, Kaposi's sarcoma and two B-cell lymphoproliferative disorders, primary effusion lymphoma (PEL), also known as body cavity-based lymphoma [2], and a plasmablastic variant of multicentric Castleman's disease (MCD) [3]. Additionally, KSHV has been linked to different lymphomas, including Burkitt's lymphoma, Germinotropic Lymphoproliferative Disorder (GLD), multiple myeloma, angio-sarcomas, malignant skin tumors, angio-immunoblastic lymphoma and primary pulmonary hypertension [4–6]. There have also been reports of a new KSHV/HHV8-associated germinotropic lymphoproliferative disorder in HIV-seronegative individuals [7].

1.1. Clinical Diseases Associated with KSHV Infection

1.1.1. Kaposi's Sarcoma (KS)

Kaposi's sarcoma is the first tumor to be associated with HIV infection and remains the most common cancer in Sub-Saharan Africa and the second most common cancer in HIV-infected patients [8]. KS is a highly vascular, non-classical tumor of endothelial lymphatic origin clinically characterized by dark red, brown or purple patches or plaques found cutaneously, mucosally or viscerally [9]. KS lesions are characterized by the presence of spindle shaped, poorly differentiated and highly proliferative cells and by infiltration of inflammatory cells and extensive neo-angiogenesis [10]. Several studies indicate that KS spindle cells are of endothelial lineage as they express the vascular endothelial cell markers CD31, CD34, CD36 [11]. More recently, KS spindle cells are thought to be of lymphatic endothelial cell (LECs) origin because they express LYVE-1, VEGFR-3 and podoplanin, markers of the lymphatic endothelium, making it difficult to identify the precursor cell type [12,13]. KSHV is required for the development of KS with greater than 95% of KS lesions harboring KSHV viral DNA in latent phase [14]. The role of KSHV in KS development is complex and involves both latent and lytic genes, many of which are pirated versions of cellular genes. The virus is found in all epidemiologic-clinical forms of the disease, including classic, African (endemic), HIV-associated (epidemic) and iatrogenic (transplant associated) KS (reviewed in [15]). Classic KS (indolent form) usually is present as lesions in the lower and upper extremities without the involvement of lymph nodes and internal organs [16]. Endemic KS, on the other hand, can be indolent or aggressive and transplant-related that represents a relatively indolent and chronic condition with a rapidly progressive course involving lymph nodes, mucosa and inner organs [17]. HIV-related KS is the most frequent and aggressive form that includes the lymph nodes and visceral spreading, though the role of HIV infection in KS development is not very well understood [18]. Since the introduction of highly active antiretroviral therapy (HAART), there has been a decline in KS incidence. However, Kaposi's sarcoma continues to be diagnosed in HIV-infected patients.

1.1.2. Primary Effusion Lymphoma (PEL)

PEL, also referred to as body cavity-based lymphoma (BCBL), is an aggressive form of non-Hodgkin's B-cell lymphoma and is linked to KSHV infection and commonly found in late stage immunocompromised AIDS patients [19]. Evidence for the contributing role of KSHV in PEL development is attributed to detection of approximately 50–150 copies of KSHV latent genomes per cell with less than 1% of cells entering the lytic cycle [20,21]. Additionally, PEL cell survival has been shown to depend on the expression of CD138/syndecan-1, the KSHV latent genes (primarily ORF73, LANA) and viral microRNAs, highlighting the association between KSHV infection and PEL development [22]. Approximately 50% of PEL patients are KSHV-positive and found to be co-infected with Epstein-Barr virus (EBV), although cases of KSHV and EBV-negative PEL have also been reported [23,24]. Consistent growth of PEL cell lines in culture and easy induction of infectious KSHV virions release have made them a valuable *in vitro* infection model for understanding the molecular mechanisms of KSHV-related oncogenesis, in terms of cell transformation, signaling, cell growth, cell survival, angiogenesis and host-immune invasion, though how KSHV directly contributes to this B-cell malignancy is yet to be known [25].

1.1.3. Multicentric Castleman's Disease

The plasmablastic variant of Multicentric Castleman's disease (MCD) containing large plasmablastic cells is frequently linked to KSHV infection and is usually characterized by lymphadenopathy and immune deregulation [14,26]. MCD is a lymphoproliferative disorder that is often diagnosed in HIV-infected patients. KSHV co-infection is predominantly observed in the immunoblastic B cells within the mantle zone of germinal centers of lymph nodes in almost all HIV-seropositive MCD cases and in less than 40% HIV-seronegative MCD cases [27]. Interestingly, in contrast to KS and PEL, KSHV infection in MCD is mostly lytic and thought to be driven by an elevated levels of cytokines, interleukin-6 and 10 (IL-6, IL-10) and the vascular endothelial growth factor (VEGF) [28]. Additionally, so far the co-infection of KSHV with EBV has not been detected in MCD plasmablasts [29].

1.2. Epidemiology and KSHV Transmission

Epidemiology studies on KSHV have identified eight distinctive subtypes based on the sequence analysis of a well-conserved minor capsid gene, ORF26 [30]. Though large parts of the KSHV genome are conserved in these variants, several regions were shown to be highly variable, including the K1 and K15 gene regions. The sequence variability of the K1 gene has led to the identification of seven major viral subtypes, namely A, B, C, D, E, F and G [31,32]. General nucleotide differences between these subtypes are only 3%, however up to 60% sequence variation is observed in the two-hypervariable regions (VR1 and VR2) of the K1 gene [33]. Only two of the KSHV subtypes, A and C have diversity in the region surrounding K15 with variants designated as P (or prototype), M (or minority), N and Q. These variations are thought to arise from a recombination event with an unknown progenitor herpesvirus [34,35].

KSHV prevalence is found to correlate with geographic location. For instance, subgroup A1–4 and subtype C are predominant among individuals in North Europe, the United States and in some regions of Asia and Middle East. Subgroup B1–4 is located primarily in sub-Saharan Africa while D and E strains are found principally in Australia, the Pacific and Brazilian Amerindians [36–38]. Several serology studies have indicated that KSHV infection is widespread in sub-Saharan Africa and the Amazon basin where greater than 50% population is infected [39]. Intermediate levels of KSHV prevalence are seen in Mediterranean, Middle East and the Caribbean regions where 4%–45% population is tested as KSHV-seropositive. Lower levels of viral infection occur in Northern Europe and North America with KSHV seropositivity ranging from 3% to 10% [40,41].

Although, the transmission modes and the risk factors for KSHV infection are not well understood, the virus is reported to transmit through both sexual and non-sexual transmission routes [42,43]. In low prevalence areas, a direct link has been reported between the number of sexual partners and the risk of KSHV infection, indicating sexual transmission as the predominant transmission route [44]. Also, seroprevalence is lower for women and children than in men. The epidemiology differs significantly in the high prevalence areas with equal seroprevalence amongst children, adult men and women highlighting non-sexual routes of virus transmission. Studies in Italy, northern Sweden and Uganda suggest that the KSHV virions are mostly transmitted via saliva and sometimes through water and insect bite indicating KSHV transmission is dependent on a combination of both environmental and genetic factors [45–47].

1.3. KSHV Genome and Its Chromatinization

KSHV has a double stranded DNA (dsDNA) genome of 165–170 kb consisting of long unique coding region, which is ~140 kb in length and is flanked with highly GC-rich 801 bp long terminal repeat sequences (TRs) that encodes for nearly 86 viral open-reading frames (vORFs), 12 miRNAs and a number of non-coding RNAs (ncRNAs) and antisense RNAs [48,49]. The viral genes encoded by KSHV can be classified into three categories: (1) Herpesviruses-common genes; (2) KSHV-unique genes, and (3) Cellular-homologous genes, which may include categories (1) and (2) [50]. Studies on KSHV virion-associated proteins indicate that the virus particle is formed through several highly specific protein-protein interactions among capsid, tegument proteins and glycoproteins [51].

Each KSHV virion consists of a linear dsDNA duplex. The virion particle binds to the host cell surface receptor and penetrates into the host cell cytoplasm by a complex multistep process (reviewed in [52]). Virion capsids are then transported to the nuclear pore with concominant release of linear viral DNA. During *de novo* infection (*i.e.*, entry of the virion in the target cells) and establishment of latency, the incoming linear dsDNA is circularized using the cellular enzymatic machinery to generate a closed-circular DNA, which is further maintained in a circular episomal form tightly packed as nucleosome (Figure 1). Encapsidated virion DNA is generally naïve and shows no chromatin structure, however, the resulting circular episome gets chromatinized due to its association with cellular histones in order to ensure: (1) protection of viral DNA ends to escape the host DNA damage response; (2) stable maintenance, replication and segregation of the viral genome to daughter cells during mitosis; (3) successful completion of viral life cycle; and (4) the regulation of viral gene expression (reviewed in [53]).

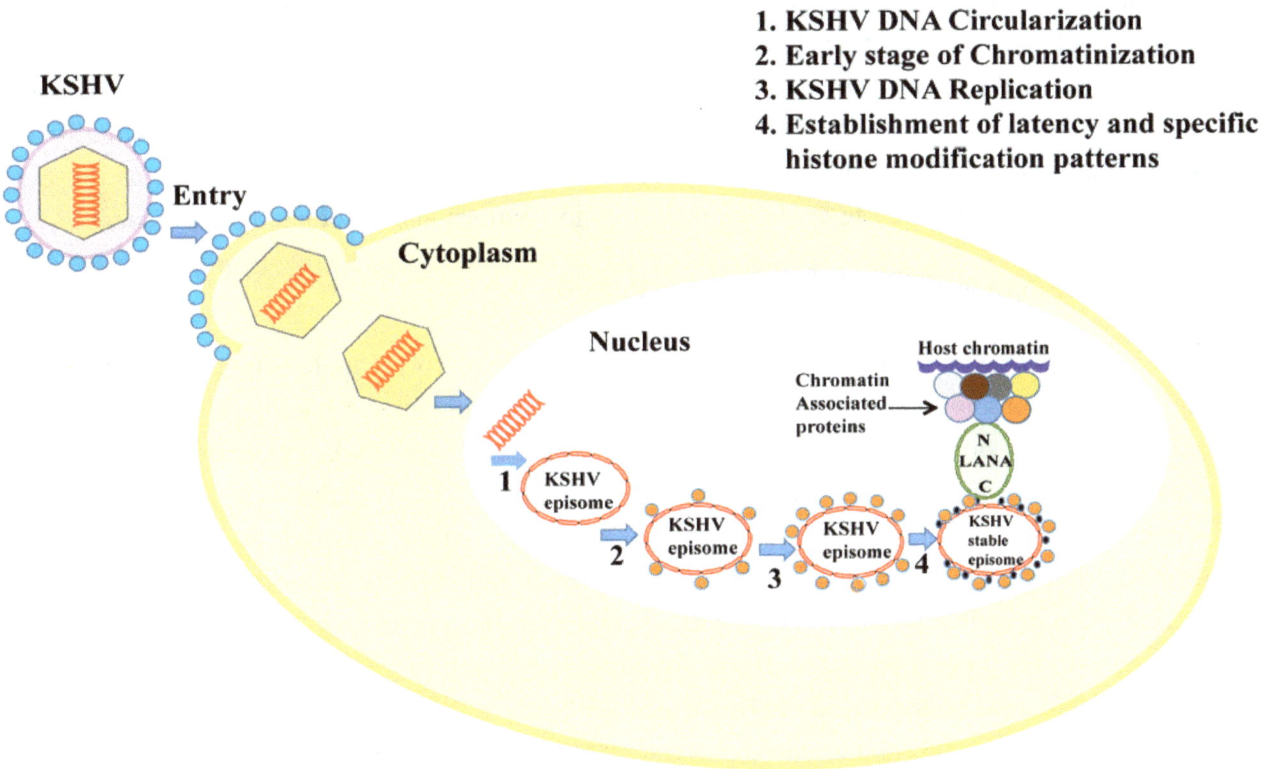

Figure 1. The chromatinization and maintenance of the KSHV genome following *de novo* infection: After the KSHV virion attaches to the host cell, the viral capsid enters the cytoplasm, followed by the ejection of viral DNA into the nucleus. Subsequently, the linear viral genome is circularized into an extrachromosomal episome to avoid detection by the host DNA damage response; (2) Circularized genome is further chromatinized using cellular histones and histone modifying factors resulting in a stable episome; (3) Viral genome, which is being maintained as multicopy chromatinized episome then replicates along with the cellular genome; (4) For the stable persistence and segregation of KSHV epigenome during latency, KSHV latent protein LANA binds to the TR region of the viral genome and tethers the viral genome to the host chromosome through its amino-terminus via interaction with histones and cellular chromatin associated proteins.

Though the processes of viral genome circularization and chromatinization are poorly understood, there are key regulatory steps in the life cycle of many viruses, which are crucial for the establishment and persistence of the viral quiescence or latency [53,54]. The viral genome upon entry into the host cell nucleus must adopt a structure similar to the host genome and interact with cellular chromatin. The chromatinized viral DNA is influenced by the same epigenetic factors as the cellular DNA thereby generating the so-called "*viral epigenome*", which significantly impacts both latency and lytic reactivation of the viral genome. Additionally, studies have indicated that viruses that enter and hide in the host nucleus have co-evolved with numerous cellular chromatin modulation mechanisms to ensure their survival and propagation [54].

Recent studies have uncovered a wealth of information regarding the dynamic aspects of chromatin structure and the mechanisms whereby chromatin modifications regulate the viral gene expression and viral-host chromatin interactions. Importantly, chromatin and epigenetic modulation of KSHV genome represents a novel antiviral target for blocking virus-mediated tumorigenesis. This compilation review summarizes some of the emerging concepts that will describe in the detail our current knowledge of chromatin assembly and remodeling factors, and epigenetic alterations, including DNA methylation, post-translational histone modifications, and nucleosome occupancy of KSHV genome, as the master controllers of KSHV's biphasic life cycle, gene expression pattern and associated pathogenesis.

2. Chromatin Regulation and Gene Expression Pattern

The eukaryotic DNA is wrapped around histone proteins to form nucleosomes, the fundamental repeating units of chromatin. The nucleosome consists of an octameric histone core containing two H2A-H2B dimers and one H3-H4 tetramer with 147-bp segment of DNA wrapped in 1.65 turns and ~50 bp of free DNA separating the neighboring nucleosomes [55]. Together with linker histone H1, nucleosomes can compact to form condensed chromatin. The histone tails that protrudes out from the nucleosome undergoes different posttranslational modifications such as lysine acetylation, lysine and arginine methylation, serine, tyrosine and threonine phosphorylation and lysine ubiquitination to provide coding mechanism for protein recognition and signaling (reviewed in [56,57]).

Acetylation of histone tails, carried out by histone acetyltransferases (HAT's) results in the relaxation of the chromatin structure through increased charge repulsions and is primarily associated with active gene expression [58]. Higher-order folding of the nucleosomal DNA can give rise to either less condensed, *actively transcribed euchromatin* or to highly condensed, *transcriptionally silent heterochromatin* and histone modifications can be found in both varieties of the chromatin. Euchromatin state is characterized by high levels of histone acetylation and methylation of lysine residues at 4, 36 and 79 of histone H3. Alternatively, the heterochromatin has low levels of acetylation and high levels of methylation of lysine residues at 9 and 27 of histone H3. Genes that are transcriptionally active possess high levels of H3K4me3, H3K27ac, H2BK5ac and H4K20me1 histone marks in their promoter region and H3K79me1 and H4K20me1 along the gene body [59]. These patterns of histone modifications that trigger activation or silencing of the gene can potentially be transmitted to the daughter cells and thus referred to as sequence-independent heritable changes of the genome (*epigenome*). Several well defined "*epigenomic marks*" on chromatin range from chemical modifications on DNA, histone proteins and 3D chromatin organization.

Structure of chromatin is highly variable and dynamic and their structures vary among different cell types. Analysis of the chromatin structure at the genomic level leads to characterization of the landscape of the epigenome that helps to define the gene expression pattern of any cell. Advances in next-generation sequencing technologies have enabled a high-resolution genome-wide investigation of the viral and cellular epigenomic landscape in various cell types. Powerful sequencing-based methods are used as excellent tools to interrogate the interplay between genomic locations of open chromatin regions, DNA-binding factors, nucleosomes and chromatin conformations at a single nucleotide resolution [60,61].

Chromatin Immunoprecipitation (ChIP) analysis of DNA-histone complexes is one of the efficient methods for the elucidation of chromatin structure and histone modifications. ChIP assays combined with DNA microarrays (ChIP-on-Chip) or high-throughput sequencing of purified DNA fragments

(ChIP-seq) and chromatin conformation capture assays (3C) are primarily used to characterize endogenous chromatin structure together with mapping the genomic locations of DNA-associated proteins. In the context of the KSHV genome, prior studies conducted on KSHV infected cell lines at nucleotide resolution using ChIP-seq established the presence of histones, DNA methylation, DNA-protein interactions such as RNA polymerase II binding, LANA and CTCF-cohesin occupancy and nucleosome depletion on the latent KSHV episome [62–64]. More recently FAIRE (Formaldehyde-Assisted Isolation of Regulatory Elements) has been utilized as an alternative and robust approach than antibody-dependent ChIP-sequencing, to depict several regions of open chromatin in the latent KSHV genome. FAIRE, followed by next-generation sequencing (FAIRE-seq), together with previously identified nucleosome depletion and histone modification data, has led to the identification of the regulatory elements in KSHV genome, adding to our existing knowledge on the whole genome landscape of latent KSHV chromatin [65].

3. KSHV Latent Gene Expression Profile

During latent infection, the KSHV genome persists in a relatively quiescent state as multicopy chromatinized "*minichromosomes* or *episomes*" that transcribes and replicates simultaneously with the cellular chromosome thereby evades host's immune surveillance [66]. Major latent genes are located between ORF 69 and K14 in the KSHV genome in the latency locus with their gene expression under the control of a few promoters, whereas the other viral genes are silenced during latency (reviewed in [67]). Viral latency is, however, reversible and can be periodically reactivated into lytic replication by specific environmental and physiological stimuli, thereby expressing all of the viral lytic genes in an ordered cascade resulting in the production of viral progeny. Both latent and lytic cycle replications are essential for the long-term persistence of the virus, and the gene products of these transcriptional programs contribute to KSHV-induced pathogenesis [49,67].

Majority of the KS biopsy samples and PEL cell lines exhibits latent gene expression profiles, thus provides a remarkable tumor model for better understanding of the mechanisms that regulate the expression of viral genes during latency. These latency models express a restricted yet variable pattern of viral latency-associated genes that modulate both viral and cellular gene expressions to establish and maintain latency. KSHV latent genes or transcripts include the latency-associated nuclear antigen LANA encoded by ORF73, viral cyclinD homologue, v-Cyclin encoded by ORF72, a viral homologue of a FLICE-inhibitory protein v-FLIP encoded by ORF71, Kaposin encoded by K12, and a cluster of 12 viral microRNAs [68–72], mRNA of several other viral genes including viral G protein-coupled receptor v-GPCR encoded by ORF74, K1, vIL-6 and ORF59 encoded by ORF59 have also been detected in most KS and PEL-tumor models [14]. Together, these latency-associated viral proteins are required for constant latent infection and survival of the infected cell.

For most of the KSHV positive PEL-derived cell lines studied so far the expression of the major viral latent proteins: LANA, v-Cyclin and v-FLIP is limited to a single multi-cistronic latent transcript [66]. LANA, functional orthologue of Epstein-Barr virus encoded EBNA1, binds to multiple sites on the KSHV genome, preferentially in the TR region, which helps in tethering of the viral genome to the host chromosome and maintenance of the replicated episomal copies after duplication of the tumor cells during latency [73]. The v-Cyclin and v-FLIP play key roles in host cell proliferation and survival [74–76]. The Kaposin transcript is expressed either from promoters downstream of LANA or the ones within the repeat region upstream of Kaposin [77]. Along with ORF74, K14 is expressed as a bi-cistronic transcript from the promoter downstream of LANA-v-Cyclin-v-FLIP RNA [78]. The ORF74-K14 transcript initiates from the 5' UTR of the LANA-v-Cyclin-v-FLIP and is expressed in latently infected cells along with LANA-v-Cyclin-v-FLIP gene expression [79]. More sensitive methods using micro-arrays and proteomics have identified several viral transcripts and peptide motifs that further provide valuable knowledge regarding viral latent gene expression [80].

Latency-associated Nuclear Antigen (LANA): LANA, a large nuclear protein of 220–230 kDa with DNA binding and chromatin binding domains in carboxy and amnio terminal domains, respectively is encoded by ORF73 and is critical for the establishment of latent infection [73,81,82]. LANA, a multifunctional protein can regulate transcription of cellular and viral genes through activation or repression of various cellular and viral promoters [83]. Additionally, LANA has also been shown to deregulate the expressions many oncogenes (by stabilizing) and tumor suppressors (by degrading) to induce tumor growth and these includes c-Myc, p53, hypoxia-inducible factor 1 (HIF-1), glycogen synthase kinase 3 (GSK3), von Hippel-Lindau protein (pVHL) and β-catenin [84–89]. LANA also controls lytic origin dependent DNA synthesis by interacting with origin binding protein (OBP), K-bZIP [90]. LANA promotes tumorigenesis and cell growth by inducing chromosome instability and upregulation of cellular IAP expression in KSHV-infected cells [91]. LANA plays a critical role in maintaining the KSHV genome in infected cells by ensuring faithful segregation of the newly synthesized viral genome into the divided cells by interacting with cellular proteins, Bub-1 and CENP-F [92]. Additionally, LANA inhibits interleukin-4 (IL-4)-mediated STAT6 phosphorylation, which helps in blocking apoptosis to maintain latency [93].

The role of LANA in the persistence of the KSHV genome was identified by using the 33-kb left-end of KSHV in a persistence assay in BJAB cells expressing LANA [73]. Additional studies identified the LANA binding sites, named LBS1 in the TR region of the KSHV genome [81,94,95]. Minimal LANA binding sequence in TR was identified by *in vitro* binding assays to be a 13 bp sequence within the TR [95]. Additional studies identified another LANA binding site (LBS2), which has lower affinity than LBS1 and is located right next to the first LANA binding site (LBS1) in the TRs [96]. The first LANA binding site lies between positions 571 and 589 of the 801bp long TR and is termed as LANA binding sequence 1 (LBS1) [96]. Binding of LANA to these two LANA Binding Sequences (LBS1/2) of the TR creates DNA bending and suppresses transcriptional activities when fused to a reporter plasmid [94,97].

The DNA binding domain of LANA is mapped to the C-terminal domain between amino acids 996 and 1139 [98]. Scanning of this region for identifying the exact residues in DNA binding by generating substitution mutants determined that amino acids between 1007 and 10021aa may be the DNA contact residues as the mutants of this region abolished DNA binding as well as replication and episome persistence abilities of LANA [98]. The amino terminal domain of LANA binds to the host chromatin through nucleosomal histones and tethers the viral genome bound to the C-terminus of LANA to the host chromosomes. Along with histones various other chromatin-associated proteins including RING3, which colocalizes to heterochromatin and heterochromatin proteins 1 (HP1) was also detected as LANA binding proteins by various biochemical assays [99]. A model for tethering of LANA to the host chromatin either through N-terminus binding proteins such as linker histone H1, core histones H2A/H2B, budding uninhibited by benzimidazole 1 (Bub1) and centromeric protein F (CENP-F) or C-terminus binding proteins including 43-kDa protein DEK, methyl CpG binding protein (MeCP2), bromodomain proteins Brd2/Brd4, nuclear mitotic apparatus protein CENP-F and Bub1 has been proposed [100].

A number of studies have demonstrated the role of LANA in modulating the activities of various cellular pathways by directly interacting with the major players of the pathways or complexing with additional proteins to favor cell growth (reviewed in [101]). LANA does not seem to possess enzymatic activities required for DNA replication but is critical for the replication of TR-containing plasmids [102]. LANA achieves this by recruiting host cellular replication factors to the TR in a cell cycle dependent manner (reviewed in [101,103]. Studies from others as well as our lab have shown the involvement of host cellular replication proteins in the replication of KSHV episomal DNA [104–107]. The replication of host genome occurs in a very precise manner in order to maintain genetic integrity, which is achieved by ensuring that no segment of DNA replicates more than once per cell cycle [108]. Replication process starts during the late G_1 and early S phase by licensing of the replication origin sites by sequential loading of ORCs, cdc6, Cdt1, and the heterohexameric complex MCM2-7 (minichromosome maintenance proteins 2 to 7) to the origins to be used during the S phase [109]. Upon loading of these licensing factors, origins are licensed to form a pre-replicative complex (pre-RC) for replication initiation [107,110].

LANA has also been shown to upregulate the proteins important for the immortalization of infected cells, which includes modulation of hTERT and E2F1 responsive promoters [111,112]. LANA also promotes cell cycle progression through redistribution of the cellular pool of glycogen synthase kinase-3 beta (GSK-3b) to the nucleus, which leads to an accumulation of β-catenin in the cytoplasm. Increased levels of β-catenin in the cytoplasm are translocated to the nucleus, which in turns upregulates the β-catenin responsive, Lef-Tcf promoters. Increased levels of Lef-Tcf enhance the transcription of S-phase entry genes such as *MYC, JUN and CCND1* (Cyclin D1), which drive cell cycle progression [85]. Additionally, LANA modulates apoptotic pathways as the LANA expressing cells are resistant to p53-dependent apoptosis but not the p53-independent apoptosis confirming specificity to p53 [112]. LANA also modulates the activity of another tumor suppressor, pRb, which was determined by the fact that expression of LANA overcame the flat-cell (growth arrested) phenotype in RB1 negative cells. Saos2 (deletion mutant of *RB1*) cells enter cell cycle arrest upon exogenous expression of pRb, but the interaction of LANA with pRb overcomes this phenotype, suggesting re-entry of these cells into the S-phase of cell cycle. LANA expressing cells inhibits pRb and p53 pathways that enable these cells to circumvent the G1/S checkpoint and the apoptotic pathway, respectively, which leads to the immortalization and tumorigenesis of LANA expressing cells [113].

v-*Cyclin:* It is encoded by ORF72 and is the homologue of cellular D-cyclin which acts like a constitutive activator of cellular cyclin-dependent kinase 6 (CDK6) to regulate cellular proliferation and viral replication [114]. The v-Cyclin-CDK6 complex can phosphorylate its cellular counterpart pRb protein, Histones H1, CDK inhibitor (cdki) and p27 (Kip1) [115]. The exact role of this viral protein in regulating KSHV life cycle is not fully understood but studies indicate that v-Cyclin-CDK6 complex mediated phosphorylation of nucleophosmin (NPM) facilitates NPM-LANA interaction and recruitment of HDAC1 to promote KSHV latency [116]. Additionally, KSHV v-Cyclin shares close functional relationship with murine gammaherpesvirus 68 (MHV68) v-Cyclin that is known to mediate efficient lytic reactivation from latency [117].

v-*FLIP/K13:* ORF71 encodes the KSHV homologue of cellular FLICE like inhibitory protein v-FLIP, also known as K13. KSHV v-FLIP is likely to contribute to latency by promoting cell survival [74,118]. The v-FLIP can block apoptosis by binding to the inhibitor of kB-kinase γ (IKK γ), leading to the activation of the NF-*k*B pathway [119]. NF-*k*B pathway activation by v-FLIP has been linked to KSHV lytic replication as the KSHV mutant deficient in v-FLIP inhibits ORF50/RTA lytic gene expression [120]. Additionally, v-FLIP regulates the activation of a key cellular survival pathway to promote cell proliferation and survival during latency (reviewed in [121]).

Kaposins: The Kaposin locus (K12) and surrounding direct repeat regions DR1 and DR2 encode for 3 proteins, namely, Kaposin A, B and C [122]. Kaposin A is a hydrophobic latent protein with transforming potential in Rat-1 fibroblasts whereas Kaposin B is a small soluble nuclear protein, which affects signaling by binding to a mitogen-activated protein (MAP) kinase 2 (MK2) [123]. Kaposin C is a trans-membrane protein, however the biological function of this protein is not yet known [122]. All of these proteins are shown to contribute to the inflammatory microenvironment of KS [122].

LANA2/vIRF-3: The KSHV genome encodes four viral homologues of cellular interferon regulatory protein (vIRFs) to counteract the interferon system (IFN) for evading the host's immune response. One such protein predominantly expressed during KSHV latency is K10.5/LANA2 that is considered as a KSHV defense protein against IFN [124]. LANA2 is exclusively expressed in both PEL and MCD cell lines and has been linked to the disruption of cellular IRF-7, IRF-3 and IRF-5 mediated signaling and cellular PKR signaling [125]. LANA2 also inhibits p53 and NF-*k*B, which suggests its role in KSHV infection and pathogenesis [126].

Viral microRNAs: KSHV encodes 12 pre-miRNAs, of which 10 miRNA (miR-K1-9 and -K11) are encoded between the kaposin and ORF71/K13 region while the other two miRNAs, miR-K10 and -K12 are located in the coding and 3' untranslated region of K12, respectively [127–131]. All miRNAs are expressed in cells latently infected with KSHV and regulate latency while suppressing lytic reactivation of the virus [132–135]. Among these miRNAs, miR-K1 represses the expression of IκBα-an inhibitor of the pro-survival NF-κB pathway and inhibits the activation of lytic viral promoters. Since the NF-κB pathway is involved in cell growth and survival, miR-K1 might directly affect KSHV-mediated pathogenesis [136,137]. KSHV miR-K10 targets TNF-like weak inducer of apoptosis (TWEAKR) and is shown to protect cell from apoptosis and suppress pro-inflammatory responses, which might contribute to KSHV latent infection [136,138]. Several other miRNAs such as miR-K3, -K4, -K5 and -K9 target nuclear factor I/B, Rbl2 protein, Bcl-2 associated factor, BCLAF1 and activates the 3'UTR region of RTA protein respectively, to inhibit cell death and regulate lytic replication [139].

Chromatin Organization of KSHV Genome during Latent Infection

LANA-dependent DNA Replication and Epigenetic Modifications at the KSHV TR: KSHV LANA, a DNA binding nuclear protein acts as an initiator of DNA replication by specifically binding to a ~60 bp motif in the KSHV TRs [102]. A DNA-LANA protein complex is formed between LANA, trans-acting protein, and the LANA binding, cis-elements of KSHV TR [94,95,140]. Two or more copies of the TR are required for maintenance of the plasmid while a single copy of TR and the minimal replicator element is sufficient to initiate DNA replication [98,107,141,142]. Despite the absence of any enzymatic activity in LANA required for DNA replication, LANA supports DNA replication via its interaction with the host cellular replication factors including the origin recognition complexes (ORCs), Topoismerase IIβ, replication protein A (RPA) and proliferating cell nuclear antigen (PCNA) [104,106,110]. A recent study has demonstrated that LANA mediates KSHV DNA replication and virus persistence by recruiting replication factor C (RFC), the DNA polymerase clamp, proliferating cell nuclear antigen (PCNA) loader.

LANA mutant with deleted RFC binding domain was found to have a negative impact on LANA-mediated DNA replication and episome persistence [110]. However, the detailed mechanism by which LANA interacts with ORCs and other replication proteins to initiate replication needs to be explored. Although, the LANA-dependent TR replication is believed to be the primary site of replication initiation but, KSHV DNA synthesis can also occur outside of the TR by the autonomously replicating element in the long unique region (LUR) of the viral genome.

During the G_1/S transition phases of the cell cycle, chromatin structure at the TR (nucleosomes and two LANA binding sites) is modified to make the viral DNA more accessible to the host cell DNA replication machinery. Two independent new studies [143,144] have utilized chromatin immunoprecipitation data together with KSHV specific microarrays (CHIP-on-chip) to generate high-resolution profiles of the chromatin structure of the entire KSHV episomes in latently-infected cell lines, providing novel genome-wide sequencing of the epigenetic landscape of KSHV genome. Characteristic DNA methylation patterns were found throughout the KSHV genome, though KSHV is not subjected to extensive DNA methylation. Various peaks of CpG methylation were observed with remarkable similarity among different cell lines, ranging from PELs and infected SLKs. In all cases, regions immediately upstream of LANA and several locations including K9, ORF45/50, K7 and ORF8 were deprived of CpG methylation [143,144].

Studies so far clearly show that latent KSHV genome is extensively chromatinized with both the activating (H3ac and H3K4me3) and repressive (H3K9me3 and H3K27me3) histone marks among them the Latency-associated genes possess activating histone marks as well as colocalize with transcriptionally active RNA polymerase II (RNAPII). Immediate early (IE) and early genes (E) have bivalent chromatin marks (acH3, H3K4me3 and H3K27me3) or active chromatin marks (acH3/H3K4me3-rich) whereas all of the late genes have H3K9me3- and H3K27me3-marked heterochromatin. Also, two of the chromatin modifying enzymes: EZH2 (H3K27me3 histone methyltransferase) of the Polycomb Repressive Complex 2 (PRC2) family and JMJD2A (H3K9me3 histone demethylase) have been shown to associate with the latent KSHV genome [143,145,146]. EZH2, which ubiquitously binds on the viral genome represses the lytic gene expression program during latency and JMJD2 that binds to the acH3/H3K4me3 chromatin regions of KSHV genome, guards the methylation of H3K9. Overall, the whole KSHV genome epigenetic analysis indicates that KSHV genome chromatinization regulates the expression of latent and lytic genes in a systematic manner.

Additionally, the DNA replication is governed by various epigenetic modifications including DNA methylation, post-synthesis histone modification patterns and nucleosome occupancy [147]. DNA methylation slowly builds up over the entire KSHV genome following the *de novo* infection and typically represses the viral gene expression [148] (Figure 2). For KSHV, DNA methylation does not exist at transcriptionally active LANA promoters, however it is found at several transcriptionally silent regions [53]. Though the factors governing the locus-specific methylation of DNA are not clearly understood, it is predicted that some sites are methylated due to a lack of transcriptional activity whereas others lack DNA methylation due to the inhibitory effects by DNA-binding proteins. Chromatin immunoprecipitation assays suggest that KSHV TR is associated with stable positioned nucleosomes that are further subjected to cell cycle regulation and nucleosome remodeling [104].

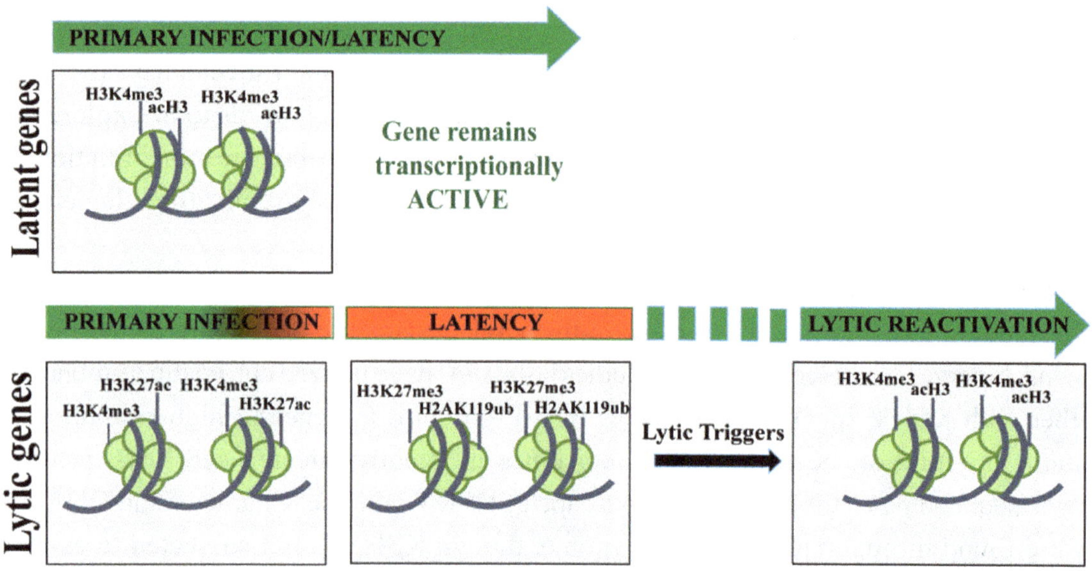

Figure 2. The chromatin landscape of the KSHV genome during various phases of viral life cycle. Following primary infection, promoters of the key latent genes get epigenetically modified with activating histone marks (H3K4me3/acH3) resulting in the expression of those genes throughout the viral life cycle. In contrast, KSHV lytic gene promoters possess either H3K27Ac/H3K4Me3-rich, active chromatin or H3Ac/H3K4Me3/H3K27Me3-rich bivalent chromatin. During latency, the lytic gene promoters are epigenetically modified with H3K9Me3/H3K27Me3 marks to form a heterochromatin. However, upon reactivation these repressive histone marks are enzymatically removed and gets modified with the activating histone marks (H3K4Me3/H3Ac).

CTCF-cohesin Binding and Higher-order Chromatin Conformation: The association of architectural proteins, cellular chromatin boundary factor (CTCF) and cohesin plays an integral role in sister-chromatid cohesion and chromosome segregation during mitosis [149]. CTCF/cohesin binds to the first intron of the LANA-vCyclin-vFLIP multicistronic latent transcript in KSHV, nearly 15 kb from the TR [150]. Depletion of the CTCF, cohesin or the CTCF-cohesin binding sites in the KSHV bacmid leads to dysregulated gene expression [150,151]. This suggests that CTCF-cohesin complex provides a chromosome-organizing center that facilitates stable episome maintenance [150]. Genome-wide ChIP analysis combined with next generation sequencing of the KSHV genome indicate cohesin binding sites are colocalized with CTCF binding sites at several sites throughout the latent KSHV genomes [62,150]. These studies support that the DNA-binding factor CTCF/CTCF cluster is important for the control of latent transcription. A recent study further demonstrated that CTCF and cohesion binding on the viral genome dynamically changes during viral reactivation and depletion of these chromatin insulators positively regulate the transcription of lytic genes [152]. The molecular functions of these CTCF-cohesin clusters are beginning to understand and it is likely that during mitotic cell division these clusters correlate with chromosome for segregation and gene transcription [153].

Higher order DNA structure is likely to be a heritable epigenetic regulatory factor. Higher order DNA structures like those involving DNA looping have been identified for the CTCF binding sites in the KSHV LANA promoter region [154]. A loop was formed with the 3' end of the KSHV latency transcripts ending at the K12 gene suggesting that the entire latency transcription area is restrained to a DNA loop mediated in part by CTCF binding. Using the viral genome-wide chromatin conformation capture method (3C), chromatin conformation of the latent EBV and KSHV genomes has been depicted recently and CTCF/cohesin binding sites have been found to be physically linked to other regions of the viral genomes *via* extensive DNA-loop formation [150]. For KSHV, a long DNA loop is found between the LANA and RTA control regions and these loops are stabilized by cohesin subunits primarily SMC1, SMC3 and Rad21 and SA1/SA2 [62]. Depletion of cohesin subunits disrupts the DNA loop between the latency and lytic promoter regions and a robust reactivation of lytic cycle gene transcription, indicating an important role of chromatin organizing factors and chromosome conformation in maintenance of stable gene programs during KSHV latent infection [150].

Recently, MAPit (Methylation Accessibility Probing for individual templates) single-molecule footprinting assays were employed to characterize several chromatin states at selected loci within mammalian nuclei [155,156]. The chromatin structures of the latency promoter and immediate early lytic genes, RTA and K2 promoter were investigated. The results indicated a heterogeneous chromatin structure with both fully closed and open conformations being present at investigated promoter regions in the KSHV genome. In addition, the epigenetic drift, *i.e.*, imperfect maintenance of the chromatin states was found to coordinate the latent and lytic gene control [156].

4. KSHV Lytic Gene Expression Profile

Within the predominantly latent population of KS spindle cells a few percent of the latent cells express markers of lytic replication [157,158]. During lytic DNA replication, a linear form of dsDNA molecule is generated and one copy of viral DNA is packaged per virion. For KSHV, viral lytic genes promote cell proliferation, survival and angiogenesis leading to onset and progression of KS lesions [15,159].

During lytic phase, viral gene expression is time-controlled and tightly regulated in order to allow a systematic synthesis of viral gene products. Lytic genes are widely distributed across the whole KSHV genome with their expression been controlled by several different promoters. Genes expressed during the lytic cycle can be grouped according to their timing and expression in response to the protein synthesis/DNA replication inhibitors as immediate early (IE), early (E) and late (L) genes [160–163]. IE genes include RTA/ORF50, ORF45 and K4.2, the primary genes expressed during lytic replication and encode regulatory proteins for viral replication. The latent to lytic switch of KSHV is regulated by the Replication and Transcription Activator, RTA, a 110 kDa protein, encoded by the ORF50 gene, which is capable of inducing the cascade of lytic gene expression including viral microphage inflammatory protein-I, viral interleukin 6 (vIL-6), ORF59, ORF65 and K8.1 and the production of DNase-resistant encapsidated viral DNA. Interestingly, the over-expression of RTA protein alone is necessary and sufficient to disrupt KSHV latency and initiate the lytic replication cascade [164–167]. Many early genes (E) have enzymatic functions (ORF59), regulation of gene expression (MTA protein), modulation of the immune system (MIR1/2) and selective accelerated turnover of host mRNA (ORF37) [168–170]. The expression of early genes (E) is controlled by the IE genes and include the polyadenylated nuclear RNA (PAN RNA), Kaposin, ORF57, k-bZIP (K8), K5, K9, K14, K15 ORF6, ORF21 and ORF74 [15], followed by expression of the late genes including major capsid protein

(MCP) encoded by ORF25 and the small viral capsid (sVCA). Late genes are transcribed following DNA replication and they are the structural genes for virus assembly [160,161].

Recently, anem's group performed a comprehensive genome analysis of transcriptional and translational profiles of the KSHV genome during the productive/lytic infection in epithelial iSLK-219 cell line using a combination of mRNA-sequencing (mRNA-seq) and ribosome profiling (Ribo-seq) [171]. This showed that ribosomes promptly bind to the transcripts of lytic genes during reactivation, suggesting that they are regulated at the transcriptional level. These modern approaches also revealed a wealth of additional information including occupancy of ribosomes on viral non coding RNA, numerous small open reading frames (ORFs), alternative splicing sites and alternative translation initiation sites to expand the coding potential of the viral genome. These new features of the KSHV genome led to a new annotation, which is termed, KSHV 2.0 [171].

4.1. Chromatin Organization of the KSHV Genome during Lytic Reactivation

The Lytic reactivation is regulated by alteration in the histone modifications of the viral genome including acetylation of core histone tails by histone acetyltransferases (HATs) and making the chromatin transcriptionally active. On the other hand, deacetylation of histone tails by histone acetyltransferases (HDACs) condenses the chromatin to make it transcriptionally silent [172]. During latency, HDACs attach to the RTA promoter resulting in hypoacetylation of histones and an inactive promoter [173,174]. However, the RTA promoter can be activated by physiological conditions, such as hypoxia, or in latently infected cell cultures by treatment with HDAC inhibitors, sodium butyrate (NaB) or the HAT inducer tetradecanoylphorbol acetate (TPA) leading to hyperacetylation of histones [175]. Additionally, DNA methylation plays an important role in controlling lytic reactivation as the inhibitor of enzyme DNA methyltransferases, 5-azacytidine (5-AzaC) triggers the KSHV lytic cycle [176]. The KSHV genome is subjected to methylation at CpG dinucleotides and shows CpG suppression at the RTA promoter during latency [144]. Together, these facts indicate that epigenetic modifications play an important role in the lytic reactivation process.

KSHV viral long non-coding PAN RNA and gene regulation: Among the early gene transcripts, PAN RNA is the most abundant lytic cycle transcript of KSHV [158,161]. New insights suggest an important role for long non-coding RNAs (lncRNAs) in the regulation of gene expression patterns via modulation of the lytic switch [177]. Long non-coding RNAs often referred to as "junk-regions" are RNAs which are typically longer than 200 bases that do not code for any protein [178]. KSHV expresses an unusual ncRNA called Polyadenylated nuclear non-coding RNA, abbreviated as PAN RNA in the nucleus during lytic induction that down regulates the expression of many immunomodulatory genes [176,179]. PAN RNA is transcribed by Pol II, is capped at its 5' end and ends with a 3' polyadenylate tail [180]. The expression of PAN RNA appears to be tightly regulated by RTA through a *cis*-acting RTA Response Element (RRE) present in the PAN RNA promoter region and by ORF57, which further stabilizes PAN RNA [181–183]. Although PAN RNA interacts with several viral and cellular encoded proteins to suppress gene expression, the exact role of PAN RNA in virus replication and KSHV growth is yet to be elucidated owing to the difficulty of generating a recombinant virus lacking the PAN RNA.

In order to elucidate the role of PAN RNA in the KSHV life cycle, recent studies on a recombinant BACmid with a deleted PAN RNA locus showed decreased RTA expression in the induced cells at both the early and late induction time points [177]. The RTA promoter is enriched in both activating (H3K4me3) and repressive (H3K27me3) histone marks. As a result, the chromatin of RTA promoter is often referred to as a bivalent promoter [144]. H3K27me3 is deposited by one of the Polycomb-group proteins, namely Polycomb Repressive Complex 2 (PRC2) that consists of subunit: EZH2, SUZ12, EED and the histone binding proteins RbAp48/46. Upon reactivation, chromatin remodeling proteins, JMJD3 and UTX H3K27me3 histone demethylases and H3K4me3 histone methyltransferase are recruited to the RTA promoter via KSHV-encoded Polyadenylated nuclear non-coding PAN RNA that disrupts polycomb mediated chromatin repression [177]. RTA binds to its own promoter through the cellular transcription factor CBF1 and recruits histone acetyltransferases (CBP/p300) and chromatin remodeling factors (SWI/SNF2) to modify the viral chromatin structure to a transcriptionally active state allowing a complete cycle of viral reactivation (Figure 3). RNA ChIP assays show that PAN RNA interacts with histone H3K27 demethylases JMJD3, UTX and methylases MLL2 to reverse the Polycomb-mediated repression of viral IE RTA transcripts through an interaction with the viral genome [177]. These studies further establish that PAN RNA is a multifunctional regulatory transcript that controls KSHV gene expression by mediating chromatin-modulations of the KSHV repressed genome.

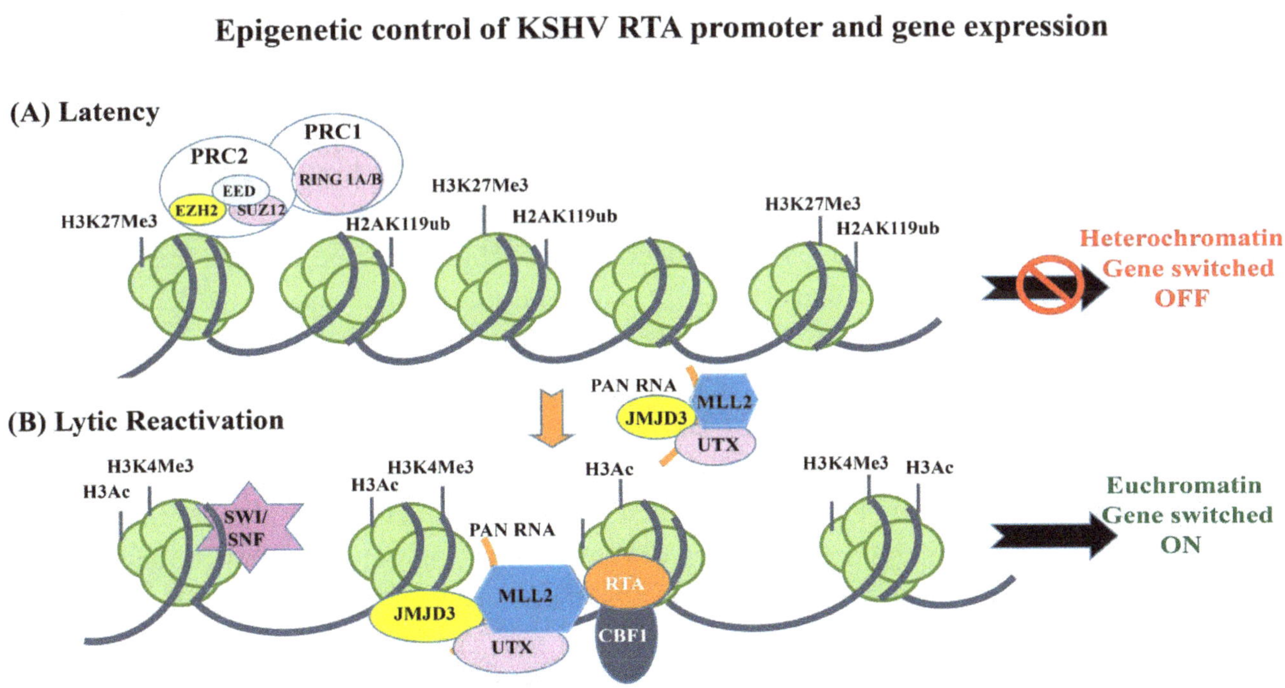

Figure 3. Polycomb repressive complexes (PRC1 and PRC2) and Polyadenylated RNA-mediated control of KSHV RTA promoter during latency and lytic reactivation. (**A**) During latency, the histone methyltransferase EZH2 subunit of PRC2 and RING 1A/B subunit of PRC1 bind to the KSHV genome and colocalizes with corresponding repressive histone marks H3K27me3 and H2AK119ub, respectively, leading to silencing of the target genes; (**B**) Lytic reactivation, triggered by the dissociation of PRC2 and PRC1 from the viral genome or inhibition of EZH2 by chemical compounds, leads to the enrichment of activating histone marks on the viral genome and the activation of gene transcription. PAN RNA, which is highly expressed during lytic reactivation, recruits several cellular and viral chromatin factors (MLL2, JMJD3 and UTX) to the RTA promoter and triggers the expression of immediate early, RTA protein.

4.2. Chromatin Organization of KSHV Genome during de Novo Infection

PEL cell lines are latently infected by KSHV and can be induced to trigger lytic cycle and produce infectious virions. However, PEL cells being lymphoid in nature do not support *de novo* KSHV infection, viral replication or serial propagation. Similarly, many other standard established cell lines such as 293 cells have been reported to support a very low level of KSHV infection with limited release of infectious virus [184,185]. These limitations have impacted the development of systems for the genetic analysis of KSHV and in turn a deeper understanding of early events of KSHV infection.

The process of KSHV *de novo* or primary infection involves attachment of the viral envelope proteins to host cell receptors and entry in the target cells by a multistep complex process [186]. Several transmembrane glycoproteins, encoded by KSHV have been found to be involved in the attachment and entry of KSHV in the target cells including gB (ORF8), gH (ORF22), gL (ORF 47), gM (ORF39) and gN (ORF53) [187–189]. Following the entry of viral genome into the nucleus, the viral genome undergoes extensive modification including circularization and chromatinization to escape the host cell defenses [53,190]. KSHV encoded ORF75 protein, which belongs a formylglycineamide ribotide amidotransferase (FGARAT), blocks cellular defenses by antagonizing the ND10 (nuclear domain 10) components [190]. Since chromatin association of the genome restricts the access of transcription factors to the viral promoter regions, modifications of the viral chromatin play an integral role in controlling viral gene expression [191].

Two independent studies have used ChIP-on-chip assays to provide the first unbiased and genome-wide views of the latent KSHV chromatin in infected BCBL-1 and SLK cells indicating a uniform distribution of total histone H3 and genomic localization of its modified forms, *i.e.*, activated H3K4me3 and acetylated H3K9 (acH3) and repressive histone marks [143,144]. Latent genes, IE and E lytic genes are found to be rich in H3K4me3/H3K9 (acH3) during latency and reactivation whereas the genomic regions of KSHV that encode for many late lytic genes display high levels of H3K9me3 /H3K27me3 during latency and early lytic reactivation [67].

In order to provide an overall description of the pre-latency phase of KSHV infection, a comprehensive epigenetic study was performed by Dr. Jae Jung's group on SLK cells using ChIP-on-chip and FAIRE analysis [192]. During the onset of infection, the KSHV epigenome develops a transcriptionally active chromatin structure (euchromatin) with a high level of activating histone marks H3K4me3 and H3K27ac, accompanied by the temporary induction of a limited number of lytic genes, which further increase the activating histone marks on the viral genome. Between 24 and 72 h post-infection, levels of activating histone marks decrease due to the Polycomb group protein (PcG protein)-mediated increase in the amount of repressive histone marks H3K27me3 and H2AK119ub, thereby inhibiting lytic gene expression. PcG proteins are cellular transcription silencing proteins that form enzymatic complexes with cellular Polycomb Repressive Complex 1 (PRC1) and PRC2 [193]. *De novo* acquisition of H3K27me3 marks is catalyzed by EZH2, which together with SUZ12 and EED form the subunits of the PRC2 complex. Both PRC1 and PRC2 are recruited to the KSHV genome leading to the temporally ordered biphasic euchromatin to heterochromatin transition in SLK and TIME cells, following *de novo* infection [192]. In contrast, KSHV is proposed to exist in a transcriptionally active euchromatin form in oral epithelial cells, resulting in efficient and robust lytic gene expression. Thus, the differential epigenetic modification of the KSHV genome in distinct cell types is a potential determining factor for latent infection *versus* lytic replication [192].

During the past years, components of distinct nuclear compartments called Promyelocytic leukemia nuclear bodies (PML-NB) have been found to regulate viral chromatin and viral gene expression [194]. PML-NB, also called nuclear domain 10 (ND10s) are nuclear multi-protein complexes that are 0.2–1.0 μm in size and include several subunits like Daxx (Death domain associated protein, Sp100 (speckled protein of 100 kDa), SUMO (small ubiquitin-related modifier) and 53 kDa protein associated with the nuclear matrix [195,196]. ND10s are the mediators of the innate antiviral defense mechanism and many viruses have developed strategies to counteract repressive properties of ND10s [196,197]. A systematic study by Grundhoff's group reported the role of ND10s and its core components on the establishment of KSHV latency during the early infection phase in *de novo* infected SLK, established from tumor biopsy of oral mucosa, cells [148]. The KSHV episome/LANA in iSLK cells is found not to directly or transiently interact with ND10s during the establishment of latency (between 24 and 48 h post infection) *i.e.*, the time period when H3K27me3 marks accumulate on the KSHV episome. However, KSHV infection is reported to influence relocalization of ND10s components especially Sp100 protein, which is efficiently and permanently relocalized from nucleoplasmic and chromatin-associated fractions into the insoluble matrix by LANA, which induces SUMOylation of Sp100. Depletion of ND10s core components, Sp100, PML or Daxx did not interfere with latency establishment, though depletion of Sp100 accelerates the occupancy of the repressive histone mark H3K27me3 on viral episomes indicating that Sp100 acts as a negative regulator of PRC2 recruitment onto the KSHV genome [148].

5. Conclusions

KSHV is a complex and sophisticated oncogenic virus that developed numerous regulatory mechanisms to modulate the host-cell proliferation, apoptosis and host immune evasion, enabling the prolonged survival of the infected cell with the following latent infection and lytic reactivation. Despite the enormous wealth of information available about the mechanisms of how gammaherpesviruses persist in tumor cells, we are far from fully understanding the mechanism of latency establishment by KSHV, and the key cellular and viral factors that are responsible for restricted lytic gene expression during primary infection. Undoubtedly, the chromatin remodeling and epigenetic modifications of both viral and host genomes play crucial roles in determining the expression pattern of genes, that will lead to abortive or persistent infection. These epigenetic modifications include DNA methylation, histones post-translational modifications and higher-order chromosome conformations, including long intervening DNA loops. More importantly, prior to the chromatinization of incoming viral genomes, function of the cellular chromatin modifying enzymes is deregulated by a combination of viral proteins in order to re-program the cellular gene expression profiles and generate an altered chromatin landscape of KSHV genome favoring latency establishment [198,199]. Although the advances in technological development has enabled extremely high-resolution whole-epigenome analysis of KSHV on a large scale and provided us with a better picture of the chromatin regulation of the KSHV latent and lytic genomes, much remains to be discovered for understanding the complex orchestration of various epigenetic players that regulate KSHV chromatin remodeling by site-specific recruitment of histone-modifying machinery during various stages of viral infection. Therefore, further investigations of significant cellular and viral factors along with most important epigenetic regulatory factors, including histone-modifying enzymes, HDAC inhibitors and demethylating agents that alter the chromatin status of KSHV towards the formation of unique latent epigenomes need to be performed in order (1) to generate a detailed and complete epigenomic map for KSHV; and (2) to provide novel therapeutic strategies that can be exploited for controlling KSHV infection and KSHV-driven carcinogenesis.

Acknowledgments

We sincerely apologize to the authors whose important work could not be cited here owing to space limitations. This work was supported by the public health grants from NIH (CA174459 and AI105000) to Subhash C. Verma and CA137894, CA171979, CA174439, CA177423, P30-DK-050306 and P01-CA-174439 to Erle S. Robertson.

Author Contributions

This review was conceptualized and written through the combined efforts of all the authors.

References

1. Chang, Y.; Cesarman, E.; Pessin, M.S.; Lee, F.; Culpepper, J.; Knowles, D.M.; Moore, P.S. Identification of herpesvirus-like DNA sequences in aids-associated Kaposi's sarcoma. *Science* **1994**, *266*, 1865–1869.
2. Cesarman, E.; Chang, Y.; Moore, P.S.; Said, J.W.; Knowles, D.M. Kaposi's sarcoma-associated herpesvirus-like DNA sequences in AIDS-related body-cavity-based lymphomas. *N. Engl. J. Med.* **1995**, *332*, 1186–1191.
3. Soulier, J.; Grollet, L.; Oksenhendler, E.; Cacoub, P.; Cazals-Hatem, D.; Babinet, P.; d'Agay, M.F.; Clauvel, J.P.; Raphael, M.; Degos, L.; *et al.* Kaposi's sarcoma-associated herpesvirus-like DNA sequences in multicentric castleman's disease. *Blood* **1995**, *86*, 1276–1280.
4. Deloose, S.T.; Smit, L.A.; Pals, F.T.; Kersten, M.J.; van Noesel, C.J.; Pals, S.T. High incidence of Kaposi sarcoma-associated herpesvirus infection in HIV-related solid immunoblastic/plasmablastic diffuse large B-cell lymphoma. *Leukemia* **2005**, *19*, 851–855.
5. Cool, C.D.; Rai, P.R.; Yeager, M.E.; Hernandez-Saavedra, D.; Serls, A.E.; Bull, T.M.; Geraci, M.W.; Brown, K.K.; Routes, J.M.; Tuder, R.M.; *et al.* Expression of human herpesvirus 8 in primary pulmonary hypertension. *N. Engl. J. Med.* **2003**, *349*, 1113–1122.
6. Carbone, A.; Gloghini, A.; Vaccher, E.; Cerri, M.; Gaidano, G.; Dalla-Favera, R.; Tirelli, U. Kaposi's sarcoma-associated herpesvirus/human herpesvirus type 8-positive solid lymphomas: A tissue-based variant of primary effusion lymphoma. *J. Mol. Diagn.* **2005**, *7*, 17–27.
7. Du, M.Q.; Diss, T.C.; Liu, H.; Ye, H.; Hamoudi, R.A.; Cabecadas, J.; Dong, H.Y.; Harris, N.L.; Chan, J.K.; Rees, J.W.; *et al.* KSHV- and EBV-associated germinotropic lymphoproliferative disorder. *Blood* **2002**, *100*, 3415–3418.
8. Gbabe, O.F.; Okwundu, C.I.; Dedicoat, M.; Freeman, E.E. Treatment of severe or progressive Kaposi's sarcoma in HIV-infected adults. *Cochrane Database Syst. Rev.* **2014**, *8*, CD003256.

9. Cornali, E.; Zietz, C.; Benelli, R.; Weninger, W.; Masiello, L.; Breier, G.; Tschachler, E.; Albini, A.; Sturzl, M. Vascular endothelial growth factor regulates angiogenesis and vascular permeability in Kaposi's sarcoma. *Am. J. Pathol.* **1996**, *149*, 1851–1869.
10. Gessain, A.; Duprez, R. Spindle cells and their role in Kaposi's sarcoma. *Int. J. Biochem. Cell Biol.* **2005**, *37*, 2457–2465.
11. Gasperini, P.; Espigol-Frigole, G.; McCormick, P.J.; Salvucci, O.; Maric, D.; Uldrick, T.S.; Polizzotto, M.N.; Yarchoan, R.; Tosato, G. Kaposi sarcoma herpesvirus promotes endothelial-to-mesenchymal transition through notch-dependent signaling. *Cancer Res.* **2012**, *72*, 1157–1169.
12. Wang, H.W.; Trotter, M.W.; Lagos, D.; Bourboulia, D.; Henderson, S.; Makinen, T.; Elliman, S.; Flanagan, A.M.; Alitalo, K.; Boshoff, C. Kaposi sarcoma herpesvirus-induced cellular reprogramming contributes to the lymphatic endothelial gene expression in Kaposi sarcoma. *Nat. Genet.* **2004**, *36*, 687–693.
13. Hong, Y.K.; Foreman, K.; Shin, J.W.; Hirakawa, S.; Curry, C.L.; Sage, D.R.; Libermann, T.; Dezube, B.J.; Fingeroth, J.D.; Detmar, M. Lymphatic reprogramming of blood vascular endothelium by Kaposi sarcoma-associated herpesvirus. *Nat. Genet.* **2004**, *36*, 683–685.
14. Wen, K.W.; Damania, B. Kaposi sarcoma-associated herpesvirus (KSHV): Molecular biology and oncogenesis. *Cancer Lett.* **2010**, *289*, 140–150.
15. Dourmishev, L.A.; Dourmishev, A.L.; Palmeri, D.; Schwartz, R.A.; Lukac, D.M. Molecular genetics of Kaposi's sarcoma-associated herpesvirus (human herpesvirus-8) epidemiology and pathogenesis. *Microbiol Mol. Biol. Rev.* **2003**, *67*, 175–212.
16. Pantanowitz, L.; Dezube, B.J. Kaposi sarcoma in unusual locations. *BMC cancer* **2008**, *8*, 190.
17. DeVita, V.T.; Lawrence, T.S.; Rosenberg, S.A. *Cancer: Principles and Practice of Oncology*, 8th ed.; Lippincott Williams & Wilkins: Philadelphia, PA, USA, 2008; Volume 2, pp. 3151.
18. Wool, G.M. Aids-related malignancies. *Oncologist* **1998**, *3*, 279–283.
19. Ablashi, D.V.; Chatlynne, L.G.; Whitman, J.E., Jr.; Cesarman, E. Spectrum of Kaposi's sarcoma-associated herpesvirus, or human herpesvirus 8, diseases. *Clin. Microbiol. Rev.* **2002**, *15*, 439–464.
20. Nador, R.G.; Cesarman, E.; Chadburn, A.; Dawson, D.B.; Ansari, M.Q.; Sald, J.; Knowles, D.M. Primary effusion lymphoma: A distinct clinicopathologic entity associated with the Kaposi's sarcoma-associated herpes virus. *Blood* **1996**, *88*, 645–656.
21. Edelman, D.C. Human herpesvirus 8—A novel human pathogen. *Virol. J.* **2005**, *2*, 78.
22. Haecker, I.; Gay, L.A.; Yang, Y.; Hu, J.; Morse, A.M.; McIntyre, L.M.; Renne, R. Ago HITS-clip expands understanding of Kaposi's sarcoma-associated herpesvirus miRNA function in primary effusion lymphomas. *PLOS Pathog.* **2012**, *8*, e1002884.
23. Fan, W.; Bubman, D.; Chadburn, A.; Harrington, W.J., Jr.; Cesarman, E.; Knowles, D.M. Distinct subsets of primary effusion lymphoma can be identified based on their cellular gene expression profile and viral association. *J. Virol.* **2005**, *79*, 1244–1251.
24. Ueda, K.; Ohsaki, E.; Nakano, K.; Zheng, X. Characterization of Kaposi's sarcoma-associated herpesvirus-related lymphomas by DNA microarray analysis. *Leuk. Res. Treat.* **2011**, *2011*, 726964.
25. Dittmer, D.P.; Damania, B. Kaposi sarcoma associated herpesvirus pathogenesis (KSHV)—An update. *Curr. Opin. Virol.* **2013**, *3*, 238–244.

26. Curioni, S.; D'Amico, M.; Quartagno, R.; Martino, S.; Dell'Antonio, G.; Cusi, D. Castleman's disease with nephrotic syndrome, amyloidosis and autoimmune manifestations. *Nephrol. Dial. Transplant.* **2001**, *16*, 1475–1478.
27. Dupin, N.; Fisher, C.; Kellam, P.; Ariad, S.; Tulliez, M.; Franck, N.; van Marck, E.; Salmon, D.; Gorin, I.; Escande, J.P.; *et al.* Distribution of human herpesvirus-8 latently infected cells in kaposi's sarcoma, multicentric castleman's disease, and primary effusion lymphoma. *Proc. Natl. Acad. Sci. USA* **1999**, *96*, 4546–4551.
28. Carbone, A.; Cesarman, E.; Spina, M.; Gloghini, A.; Schulz, T.F. HIV-associated lymphomas and gamma-herpesviruses. *Blood* **2009**, *113*, 1213–1224.
29. Nishi, J.; Arimura, K.; Utsunomiya, A.; Yonezawa, S.; Kawakami, K.; Maeno, N.; Ijichi, O.; Ikarimoto, N.; Nakata, M.; Kitajima, I.; *et al.* Expression of vascular endothelial growth factor in sera and lymph nodes of the plasma cell type of castleman's disease. *Br. J. Haematol.* **1999**, *104*, 482–485.
30. Zong, J.C.; Kajumbula, H.; Boto, W.; Hayward, G.S. Evaluation of global clustering patterns and strain variation over an extended ORF26 gene locus from Kaposi's sarcoma herpesvirus. *J. Clin. Virol.* **2007**, *40*, 19–25.
31. Hayward, G.S. KSHV strains: The origins and global spread of the virus. *Semin. Cancer Biol.* **1999**, *9*, 187–199.
32. Hayward, G.S.; Zong, J.C. Modern evolutionary history of the human KSHV genome. *Curr. Top. Microbiol. Immunol.* **2007**, *312*, 1–42.
33. Stebbing, J.; Bourboulia, D.; Johnson, M.; Henderson, S.; Williams, I.; Wilder, N.; Tyrer, M.; Youle, M.; Imami, N.; Kobu, T.; *et al.* Kaposi's sarcoma-associated herpesvirus cytotoxic T lymphocytes recognize and target darwinian positively selected autologous K1 epitopes. *J. Virol.* **2003**, *77*, 4306–4314.
34. Poole, L.J.; Zong, J.C.; Ciufo, D.M.; Alcendor, D.J.; Cannon, J.S.; Ambinder, R.; Orenstein, J.M.; Reitz, M.S.; Hayward, G.S. Comparison of genetic variability at multiple loci across the genomes of the major subtypes of Kaposi's sarcoma-associated herpesvirus reveals evidence for recombination and for two distinct types of open reading frame K15 alleles at the right-hand end. *J. Virol.* **1999**, *73*, 6646–6660.
35. Zong, J.; Ciufo, D.M.; Viscidi, R.; Alagiozoglou, L.; Tyring, S.; Rady, P.; Orenstein, J.; Boto, W.; Kalumbuja, H.; Romano, N.; *et al.* Genotypic analysis at multiple loci across Kaposi's sarcoma herpesvirus (KSHV) DNA molecules: Clustering patterns, novel variants and chimerism. *J. Clin. Virol.* **2002**, *23*, 119–148.
36. Cook, P.M.; Whitby, D.; Calabro, M.L.; Luppi, M.; Kakoola, D.N.; Hjalgrim, H.; Ariyoshi, K.; Ensoli, B.; Davison, A.J.; Schulz, T.F. Variability and evolution of Kaposi's sarcoma-associated herpesvirus in Europe and Africa. International collaborative group. *AIDS* **1999**, *13*, 1165–1176.
37. Meng, Y.X.; Spira, T.J.; Bhat, G.J.; Birch, C.J.; Druce, J.D.; Edlin, B.R.; Edwards, R.; Gunthel, C.; Newton, R.; Stamey, F.R.; *et al.* Individuals from North America, Australasia, and Africa are infected with four different genotypes of human herpesvirus 8. *Virology* **1999**, *261*, 106–119.
38. Biggar, R.J.; Whitby, D.; Marshall, V.; Linhares, A.C.; Black, F. Human herpesvirus 8 in Brazilian amerindians: A hyperendemic population with a new subtype. *J. Infect. Dis.* **2000**, *181*, 1562–1568.

39. Engels, E.A.; Sinclair, M.D.; Biggar, R.J.; Whitby, D.; Ebbesen, P.; Goedert, J.J.; Gastwirth, J.L. Latent class analysis of human herpesvirus 8 assay performance and infection prevalence in sub-Saharan Africa and Malta. *Int. J. Cancer* **2000**, *88*, 1003–1008.
40. Serraino, D.; Toma, L.; Andreoni, M.; Butto, S.; Tchangmena, O.; Sarmati, L.; Monini, P.; Franceschi, S.; Ensoli, B.; Rezza, G. A seroprevalence study of human herpesvirus type 8 (HHV8) in Eastern and Central Africa and in the mediterranean area. *Eur. J. Epidemiol.* **2001**, *17*, 871–876.
41. Pellett, P.E.; Wright, D.J.; Engels, E.A.; Ablashi, D.V.; Dollard, S.C.; Forghani, B.; Glynn, S.A.; Goedert, J.J.; Jenkins, F.J.; Lee, T.H.; *et al.* Multicenter comparison of serologic assays and estimation of human herpesvirus 8 seroprevalence among us blood donors. *Transfusion* **2003**, *43*, 1260–1268.
42. Vitale, F.; Viviano, E.; Perna, A.M.; Bonura, F.; Mazzola, G.; Ajello, F.; Romano, N. Serological and virological evidence of non-sexual transmission of human herpesvirus type 8 (HHV8). *Epidemiol. Infect.* **2000**, *125*, 671–675.
43. Mbulaiteye, S.; Marshall, V.; Bagni, R.K.; Wang, C.D.; Mbisa, G.; Bakaki, P.M.; Owor, A.M.; Ndugwa, C.M.; Engels, E.A.; Katongole-Mbidde, E.; *et al.* Molecular evidence for mother-to-child transmission of Kaposi sarcoma-associated herpesvirus in uganda and K1 gene evolution within the host. *J. Infect. Dis.* **2006**, *193*, 1250–1257.
44. Mesri, E.A.; Cesarman, E.; Boshoff, C. Kaposi's sarcoma and its associated herpesvirus. *Nat. Rev. Cancer* **2010**, *10*, 707–719.
45. Coluzzi, M.; Manno, D.; Guzzinati, S.; Tognazzo, S.; Zambon, P.; Arca, B.; Costantini, C.; Ascoli, V. The bloodsucking arthropod bite as possible cofactor in the transmission of human herpesvirus-8 infection and in the expression of Kaposi's sarcoma disease. *Parassitologia* **2002**, *44*, 123–129.
46. Ascoli, V.; Facchinelli, L.; Valerio, L.; Manno, D.; Coluzzi, M. Kaposi's sarcoma, human herpesvirus 8 infection and the potential role of promoter-arthropod bites in Northern Sweden. *J. Med. Virol.* **2006**, *78*, 1452–1455.
47. Mbulaiteye, S.M.; Biggar, R.J.; Pfeiffer, R.M.; Bakaki, P.M.; Gamache, C.; Owor, A.M.; Katongole-Mbidde, E.; Ndugwa, C.M.; Goedert, J.J.; Whitby, D.; *et al.* Water, socioeconomic factors, and human herpesvirus 8 infection in ugandan children and their mothers. *J. Acquir. Immune Defic. Syndr.* **2005**, *38*, 474–479.
48. Renne, R.; Lagunoff, M.; Zhong, W.; Ganem, D. The size and conformation of Kaposi's sarcoma-associated herpesvirus (human herpesvirus 8) DNA in infected cells and virions. *J. Virol.* **1996**, *70*, 8151–8154.
49. Russo, J.J.; Bohenzky, R.A.; Chien, M.C.; Chen, J.; Yan, M.; Maddalena, D.; Parry, J.P.; Peruzzi, D.; Edelman, I.S.; Chang, Y.; *et al.* Nucleotide sequence of the Kaposi sarcoma-associated herpesvirus (HHV8). *Proc. Natl. Acad. Sci. USA* **1996**, *93*, 14862–14867.
50. Wong, E.L.; Damania, B. Linking KSHV to human cancer. *Curr. Oncol. Rep.* **2005**, *7*, 349–356.
51. Zhu, F.X.; Chong, J.M.; Wu, L.; Yuan, Y. Virion proteins of Kaposi's sarcoma-associated herpesvirus. *J. Virol.* **2005**, *79*, 800–811.
52. Spear, P.G.; Longnecker, R. Herpesvirus entry: An update. *J. Virol.* **2003**, *77*, 10179–10185.
53. Lieberman, P.M. Keeping it quiet: Chromatin control of gammaherpesvirus latency. *Nat. Rev. Microbiol.* **2013**, *11*, 863–875.
54. Lieberman, P.M. Chromatin regulation of virus infection. *Trends Microbiol.* **2006**, *14*, 132–140.

55. Luger, K.; Mader, A.W.; Richmond, R.K.; Sargent, D.F.; Richmond, T.J. Crystal structure of the nucleosome core particle at 2.8 a resolution. *Nature* **1997**, *389*, 251–260.
56. Choudhuri, S.; Cui, Y.; Klaassen, C.D. Molecular targets of epigenetic regulation and effectors of environmental influences. *Toxicol. Appl. Pharmacol.* **2010**, *245*, 378–393.
57. Campos, E.I.; Reinberg, D. Histones: Annotating chromatin. *Annu. Rev. Genet.* **2009**, *43*, 559–599.
58. Knipe, D.M.; Cliffe, A. Chromatin control of herpes simplex virus lytic and latent infection. *Nat. Rev. Microbiol.* **2008**, *6*, 211–221.
59. Karlic, R.; Chung, H.R.; Lasserre, J.; Vlahovicek, K.; Vingron, M. Histone modification levels are predictive for gene expression. *Proc. Natl. Acad. Sci. USA* **2010**, *107*, 2926–2931.
60. Hirst, M.; Marra, M.A. Next generation sequencing based approaches to epigenomics. *Brief. Funct. Genomics* **2010**, *9*, 455–465.
61. Sarda, S.; Hannenhalli, S. Next-generation sequencing and epigenomics research: A hammer in search of nails. *Genomics Inf.* **2014**, *12*, 2–11.
62. Chen, H.S.; Wikramasinghe, P.; Showe, L.; Lieberman, P.M. Cohesins repress Kaposi's sarcoma-associated herpesvirus immediate early gene transcription during latency. *J. Virol.* **2012**, *86*, 9454–9464.
63. Kang, H.; Cho, H.; Sung, G.H.; Lieberman, P.M. CTCF regulates Kaposi's sarcoma-associated herpesvirus latency transcription by nucleosome displacement and RNA polymerase programming. *J. Virol.* **2013**, *87*, 1789–1799.
64. Kang, H.; Lieberman, P.M. Cell cycle control of Kaposi's sarcoma-associated herpesvirus latency transcription by CTCF-cohesin interactions. *J. Virol.* **2009**, *83*, 6199–6210.
65. Hilton, I.B.; Simon, J.M.; Lieb, J.D.; Davis, I.J.; Damania, B.; Dittmer, D.P. The open chromatin landscape of Kaposi's sarcoma-associated herpesvirus. *J. Virol.* **2013**, *87*, 11831–11842.
66. Greene, W.; Kuhne, K.; Ye, F.; Chen, J.; Zhou, F.; Lei, X.; Gao, S.J. Molecular biology of KSHV in relation to AIDS-associated oncogenesis. *Cancer Treat. Res.* **2007**, *133*, 69–127.
67. Toth, Z.; Brulois, K.; Jung, J.U. The chromatin landscape of Kaposi's sarcoma-associated herpesvirus. *Viruses* **2013**, *5*, 1346–1373.
68. Dittmer, D.; Lagunoff, M.; Renne, R.; Staskus, K.; Haase, A.; Ganem, D. A cluster of latently expressed genes in Kaposi's sarcoma-associated herpesvirus. *J. Virol.* **1998**, *72*, 8309–8315.
69. Sturzl, M.; Hohenadl, C.; Zietz, C.; Castanos-Velez, E.; Wunderlich, A.; Ascherl, G.; Biberfeld, P.; Monini, P.; Browning, P.J.; Ensoli, B. Expression of K13/V-FLIP gene of human herpesvirus 8 and apoptosis in Kaposi's sarcoma spindle cells. *J. Natl. Cancer Inst.* **1999**, *91*, 1725–1733.
70. Davis, M.A.; Sturzl, M.A.; Blasig, C.; Schreier, A.; Guo, H.G.; Reitz, M.; Opalenik, S.R.; Browning, P.J. Expression of human herpesvirus 8-encoded cyclin D in Kaposi's sarcoma spindle cells. *J. Natl. Cancer Inst.* **1997**, *89*, 1868–1874.
71. Muralidhar, S.; Veytsmann, G.; Chandran, B.; Ablashi, D.; Doniger, J.; Rosenthal, L.J. Characterization of the human herpesvirus 8 (Kaposi's sarcoma-associated herpesvirus) oncogene, kaposin (ORF K12). *J. Clin. Virol.* **2000**, *16*, 203–213.
72. Cai, X.; Lu, S.; Zhang, Z.; Gonzalez, C.M.; Damania, B.; Cullen, B.R. Kaposi's sarcoma-associated herpesvirus expresses an array of viral micrornas in latently infected cells. *Proc. Natl. Acad. Sci. USA* **2005**, *102*, 5570–5575.

73. Ballestas, M.E.; Chatis, P.A.; Kaye, K.M. Efficient persistence of extrachromosomal KSHV DNA mediated by latency-associated nuclear antigen. *Science* **1999**, *284*, 641–644.
74. Ye, F.C.; Zhou, F.C.; Xie, J.P.; Kang, T.; Greene, W.; Kuhne, K.; Lei, X.F.; Li, Q.H.; Gao, S.J. Kaposi's sarcoma-associated herpesvirus latent gene vFLIP inhibits viral lytic replication through NF-kappaB-mediated suppression of the AP-1 pathway: A novel mechanism of virus control of latency. *J. Virol.* **2008**, *82*, 4235–4249.
75. Thome, M.; Schneider, P.; Hofmann, K.; Fickenscher, H.; Meinl, E.; Neipel, F.; Mattmann, C.; Burns, K.; Bodmer, J.L.; Schroter, M.; *et al.* Viral flice-inhibitory proteins (FLIPS) prevent apoptosis induced by death receptors. *Nature* **1997**, *386*, 517–521.
76. Godden-Kent, D.; Talbot, S.J.; Boshoff, C.; Chang, Y.; Moore, P.; Weiss, R.A.; Mittnacht, S. The cyclin encoded by Kaposi's sarcoma-associated herpesvirus stimulates CDK6 to phosphorylate the retinoblastoma protein and histone H1. *J. Virol.* **1997**, *71*, 4193–4198.
77. Li, H.; Komatsu, T.; Dezube, B.J.; Kaye, K.M. The Kaposi's sarcoma-associated herpesvirus K12 transcript from a primary effusion lymphoma contains complex repeat elements, is spliced, and initiates from a novel promoter. *J. Virol.* **2002**, *76*, 11880–11888.
78. Bieleski, L.; Talbot, S.J. Kaposi's sarcoma-associated herpesvirus vcyclin open reading frame contains an internal ribosome entry site. *J. Virol.* **2001**, *75*, 1864–1869.
79. Tempera, I.; Lieberman, P.M. Chromatin organization of gammaherpesvirus latent genomes. *Biochim. Biophys. Acta* **2010**, *1799*, 236–245.
80. Maxwell, K.L.; Frappier, L. Viral proteomics. *Microbiol. Mol. Biol. Rev.* **2007**, *71*, 398–411.
81. Cotter, M.A., 2nd; Robertson, E.S. The latency-associated nuclear antigen tethers the Kaposi's sarcoma-associated herpesvirus genome to host chromosomes in body cavity-based lymphoma cells. *Virology* **1999**, *264*, 254–264.
82. Si, H.; Verma, S.C.; Lampson, M.A.; Cai, Q.; Robertson, E.S. Kaposi's sarcoma-associated herpesvirus-encoded LANA can interact with the nuclear mitotic apparatus protein to regulate genome maintenance and segregation. *J. Virol.* **2008**, *82*, 6734–6746.
83. Kelley-Clarke, B.; de Leon-Vazquez, E.; Slain, K.; Barbera, A.J.; Kaye, K.M. Role of Kaposi's sarcoma-associated herpesvirus C-terminal LANA chromosome binding in episome persistence. *J. Virol.* **2009**, *83*, 4326–4337.
84. Fujimuro, M.; Hayward, S.D. The latency-associated nuclear antigen of Kaposi's sarcoma-associated herpesvirus manipulates the activity of glycogen synthase kinase-3beta. *J. Virol.* **2003**, *77*, 8019–8030.
85. Fujimuro, M.; Wu, F.Y.; ApRhys, C.; Kajumbula, H.; Young, D.B.; Hayward, G.S.; Hayward, S.D. A novel viral mechanism for dysregulation of beta-catenin in Kaposi's sarcoma-associated herpesvirus latency. *Nat. Med.* **2003**, *9*, 300–306.
86. Cai, Q.; Lan, K.; Verma, S.C.; Si, H.; Lin, D.; Robertson, E.S. Kaposi's sarcoma-associated herpesvirus latent protein LANA interacts with HIF-1 alpha to upregulate RTA expression during hypoxia: Latency control under low oxygen conditions. *J. Virol.* **2006**, *80*, 7965–7975.
87. Liu, J.; Martin, H.J.; Liao, G.; Hayward, S.D. The Kaposi's sarcoma-associated herpesvirus LANA protein stabilizes and activates C-myc. *J. Virol.* **2007**, *81*, 10451–10459.

88. Cai, Q.; Murakami, M.; Si, H.; Robertson, E.S. A potential alpha-helix motif in the amino terminus of LANA encoded by Kaposi's sarcoma-associated herpesvirus is critical for nuclear accumulation of HIF-1alpha in normoxia. *J. Virol.* **2007**, *81*, 10413–10423.
89. Cai, Q.L.; Knight, J.S.; Verma, S.C.; Zald, P.; Robertson, E.S. Ec5s ubiquitin complex is recruited by KSHV latent antigen LANA for degradation of the VHL and P53 tumor suppressors. *PLOS Pathog.* **2006**, *2*, e116.
90. Rossetto, C.; Yamboliev, I.; Pari, G.S. Kaposi's sarcoma-associated herpesvirus/human herpesvirus 8 K-BZIP modulates latency-associated nuclear protein-mediated suppression of lytic origin-dependent DNA synthesis. *J. Virol.* **2009**, *83*, 8492–8501.
91. Lu, J.; Verma, S.C.; Murakami, M.; Cai, Q.; Kumar, P.; Xiao, B.; Robertson, E.S. Latency-associated nuclear antigen of Kaposi's sarcoma-associated herpesvirus (KSHV) upregulates survivin expression in KSHV-associated B-lymphoma cells and contributes to their proliferation. *J. Virol.* **2009**, *83*, 7129–7141.
92. Xiao, B.; Verma, S.C.; Cai, Q.; Kaul, R.; Lu, J.; Saha, A.; Robertson, E.S. BUB1 and CENP-F can contribute to Kaposi's sarcoma-associated herpesvirus genome persistence by targeting LANA to kinetochores. *J. Virol.* **2010**, *84*, 9718–9732.
93. Cai, Q.; Verma, S.C.; Choi, J.Y.; Ma, M.; Robertson, E.S. Kaposi's sarcoma-associated herpesvirus inhibits interleukin-4-mediated STAT6 phosphorylation to regulate apoptosis and maintain latency. *J. Virol.* **2010**, *84*, 11134–11144.
94. Garber, A.C.; Shu, M.A.; Hu, J.; Renne, R. DNA binding and modulation of gene expression by the latency-associated nuclear antigen of Kaposi's sarcoma-associated herpesvirus. *J. Virol.* **2001**, *75*, 7882–7892.
95. Cotter, M.A., 2nd; Subramanian, C.; Robertson, E.S. The Kaposi's sarcoma-associated herpesvirus latency-associated nuclear antigen binds to specific sequences at the left end of the viral genome through its carboxy-terminus. *Virology* **2001**, *291*, 241–259.
96. Garber, A.C.; Hu, J.; Renne, R. Latency-associated nuclear antigen (LANA) cooperatively binds to two sites within the terminal repeat, and both sites contribute to the ability of LANA to suppress transcription and to facilitate DNA replication. *J. Biol. Chem.* **2002**, *277*, 27401–27411.
97. Wong, L.Y.; Wilson, A.C. Kaposi's sarcoma-associated herpesvirus latency-associated nuclear antigen induces a strong bend on binding to terminal repeat DNA. *J. Virol.* **2005**, *79*, 13829–13836.
98. Komatsu, T.; Ballestas, M.E.; Barbera, A.J.; Kelley-Clarke, B.; Kaye, K.M. KSHV LANA1 binds DNA as an oligomer and residues N-terminal to the oligomerization domain are essential for DNA binding, replication, and episome persistence. *Virology* **2004**, *319*, 225–236.
99. Lim, C.; Lee, D.; Seo, T.; Choi, C.; Choe, J. Latency-associated nuclear antigen of Kaposi's sarcoma-associated herpesvirus functionally interacts with heterochromatin protein 1. *J. Biol. Chem.* **2003**, *278*, 7397–7405.
100. Verma, S.C.; Cai, Q.; Kreider, E.; Lu, J.; Robertson, E.S. Comprehensive analysis of LANA interacting proteins essential for viral genome tethering and persistence. *PLOS ONE* **2013**, *8*, e74662.
101. Cai, Q.; Verma, S.C.; Lu, J.; Robertson, E.S. Molecular biology of Kaposi's sarcoma-associated herpesvirus and related oncogenesis. *Adv. Virus Res.* **2010**, *78*, 87–142.

102. Hu, J.; Garber, A.C.; Renne, R. The latency-associated nuclear antigen of Kaposi's sarcoma-associated herpesvirus supports latent DNA replication in dividing cells. *J. Virol.* **2002**, *76*, 11677–11687.
103. Verma, S.C.; Lan, K.; Robertson, E. Structure and function of latency-associated nuclear antigen. *Curr. Top. Microbiol. Immunol.* **2007**, *312*, 101–136.
104. Stedman, W.; Deng, Z.; Lu, F.; Lieberman, P.M. Orc, mcm, and histone hyperacetylation at the Kaposi's sarcoma-associated herpesvirus latent replication origin. *J. Virol.* **2004**, *78*, 12566–12575.
105. Purushothaman, P.; McDowell, M.E.; McGuinness, J.; Salas, R.; Rumjahn, S.M.; Verma, S.C. Kaposi's sarcoma-associated herpesvirus-encoded LANA recruits topoisomerase iibeta for latent DNA replication of the terminal repeats. *J. Virol.* **2012**, *86*, 9983–9994.
106. Verma, S.C.; Choudhuri, T.; Kaul, R.; Robertson, E.S. Latency-associated nuclear antigen (LANA) of Kaposi's sarcoma-associated herpesvirus interacts with origin recognition complexes at the LANA binding sequence within the terminal repeats. *J. Virol.* **2006**, *80*, 2243–2256.
107. Verma, S.C.; Choudhuri, T.; Robertson, E.S. The minimal replicator element of the Kaposi's sarcoma-associated herpesvirus terminal repeat supports replication in a semiconservative and cell-cycle-dependent manner. *J. Virol.* **2007**, *81*, 3402–3413.
108. Nishitani, H.; Lygerou, Z. Control of DNA replication licensing in a cell cycle. *Genes Cells* **2002**, *7*, 523–534.
109. Bell, S.P.; Dutta, A. DNA replication in eukaryotic cells. *Annu. Rev. Biochem.* **2002**, *71*, 333–374.
110. Sun, Q.; Tsurimoto, T.; Juillard, F.; Li, L.; Li, S.; de Leon Vazquez, E.; Chen, S.; Kaye, K. Kaposi's sarcoma-associated herpesvirus LANA recruits the DNA polymerase clamp loader to mediate efficient replication and virus persistence. *Proc. Natl. Acad. Sci. USA* **2014**, *111*, 11816–11821.
111. Verma, S.C.; Borah, S.; Robertson, E.S. Latency-associated nuclear antigen of Kaposi's sarcoma-associated herpesvirus up-regulates transcription of human telomerase reverse transcriptase promoter through interaction with transcription factor SP1. *J. Virol.* **2004**, *78*, 10348–10359.
112. Friborg, J., Jr.; Kong, W.; Hottiger, M.O.; Nabel, G.J. P53 inhibition by the LANA protein of KSHV protects against cell death. *Nature* **1999**, *402*, 889–894.
113. Radkov, S.A.; Kellam, P.; Boshoff, C. The latent nuclear antigen of Kaposi sarcoma-associated herpesvirus targets the retinoblastoma-E2F pathway and with the oncogene HRAS transforms primary rat cells. *Nat. Med.* **2000**, *6*, 1121–1127.
114. Van Dross, R.; Yao, S.; Asad, S.; Westlake, G.; Mays, D.J.; Barquero, L.; Duell, S.; Pietenpol, J.A.; Browning, P.J. Constitutively active K-cyclin/CDK6 kinase in Kaposi sarcoma-associated herpesvirus-infected cells. *J. Natl. Cancer Inst.* **2005**, *97*, 656–666.
115. Direkze, S.; Laman, H. Regulation of growth signalling and cell cycle by Kaposi's sarcoma-associated herpesvirus genes. *Int. J. Exp. Pathol.* **2004**, *85*, 305–319.
116. Sarek, G.; Jarviluoma, A.; Moore, H.M.; Tojkander, S.; Vartia, S.; Biberfeld, P.; Laiho, M.; Ojala, P.M. Nucleophosmin phosphorylation by v-cyclin-CDK6 controls KSHV latency. *PLOS Pathog.* **2010**, *6*, e1000818.
117. Liang, X.; Paden, C.R.; Morales, F.M.; Powers, R.P.; Jacob, J.; Speck, S.H. Murine gamma-herpesvirus immortalization of fetal liver-derived B cells requires both the viral cyclin D homolog and latency-associated nuclear antigen. *PLOS Pathog.* **2011**, *7*, e1002220.

118. Guasparri, I.; Keller, S.A.; Cesarman, E. KSHV vFLIP is essential for the survival of infected lymphoma cells. *J. Exp. Med.* **2004**, *199*, 993–1003.
119. Israel, A. The IKK complex, a central regulator of NF-kappaB activation. *Cold Spring Harbor Perspect. Biol.* **2010**, *2*, a000158.
120. Field, N.; Low, W.; Daniels, M.; Howell, S.; Daviet, L.; Boshoff, C.; Collins, M. KSHV vFLIP binds to IKK-gamma to activate IKK. *J. Cell Sci.* **2003**, *116*, 3721–3728.
121. Ye, F.; Lei, X.; Gao, S.J. Mechanisms of Kaposi's sarcoma-associated herpesvirus latency and reactivation. *Adv. Virol.* **2011**, *2011*, Article ID 193860.
122. Sadler, R.; Wu, L.; Forghani, B.; Renne, R.; Zhong, W.; Herndier, B.; Ganem, D. A complex translational program generates multiple novel proteins from the latently expressed kaposin (K12) locus of Kaposi's sarcoma-associated herpesvirus. *J. Virol.* **1999**, *73*, 5722–5730.
123. McCormick, C.; Ganem, D. The kaposin B protein of KSHV activates the P38/MK2 pathway and stabilizes cytokine mrnas. *Science* **2005**, *307*, 739–741.
124. Kanno, T.; Sato, Y.; Sata, T.; Katano, H. Expression of Kaposi's sarcoma-associated herpesvirus-encoded K10/10.1 protein in tissues and its interaction with poly(A)-binding protein. *Virology* **2006**, *352*, 100–109.
125. Esteban, M.; Garcia, M.A.; Domingo-Gil, E.; Arroyo, J.; Nombela, C.; Rivas, C. The latency protein LANA2 from Kaposi's sarcoma-associated herpesvirus inhibits apoptosis induced by dsRNA-activated protein kinase but not RNase l activation. *J. Gen. Virol.* **2003**, *84*, 1463–1470.
126. Rivas, C.; Thlick, A.E.; Parravicini, C.; Moore, P.S.; Chang, Y. Kaposi's sarcoma-associated herpesvirus LANA2 is a B-cell-specific latent viral protein that inhibits p53. *J. Virol.* **2001**, *75*, 429–438.
127. Lin, Y.T.; Kincaid, R.P.; Arasappan, D.; Dowd, S.E.; Hunicke-Smith, S.P.; Sullivan, C.S. Small RNA profiling reveals antisense transcription throughout the KSHV genome and novel small RNAs. *RNA* **2010**, *16*, 1540–1558.
128. Cai, X.; Cullen, B.R. Transcriptional origin of Kaposi's sarcoma-associated herpesvirus micrornas. *J. Virol.* **2006**, *80*, 2234–2242.
129. Grundhoff, A.; Sullivan, C.S.; Ganem, D. A combined computational and microarray-based approach identifies novel micrornas encoded by human gamma-herpesviruses. *RNA* **2006**, *12*, 733–750.
130. Pfeffer, S.; Sewer, A.; Lagos-Quintana, M.; Sheridan, R.; Sander, C.; Grasser, F.A.; van Dyk, L.F.; Ho, C.K.; Shuman, S.; Chien, M.; *et al.* Identification of micrornas of the herpesvirus family. *Nat. Methods* **2005**, *2*, 269–276.
131. Samols, M.A.; Hu, J.; Skalsky, R.L.; Renne, R. Cloning and identification of a microrna cluster within the latency-associated region of Kaposi's sarcoma-associated herpesvirus. *J. Virol.* **2005**, *79*, 9301–9305.
132. Feldman, E.R.; Kara, M.; Coleman, C.B.; Grau, K.R.; Oko, L.M.; Krueger, B.J.; Renne, R.; van Dyk, L.F.; Tibbetts, S.A. Virus-encoded micrornas facilitate gammaherpesvirus latency and pathogenesis *in vivo*. *mBio* **2014**, *5*, doi:10.1128/mBio.00981-14.
133. Lei, X.; Bai, Z.; Ye, F.; Huang, Y.; Gao, S.J. Regulation of herpesvirus lifecycle by viral micrornas. *Virulence* **2010**, *1*, 433–435.

134. Lu, C.C.; Li, Z.; Chu, C.Y.; Feng, J.; Feng, J.; Sun, R.; Rana, T.M. Micrornas encoded by Kaposi's sarcoma-associated herpesvirus regulate viral life cycle. *EMBO Rep.* **2010**, *11*, 784–790.
135. Plaisance-Bonstaff, K.; Choi, H.S.; Beals, T.; Krueger, B.J.; Boss, I.W.; Gay, L.A.; Haecker, I.; Hu, J.; Renne, R. Kshv mirnas decrease expression of lytic genes in latently infected PEL and endothelial cells by targeting host transcription factors. *Viruses* **2014**, *6*, 4005–4023.
136. Moody, R.; Zhu, Y.; Huang, Y.; Cui, X.; Jones, T.; Bedolla, R.; Lei, X.; Bai, Z.; Gao, S.J. KSHV micrornas mediate cellular transformation and tumorigenesis by redundantly targeting cell growth and survival pathways. *PLOS Pathog.* **2013**, *9*, e1003857.
137. Lei, X.; Bai, Z.; Ye, F.; Xie, J.; Kim, C.G.; Huang, Y.; Gao, S.J. Regulation of NF-kappaB inhibitor ikappabalpha and viral replication by a KSHV microrna. *Nat. Cell Biol.* **2010**, *12*, 193–199.
138. Suffert, G.; Malterer, G.; Hausser, J.; Viiliainen, J.; Fender, A.; Contrant, M.; Ivacevic, T.; Benes, V.; Gros, F.; Voinnet, O.; *et al.* Kaposi's sarcoma herpesvirus micrornas target caspase 3 and regulate apoptosis. *PLOS Pathog.* **2011**, *7*, e1002405.
139. Qin, Z.; Jakymiw, A.; Findlay, V.; Parsons, C. KSHV-encoded micrornas: Lessons for viral cancer pathogenesis and emerging concepts. *Int. J. Cell Biol.* **2012**, *2012*, 603961.
140. Ballestas, M.E.; Kaye, K.M. Kaposi's sarcoma-associated herpesvirus latency-associated nuclear antigen 1 mediates episome persistence through CIS-acting terminal repeat (TR) sequence and specifically binds TR DNA. *J. Virol.* **2001**, *75*, 3250–3258.
141. Hu, J.; Renne, R. Characterization of the minimal replicator of Kaposi's sarcoma-associated herpesvirus latent origin. *J. Virol.* **2005**, *79*, 2637–2642.
142. Skalsky, R.L.; Hu, J.; Renne, R. Analysis of viral *cis* elements conferring Kaposi's sarcoma-associated herpesvirus episome partitioning and maintenance. *J. Virol.* **2007**, *81*, 9825–9837.
143. Toth, Z.; Maglinte, D.T.; Lee, S.H.; Lee, H.R.; Wong, L.Y.; Brulois, K.F.; Lee, S.; Buckley, J.D.; Laird, P.W.; Marquez, V.E.; *et al.* Epigenetic analysis of KSHV latent and lytic genomes. *PLOS Pathog.* **2010**, *6*, e1001013.
144. Gunther, T.; Grundhoff, A. The epigenetic landscape of latent Kaposi sarcoma-associated herpesvirus genomes. *PLOS Pathog.* **2010**, *6*, e1000935.
145. He, M.; Zhang, W.; Bakken, T.; Schutten, M.; Toth, Z.; Jung, J.U.; Gill, P.; Cannon, M.; Gao, S.J. Cancer angiogenesis induced by Kaposi sarcoma-associated herpesvirus is mediated by EZH2. *Cancer Res.* **2012**, *72*, 3582–3592.
146. Chang, P.C.; Fitzgerald, L.D.; Hsia, D.A.; Izumiya, Y.; Wu, C.Y.; Hsieh, W.P.; Lin, S.F.; Campbell, M.; Lam, K.S.; Luciw, P.A.; *et al.* Histone demethylase JMJD2A regulates Kaposi's sarcoma-associated herpesvirus replication and is targeted by a viral transcriptional factor. *J. Virol.* **2011**, *85*, 3283–3293.
147. Paschos, K.; Allday, M.J. Epigenetic reprogramming of host genes in viral and microbial pathogenesis. *Trends Microbiol.* **2010**, *18*, 439–447.
148. Gunther, T.; Schreiner, S.; Dobner, T.; Tessmer, U.; Grundhoff, A. Influence of ND10 components on epigenetic determinants of early KSHV latency establishment. *PLOS Pathog.* **2014**, *10*, e1004274.
149. Merkenschlager, M.; Odom, D.T. CTCF and Cohesin: Linking gene regulatory elements with their targets. *Cell* **2013**, *152*, 1285–1297.

150. Kang, H.; Wiedmer, A.; Yuan, Y.; Robertson, E.; Lieberman, P.M. Coordination of KSHV latent and lytic gene control by CTCF-cohesin mediated chromosome conformation. *PLOS Pathog.* **2011**, *7*, e1002140.
151. Stedman, W.; Kang, H.; Lin, S.; Kissil, J.L.; Bartolomei, M.S.; Lieberman, P.M. Cohesins localize with CTCF at the KSHV latency control region and at cellular C-myc and H19/IGF2 insulators. *EMBO J.* **2008**, *27*, 654–666.
152. Li, D.J.; Verma, D.; Mosbruger, T.; Swaminathan, S. CTCF and RAD21 act as host cell restriction factors for Kaposi's sarcoma-associated herpesvirus (KSHV) lytic replication by modulating viral gene transcription. *PLOS Pathog.* **2014**, *10*, e1003880.
153. Losada, A. Cohesin in cancer: Chromosome segregation and beyond. *Nat. Rev. Cancer* **2014**, *14*, 389–393.
154. Chen, H.S.; Lu, F.; Lieberman, P.M. Epigenetic regulation of EBV and KSHV latency. *Curr. Opin. Virol.* **2013**, *3*, 251–259.
155. Darst, R.P.; Haecker, I.; Pardo, C.E.; Renne, R.; Kladde, M.P. Epigenetic diversity of Kaposi's sarcoma-associated herpesvirus. *Nucl. Acids Res.* **2013**, *41*, 2993–3009.
156. Darst, R.P.; Nabilsi, N.H.; Pardo, C.E.; Riva, A.; Kladde, M.P. DNA methyltransferase accessibility protocol for individual templates by deep sequencing. *Methods Enzymol.* **2012**, *513*, 185–204.
157. Staskus, K.A.; Zhong, W.; Gebhard, K.; Herndier, B.; Wang, H.; Renne, R.; Beneke, J.; Pudney, J.; Anderson, D.J.; Ganem, D.; *et al.* Kaposi's sarcoma-associated herpesvirus gene expression in endothelial (spindle) tumor cells. *J. Virol.* **1997**, *71*, 715–719.
158. Zhong, W.; Wang, H.; Herndier, B.; Ganem, D. Restricted expression of Kaposi sarcoma-associated herpesvirus (human herpesvirus 8) genes in Kaposi sarcoma. *Proc. Natl. Acad. Sci. USA* **1996**, *93*, 6641–6646.
159. Cavallin, L.E.; Goldschmidt-Clermont, P.; Mesri, E.A. Molecular and cellular mechanisms of KSHV oncogenesis of Kaposi's sarcoma associated with HIV/AIDS. *PLOS Pathog.* **2014**, *10*, e1004154.
160. Honess, R.W.; Roizman, B. Regulation of herpesvirus macromolecular synthesis. I. Cascade regulation of the synthesis of three groups of viral proteins. *J. Virol.* **1974**, *14*, 8–19.
161. Sun, R.; Lin, S.F.; Staskus, K.; Gradoville, L.; Grogan, E.; Haase, A.; Miller, G. Kinetics of Kaposi's sarcoma-associated herpesvirus gene expression. *J. Virol.* **1999**, *73*, 2232–2242.
162. Zhu, F.X.; Cusano, T.; Yuan, Y. Identification of the immediate-early transcripts of Kaposi's sarcoma-associated herpesvirus. *J. Virol.* **1999**, *73*, 5556–5567.
163. Jenner, R.G.; Alba, M.M.; Boshoff, C.; Kellam, P. Kaposi's sarcoma-associated herpesvirus latent and lytic gene expression as revealed by DNA arrays. *J. Virol.* **2001**, *75*, 891–902.
164. Lukac, D.M.; Kirshner, J.R.; Ganem, D. Transcriptional activation by the product of open reading frame 50 of Kaposi's sarcoma-associated herpesvirus is required for lytic viral reactivation in B cells. *J. Virol.* **1999**, *73*, 9348–9361.
165. Lukac, D.M.; Renne, R.; Kirshner, J.R.; Ganem, D. Reactivation of Kaposi's sarcoma-associated herpesvirus infection from latency by expression of the ORF 50 transactivator, a homolog of the EBV R protein. *Virology* **1998**, *252*, 304–312.

166. Sun, R.; Lin, S.F.; Gradoville, L.; Yuan, Y.; Zhu, F.; Miller, G. A viral gene that activates lytic cycle expression of Kaposi's sarcoma-associated herpesvirus. *Proc. Natl. Acad. Sci. USA* **1998**, *95*, 10866–10871.
167. Xu, Y.; AuCoin, D.P.; Huete, A.R.; Cei, S.A.; Hanson, L.J.; Pari, G.S. A Kaposi's sarcoma-associated herpesvirus/human herpesvirus 8 ORF50 deletion mutant is defective for reactivation of latent virus and DNA replication. *J. Virol.* **2005**, *79*, 3479–3487.
168. Glaunsinger, B.; Ganem, D. Lytic KSHV infection inhibits host gene expression by accelerating global mrna turnover. *Mol. Cell* **2004**, *13*, 713–723.
169. Majerciak, V.; Yamanegi, K.; Zheng, Z.M. Gene structure and expression of Kaposi's sarcoma-associated herpesvirus ORF56, ORF57, ORF58, and ORF59. *J. Virol.* **2006**, *80*, 11968–11981.
170. Goto, E.; Ishido, S.; Sato, Y.; Ohgimoto, S.; Ohgimoto, K.; Nagano-Fujii, M.; Hotta, H. C-mir, a human E3 ubiquitin ligase, is a functional homolog of herpesvirus proteins MIR1 and MIR2 and has similar activity. *J. Biol. Chem.* **2003**, *278*, 14657–14668.
171. Arias, C.; Weisburd, B.; Stern-Ginossar, N.; Mercier, A.; Madrid, A.S.; Bellare, P.; Holdorf, M.; Weissman, J.S.; Ganem, D. KSHV 2.0: A comprehensive annotation of the Kaposi's sarcoma-associated herpesvirus genome using next-generation sequencing reveals novel genomic and functional features. *PLOS Pathog.* **2014**, *10*, e1003847.
172. Chen, W.Y.; Townes, T.M. Molecular mechanism for silencing virally transduced genes involves histone deacetylation and chromatin condensation. *Proc. Natl. Acad. Sci. USA* **2000**, *97*, 377–382.
173. Chen, J.; Ueda, K.; Sakakibara, S.; Okuno, T.; Parravicini, C.; Corbellino, M.; Yamanishi, K. Activation of latent Kaposi's sarcoma-associated herpesvirus by demethylation of the promoter of the lytic transactivator. *Proc. Natl. Acad. Sci. USA* **2001**, *98*, 4119–4124.
174. Lu, F.; Zhou, J.; Wiedmer, A.; Madden, K.; Yuan, Y.; Lieberman, P.M. Chromatin remodeling of the Kaposi's sarcoma-associated herpesvirus ORF50 promoter correlates with reactivation from latency. *J. Virol.* **2003**, *77*, 11425–11435.
175. Morris, T.L.; Arnold, R.R.; Webster-Cyriaque, J. Signaling cascades triggered by bacterial metabolic end products during reactivation of Kaposi's sarcoma-associated herpesvirus. *J. Virol.* **2007**, *81*, 6032–6042.
176. Pantry, S.N.; Medveczky, P.G. Epigenetic regulation of Kaposi's sarcoma-associated herpesvirus replication. *Semin. Cancer Biol.* **2009**, *19*, 153–157.
177. Rossetto, C.C.; Pari, G. KSHV PAN RNA associates with demethylases UTX and JMJD3 to activate lytic replication through a physical interaction with the virus genome. *PLOS Pathog.* **2012**, *8*, e1002680.
178. Groen, J.N.; Morris, K.V. Chromatin, non-coding RNAs, and the expression of HIV. *Viruses* **2013**, *5*, 1633–1645.
179. Majerciak, V.; Ni, T.; Yang, W.; Meng, B.; Zhu, J.; Zheng, Z.M. A viral genome landscape of RNA polyadenylation from KSHV latent to lytic infection. *PLOS Pathog.* **2013**, *9*, e1003749.
180. Steitz, J.; Borah, S.; Cazalla, D.; Fok, V.; Lytle, R.; Mitton-Fry, R.; Riley, K.; Samji, T. Noncoding RNPs of viral origin. *Cold Spring Harb. Perspect. Biol.* **2011**, *3*, doi: 10.1101/cshperspect.a005165.
181. Song, M.J.; Brown, H.J.; Wu, T.T.; Sun, R. Transcription activation of polyadenylated nuclear rna by RTA in human herpesvirus 8/Kaposi's sarcoma-associated herpesvirus. *J. Virol.* **2001**, *75*, 3129–3140.

182. Sahin, B.B.; Patel, D.; Conrad, N.K. Kaposi's sarcoma-associated herpesvirus ORF57 protein binds and protects a nuclear noncoding RNA from cellular RNA decay pathways. *PLOS Pathog.* **2010**, *6*, e1000799.
183. Massimelli, M.J.; Majerciak, V.; Kruhlak, M.; Zheng, Z.M. Interplay between polyadenylate-binding protein 1 and Kaposi's sarcoma-associated herpesvirus ORF57 in accumulation of polyadenylated nuclear RNA, a viral long noncoding RNA. *J. Virol.* **2013**, *87*, 243–256.
184. Blauvelt, A.; Herndier, B.G.; Orenstein, J.M. Propagation of a human herpesvirus from AIDS-associated Kaposi's sarcoma. *N. Engl. J. Med.* **1997**, *336*, 1837–1839.
185. Renne, R.; Blackbourn, D.; Whitby, D.; Levy, J.; Ganem, D. Limited transmission of Kaposi's sarcoma-associated herpesvirus in cultured cells. *J. Virol.* **1998**, *72*, 5182–5188.
186. Veettil, M.V.; Bandyopadhyay, C.; Dutta, D.; Chandran, B. Interaction of KSHV with host cell surface receptors and cell entry. *Viruses* **2014**, *6*, 4024–4046.
187. Luna, R.E.; Zhou, F.; Baghian, A.; Chouljenko, V.; Forghani, B.; Gao, S.J.; Kousoulas, K.G. Kaposi's sarcoma-associated herpesvirus glycoprotein K8.1 is dispensable for virus entry. *J. Virol.* **2004**, *78*, 6389–6398.
188. Chandran, B.; Bloomer, C.; Chan, S.R.; Zhu, L.; Goldstein, E.; Horvat, R. Human herpesvirus-8 ORF K8.1 gene encodes immunogenic glycoproteins generated by spliced transcripts. *Virology* **1998**, *249*, 140–149.
189. Koyano, S.; Mar, E.C.; Stamey, F.R.; Inoue, N. Glycoproteins M and N of human herpesvirus 8 form a complex and inhibit cell fusion. *J. Gen. Virol.* **2003**, *84*, 1485–1491.
190. Full, F.; Jungnickl, D.; Reuter, N.; Bogner, E.; Brulois, K.; Scholz, B.; Sturzl, M.; Myoung, J.; Jung, J.U.; Stamminger, T.; *et al.* Kaposi's sarcoma associated herpesvirus tegument protein ORF75 is essential for viral lytic replication and plays a critical role in the antagonization of ND10-instituted intrinsic immunity. *PLOS Pathog.* **2014**, *10*, e1003863.
191. Chandran, B. Early events in Kaposi's sarcoma-associated herpesvirus infection of target cells. *J. Virol.* **2010**, *84*, 2188–2199.
192. Toth, Z.; Brulois, K.; Lee, H.R.; Izumiya, Y.; Tepper, C.; Kung, H.J.; Jung, J.U. Biphasic euchromatin-to-heterochromatin transition on the KSHV genome following *de novo* infection. *PLOS Pathog.* **2013**, *9*, e1003813.
193. Morey, L.; Helin, K. Polycomb group protein-mediated repression of transcription. *Trends Biochem. Sci.* **2010**, *35*, 323–332.
194. Lallemand-Breitenbach, V.; Zhu, J.; Puvion, F.; Koken, M.; Honore, N.; Doubeikovsky, A.; Duprez, E.; Pandolfi, P.P.; Puvion, E.; Freemont, P.; *et al.* Role of promyelocytic leukemia (PML) sumolation in nuclear body formation, 11s proteasome recruitment, and AS2O3-induced PML or PML/retinoic acid receptor alpha degradation. *J. Exp. Med.* **2001**, *193*, 1361–1371.
195. Chan, J.Y.; Li, L.; Fan, Y.H.; Mu, Z.M.; Zhang, W.W.; Chang, K.S. Cell-cycle regulation of DNA damage-induced expression of the suppressor gene PML. *Biochem. Biophys. Res. Commun.* **1997**, *240*, 640–646.
196. Ishov, A.M.; Sotnikov, A.G.; Negorev, D.; Vladimirova, O.V.; Neff, N.; Kamitani, T.; Yeh, E.T.; Strauss, J.F., 3rd; Maul, G.G. PML is critical for ND10 formation and recruits the PML-interacting protein DAXX to this nuclear structure when modified by SUMO-1. *J. Cell Biol.* **1999**, *147*, 221–234.

197. Kyratsous, C.A.; Silverstein, S.J. Components of nuclear domain 10 bodies regulate varicella-zoster virus replication. *J. Virol.* **2009**, *83*, 4262–4274.
198. Gregory, S.M.; Davis, B.K.; West, J.A.; Taxman, D.J.; Matsuzawa, S.; Reed, J.C.; Ting, J.P.; Damania, B. Discovery of a viral NLR homolog that inhibits the inflammasome. *Science* **2011**, *331*, 330–334.
199. Kerur, N.; Veettil, M.V.; Sharma-Walia, N.; Bottero, V.; Sadagopan, S.; Otageri, P.; Chandran, B. IFI16 acts as a nuclear pathogen sensor to induce the inflammasome in response to Kaposi sarcoma-associated herpesvirus infection. *Cell Host Microbe* **2011**, *9*, 363–375.

3

Histone Deacetylases in Herpesvirus Replication and Virus-Stimulated Host Defense

Amanda J. Guise, Hanna G. Budayeva, Benjamin A. Diner and Ileana M. Cristea *

Department of Molecular Biology, Princeton University, Washington Road, Princeton, NJ 08544, USA; E-Mails: aguise@princeton.edu (A.J.G.); budayeva@princeton.edu (H.G.B.); bdiner@princeton.edu (B.A.D.)

* Author to whom correspondence should be addressed; E-Mail: icristea@princeton.edu;

Abstract: Emerging evidence highlights a critical role for protein acetylation during herpesvirus infection. As prominent modulators of protein acetylation, histone deacetylases (HDACs) are essential transcriptional and epigenetic regulators. Not surprisingly, viruses have evolved a wide array of mechanisms to subvert HDAC functions. Here, we review the mechanisms underlying HDAC regulation during herpesvirus infection. We next discuss the roles of acetylation in host defense against herpesvirus infection. Finally, we provide a perspective on the contribution of current mass spectrometry-based "omic" technologies to infectious disease research, offering a systems biology view of infection.

Keywords: herpesvirus; HDAC; IFI16; acetylation; NF-κB; p53; proteomics; metabolomics; chemoproteomics

1. Introduction

Protein acetylation has recently emerged as a critical regulatory factor during herpesvirus infection. Recent studies have linked chromatin remodeling and acetylation/deacetylation events to the regulation of promoter activity and maintenance of viral latency during herpesvirus infection. These studies examined herpes simplex virus 1 (HSV-1), human cytomegalovirus (HCMV), Kaposi's sarcoma-associated herpesvirus (KSHV) and Epstein-Barr virus (EBV) [1–4], thereby pointing to similarities among alpha-, beta- and gamma-herpesvirus infections. During latent infection, the HSV-1 genome is assembled into an ordered nucleosome-associated structure; however, during active lytic infection, the structure of viral chromatin exists in a more disordered state [5,6]. In lytic stages of infection, histones associate with herpesvirus promoter regions, and chromatin adopts a conformation consistent with more actively transcribed host genomic regions [6]. Moreover, it is well established that the post-translational modification of herpesvirus-associated histone tails is important for the regulation of viral gene transcription [7–11].

Given the significance of acetylation during viral infection and its requirement for essential host functions, knowledge of the regulation of the enzymes controlling protein acetylation is critical for understanding viral pathogenicity and host defense. This position is further emphasized by the recent finding that acetylation is a more prominent post-translational modification than previously thought, with several thousand host protein acetylations identified to date [12,13]. Among the enzymes involved in regulating protein acetylation are the human histone deacetylases (HDACs), which remove acetylations from their substrates [14]. Along with the numerous histone acetyltransferases (HATs) responsible for lysine acetylation, HDACs control the activity of substrates by acting as components of diverse multi-protein complexes with co-repressor functions (reviewed in [15,16]). HDACs themselves are a conserved family of proteins that evolutionarily predate histones, indicating that their interactions with non-histone proteins are integral to their cellular functions [17]. Given the array of human deacetylases, which encompasses eleven Zn^{2+}-dependent HDACs and seven NAD^{+}-dependent sirtuins (SIRTs), as well as their ability to participate in multiple protein complexes, viral interactions with members of this enzymatic family are likely to be protein-specific and individually regulated. HDACs have been linked to viral replication and pathogenesis during infection with a variety of human pathogens, including herpesviruses, hepatitis B and C, HIV-1 and HPV (reviewed in [18]). It is therefore not surprising that, during co-evolution with their hosts, viruses have gathered finely tuned mechanisms for targeting HDACs to either appropriate or inhibit their enzymatic activities. These observations highlight the importance of understanding the mechanisms of HDAC regulation during viral infection.

In this review, we summarize the mechanisms employed by herpesviruses to perturb the functions of this important family of host transcriptional regulators, the histone deacetylases. Next, we discuss the roles of acetylation in regulating host defense mechanisms against herpesvirus infection. Finally, we provide a perspective on the promise of emerging "omic" technologies for gaining a systems biology view of infection and an in-depth understanding of virus-induced changes within cellular pathways.

2. Viral Control of HDAC Complexes

Histone deacetylases are critical chromatin-associated transcriptional regulators responsible for the removal of lysine acetylations within targeted genomic regions, thereby promoting compact chromatin organization and repression of transcription. HDACs perform their repressive functions as components of numerous multi-protein co-repressor complexes, including the nucleosome remodeling and deacetylase (NuRD), co-repressor of RE1 silencing transcription factor (CoREST), mSin3A co-repressor, nuclear co-repressor (NCoR) and mitotic deacetylase (MIDAC) complexes [19–26]. The diversity of HDAC-containing complexes was clearly demonstrated by a recent proteomics-based study that profiled the interactions of all eleven human HDACs and assessed the relative stabilities of interactions within protein complexes [27]. This study demonstrated that HDACs can be part of numerous pre-assembled functional complexes that can associate with transcriptional factors for effective regulation of downstream gene expression. Moreover, these studies provided evidence that HDACs play roles not only in chromatin remodeling and transcriptional regulation, but also in diverse cellular processes, including cell cycle progression and RNA processing. Therefore, these results offer a valuable platform for examining changes in HDAC interactions during herpesvirus infection. The modulation of host protein interactions in response to infection provides both a mechanism for virus-mediated control of host protein functions for the benefit of viral replication, while also serving as a signal for the activation of host immune responses to counteract infection (summarized in Table 1 and Figure 1).

Table 1. Human histone deacetylase (HDAC) interactions with viral proteins during herpesvirus infection. HSV-1, herpes simplex virus 1; HCMV, human cytomegalovirus; EBV, Epstein-Barr virus; KSHV, Kaposi's sarcoma-associated herpesvirus.

Enzyme	Virus	Interaction	Functional consequence	Ref.
HDAC1	HSV-1	ICP8	Redistribution of HDAC1/CoREST and LSD1 to cytoplasm	[28–31]
	HSV-1	ICP0	Disrupts CoREST association; localizes HDAC1/ICP0 to ND10 bodies	[28,32–35]
	HSV-1	US3	Upstream effector of HDAC1 phosphorylation	[32,36,37]
	HCMV	pUL29/28	Associates with HDAC1/HDAC2 and NuRD to promote expression of viral genes	[38,39]
	HCMV	pUL38	Associates with HDAC1/HDAC2 and NuRD complex members via pUL29/28 bridge	[38,39]
	HCMV	IE86	Co-expression promotes MIEP repression	[40]
	EBV	ENBA3C	Represses Cp promoter via association with co-repressor complexes (e.g., mSin3A and NCoR)	[41,42]
	EBV	TRF2	Deacetylation of OriP; promotes stability of latent genome	[43]
	KSHV	ORF50 promoter	Proposed to modulate promoter acetylation status and LANA acetylation	[2,44]
HDAC2	HSV-1	US3	Upstream effector of HDAC2 phosphorylation	[32,36,37]
	HCMV	pUL29/28	Associates with HDAC1/HDAC2 and NuRD to promote expression of viral genes	[38,39]
	HCMV	IE2	De-represses pUL54 promoter; promotes localization of HDAC2 to replications sites	[45]
	HCMV	pUL38	Associates with HDAC1/HDAC2 and NuRD complex members via pUL29/28 bridge	[38,39]
	EBV	ENBA3C	Represses Cp promoter via association with co-repressor complexes (e.g., mSin3A and NCoR)	[41,42]
	EBV	TRF2	Deacetylation of OriP; promotes stability of latent genome	[43]

Table 1. *Cont.*

Enzyme	Virus	Interaction	Functional consequence	Ref.
HDAC3	HCMV	IE1	Increased acetylation at viral promoter	[46,47]
	HCMV	IE2	Increased acetylation at viral promoter	[46,47]
HDAC4	HSV-1	ICP0	Relieves MEF2-binding domain-mediated repression	[48]
HDAC5	HSV-1	ICP0	Relieves MEF2-binding domain-mediated repression	[48]
	KSHV	ORF50 promoter	Proposed to modulate promoter acetylation status and LANA acetylation	[2,44]
HDAC7	HSV-1	ICP0	Relieves MEF2-binding domain-mediated repression	[48]
	KSHV	ORF50 promoter	Proposed to modulate promoter acetylation status and LANA acetylation	[2,44]

Figure 1. Summary of HDAC functions during herpesvirus infection. (**A**) Response to alpha-herpesvirus infection (HSV-1); (**B**) response to beta-herpesvirus infection (HCMV); (**C**) response to gamma-herpesvirus infection (EBV and KSHV).

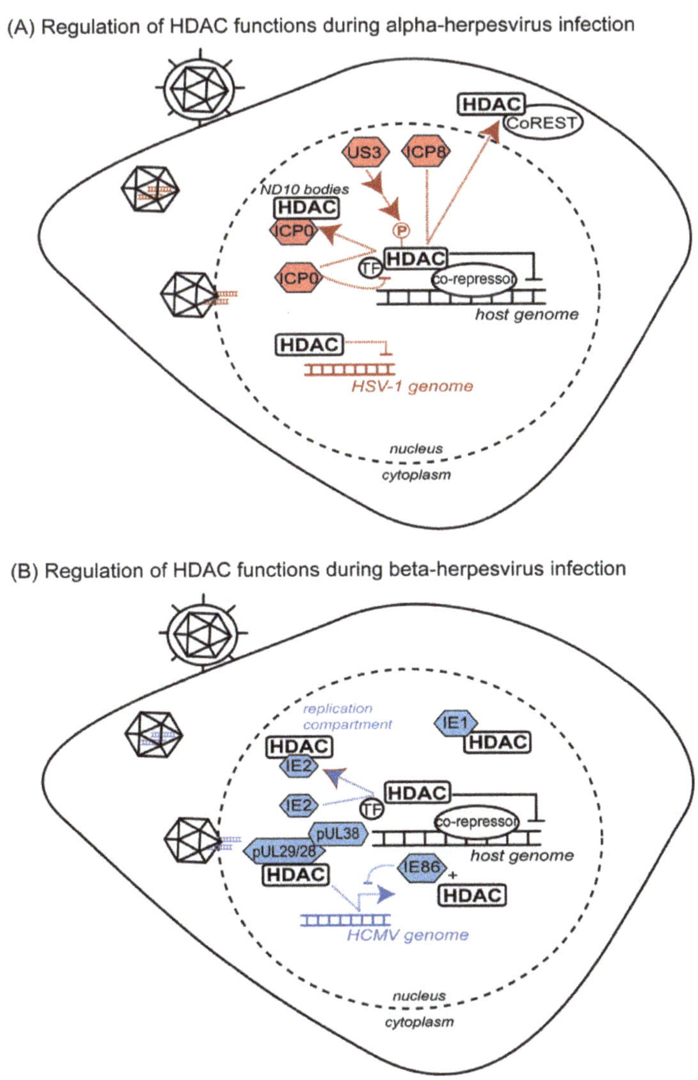

Figure 1. *Cont.*

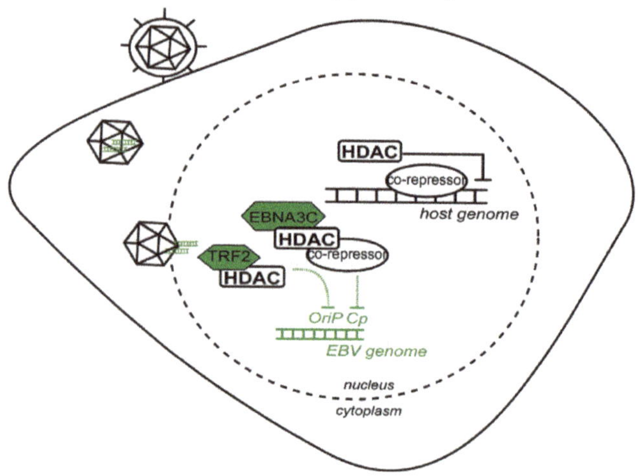

2.1. Infection with the Alpha-Herpesvirus HSV-1 Promotes Misregulation of HDAC1/HDAC2-Containing Complexes

Several studies have started to uncover the means through which HDACs are recruited to viral protein-associated complexes and to viral genomes. As components of the CoREST complex, HDAC1 and HDAC2 act as repressors of host gene transcription within the nucleus. In the absence of infection, HDAC1 is observed within distinct nuclear structures in complex with CoREST and LSD1; however, upon HSV-1 infection, the HDAC1/CoREST/LSD1 complex is redistributed to compact structures that also contain the viral protein ICP8 (Figure 1A and Table 1) [28]. Resembling viral replication compartments, these structures suggest a function for this complex in active transcription of the viral genome [28]. As LSD1 is an established histone demethylase, this association can couple demethylase and deacetylase activities for coordinated regulation of histone post-translational modifications associated with the viral genome [28–30]. It is possible that the association of separate viral factors could trigger preferential association of specific accessory demethylases with the core CoREST complex. Upon infection, components of the HDAC1/CoREST/LSD1 complex are observed to translocate to the cytoplasm, indicating that this complex or its members may adopt new functions in response to viral infection (Figure 1A) [31]. Intriguingly, the redistribution of these complex members appears to be temporally regulated, with HDAC1/CoREST accumulating in the cytoplasm at four hours post-infection (hpi) and LSD1 changing localization at 8 hpi [28]. The HDAC1-CoREST interaction also contributes to a host defense mechanism against herpesviruses, which is discussed in Section 3.2 of this review.

Interestingly, the viral protein kinase U_S3 can enhance expression of viral reporter genes, similar to the phenotype observed during HDAC inhibition, suggesting that a U_S3-mediated kinase cascade may be an upstream regulator of HDAC activity [32]. Both HDAC1 and HDAC2 hyperphosphorylation during herpesvirus infection depends on the activity of U_S3, yet HDAC phosphorylation appears to be an indirect effect of U_S3 activity, suggesting the involvement of additional viral or host kinases

(Figure 1A) [36,37]. In the absence of infection, phosphorylation is an established regulator of HDAC1 and HDAC2 activity and protein associations. Specifically, HDAC1 phosphorylation promotes binding to members of co-repressor complexes, including the Sin3a (RbAp48 and mSin3A), NuRD (RbAp48 and MTA2) and CoREST complexes [49]. Similarly, mSin3 and Mi2 (member of the NuRD complex) preferentially associate with phosphorylated HDAC2 [50]. The activity of viral kinases and perturbations in kinase signaling pathways could alter the phosphorylation landscape of these proteins, ultimately contributing to aberrant regulation of HDACs and rearrangement of HDAC complexes.

Phosphorylations can directly mediate HDAC protein interactions; however, a second level of regulation results from phosphorylation-dependent changes in HDAC localization. Class IIa HDACs (HDAC4, -5, -7 and -9) shuttle between the nucleus and the cytoplasm through a mechanism that relies on site-specific phosphorylation of 14-3-3 binding sites [51–54]. Interestingly, the subcellular distribution of class IIa HDACs has also been observed to be dynamic during infection. HDAC4, -5 and -7 co-localize with ICP0 within the nucleus during HSV-1 infection (Figure 1A) [48]. ICP0 was shown to physically interact with these enzymes via the conserved *N*-terminal extensions shared by class IIa HDACs and absent in their class I counterparts [48]. ICP0 serves to relieve repression of MEF2 induced by the binding of HDAC *N*-terminal domains to MEF2. However, transcription mediated by the HDAC *C*-terminal deacetylation domain was not relieved by ICP0, consistent with continued co-localization of HDACs with SMRT, another member of the nuclear co-repressor complex [48]. bICP0 has also been reported to interact with HDAC1 during bovine herpesvirus 1 infection to modulate Mad-dependent transcription, suggesting that this virus-host protein interaction may represent a common point of virus-mediated control of host protein complex formation [33]. Therefore, the phosphorylation status of HDACs significantly contributes to the regulation of both protein interactions and localizations in the context of infection. Recent results have demonstrated that Aurora B-dependent phosphorylation of class IIa HDACs modulates cell cycle-dependent functions of these enzymes, indicating that HDAC phosphorylations are both spatially and temporally regulated [55]. The importance of temporally regulated phosphorylations during viral infection remains to be established.

Altogether, multiple viral factors, including ICP0, ICP8 and U_S3, promote changes in the localization and functional roles of HDACs and co-repressor complexes during HSV-1 infection to promote viral reproduction. Further investigation of viral protein interactions with HDACs will contribute to development of a comprehensive understanding of the roles of individual HDAC family members during HSV-1 infection.

2.2. Beta-Herpesvirus HCMV Proteins Target Class I HDACs to Modulate Viral Gene Transcription

Modulation of HDAC complexes is also apparent during beta-herpesvirus infection. The HCMV proteins pUL29/28 and pUL38 interact with the HDAC1/HDAC2-containing NuRD complex in order to promote expression of immediate-early viral genes (Figure 1B and Table 1) [38,39] (Figure 1B). Immunoaffinity purification of pUL38 from cells infected with HCMV identified six components of the NuRD complex (Mi2β, MTA1, MTA2, HDAC1, HDAC2 and RbAp48/46 [38]), and the pUL38-NuRD interaction was shown to depend on the presence of the viral pUL29/28 protein [39]. Co-purification studies demonstrated that pUL29/28 binds to HDAC1 and MTA1 [39]. While pUL29/28 was also shown to interact with the Sin3A complex, this association seemed less stable than its interaction with NuRD, indicating preferential association of viral proteins to specific co-repressor complexes [39]. The pUL38/pUL29/28/NuRD complex forms early during infection and persists through 72 hpi, suggesting a role throughout multiple stages in the HCMV lifecycle [39]. While pUL29/28 and pUL38 exist in a complex together, these proteins also possess independent functions within the host cell. pUL38 interacts with TSC2, a component of the tuberous sclerosis tumor suppressor protein complex (TSC1/2), to maintain an active mTOR pathway during infection [38], whereas pUL29/28 was not shown to associate with TSC2 [39]. Moreover, pUL29/28 association with NuRD is independent of pUL38 and sufficient for transcriptional activation of the HCMV major immediate early promoter (MIEP). Treatment of cells infected with a pUL29/28-deficient virus with the HDAC inhibitor trichostatin A (TSA) rescued the decreased expression of immediate early genes induced by pUL29/28 depletion, demonstrating that this virus protein interaction with HDAC1/NuRD is important for stimulation of immediate early RNA production [39].

Similarly, HDAC inhibition was shown to relieve repression of other MIEP-dependent viral genes, as treatment with TSA rescued IE86-mediated autorepression [40]. IE86 interacts with HDAC1 and the histone methyltransferases G9a and Suvar(3–9)H1, likely contributing to changes in chromatin organization at the promoter region (Figure 1B) [40]. Co-expression of IE86 and HDAC1 enhanced repression of MIEP expression through both Rb-independent and -dependent mechanisms, indicating the potential involvement of multiple HDAC-containing complexes that differ in their association with Rb [40].

The immediate early proteins, IE1 and IE2, are also known to interact with HDACs to facilitate HCMV replication. IE1 and IE2 both interact with HDAC3, while IE2 was shown to also interact with HDAC2 (Figure 1B) [45,46]. Similar to the observations on IE86, HDAC inhibition rescued viral growth defects associated with IE1-deficient HCMV strains. Loss of IE1 triggers reduced histone H4 acetylation levels at the MIEP and the UL44 early promoter, indicating that HDAC activity at these regions is IE1-dependent [46]. IE2 interaction with HDAC3 is also thought to promote loss of deacetylation at viral promoter regions through a similar mechanism [46]. Intriguingly, overexpression of HDAC3 has been demonstrated to reduce activity from the MIEP and to limit HCMV infection [8]. As IE1 and IE2 are splice variants of the same mRNA sequence, domains common to both proteins could be important for association with structurally similar HDACs. Moreover, indirect association of immediate early proteins with bridge proteins could allow for interaction with multiple HDACs and HDAC-containing complexes [46,56,57]. Indeed, IE2 has been shown to associate with HDAC2 to de-repress expression from the viral polymerase (pUL54) promoter [45]. HDAC2 also exhibits altered localization during HCMV infection, co-localizing with IE2 at viral transcription and replication sites (Figure 1B); however, co-expression of IE2 alone was insufficient to induce HDAC2 redistribution, suggesting that additional viral factors contribute to its regulation during infection [45]. Interestingly, while the acetylation levels at the pUL54 promoter were observed to increase during the course of infection (from 6 hpi to 72 hpi), the acetylation at MIEP exhibited a different pattern—increasing at

24 hpi and diminishing at 48 hpi and 72 hpi. Therefore, HDAC-mediated regulation of viral promoter regions appears to be both promoter-specific and temporally regulated [45].

Careful regulation of gene expression is critical for progression through the viral lifecycle. The interaction of HCMV proteins with HDACs provides a mechanism by which viral gene programs can capitalize on the existence of an established host transcriptional regulatory system. HCMV proteins appear to display preference for individual HDAC-containing complexes, allowing for finely-tuned appropriation of host protein functions. Association of HDACs with viral promoters further allows modulation of the acetylation status of the viral genome, while simultaneously limiting the population of HDACs that would otherwise be available for interaction within typical host complexes.

2.3. The Gamma-Herpesviruses EBV and KSHV Regulate HDAC-Containing Co-Repressor Complexes through Protein Interactions and Phosphorylation-Dependent Signal Cascades

The gamma-herpesvirus EBV also modulates the activity of HDACs and HDAC complexes through the interaction of the viral Nuclear Antigen 3C (EBNA3C) protein with HDAC1 and HDAC2 (Figure 1C and Table 1) [41,42]. Careful regulation of viral gene expression is necessary for efficient replication, but also for maintenance of latency. The EBNA3C-HDAC interaction promotes the association of HDAC1 with the DNA binding protein CBF1/RPB-Jκ for both autorepression of EBNA3C and repression of Cp-responsive genes (Figure 1C) [41]. CBF1/RBP-Jκ is also reported to interact with HDAC1 and SMRT as part of a repressor complex [41,58]. As SMRT also associates with HDAC3 and class IIa HDACs, it is possible that multiple co-repressor complexes are recruited by EBNA3C to modulate complex-specific functions during infection [23,59]. Indeed, EBNA3C was subsequently shown to interact with HDAC1, HDAC2 and the co-repressor complexes mSin3A and NCoR as part of an EBNA3C-ProTα complex during EBV infection [42]. ProTα may serve as a bridge between EBNA3C and HDACs, as these co-repressor complexes were also demonstrated to associate with ProTα alone.

Viral gene transcription is further regulated by exploiting class IIa HDAC association with MEF2, which recruits HDACs 4, 5 and 7 to inhibit the viral BLZF1 promoter (Zp) [60,61]. Specifically, the de-phosphorylation of MEF2D has been shown to be important for regulating HDAC-mediated repression of Zp [61]. A consequence of this interaction is limited production of the immediate early viral protein BLZF1, which is a transcriptional activator important for exit from latency [60,61]. The temporal regulation of EBV gene expression is not only connected to HDAC transcriptional repressive functions (as in the case of MEF2), but also to deacetylation activity. HDAC1 and HDAC2 stably associate with the telomere repeat factor 2 (TRF2), which binds the EBV origin of plasmid replication (OriP) (Figure 1C) [43]. Based on the loss of HDAC/TRF2 binding to OriP during G1/S, along with a loss of deacetylation at OriP upon HDAC inhibition, this HDAC/TRF2 complex has been proposed to delay replication initiation from OriP in order to promote the stability of the latent EBV genome [43]. Thus, the temporal regulation of genome acetylation status and gene expression by HDACs is important for the preservation of latent stores of EBV within the host cell.

In addition to protein interactions, signaling pathways activated by viral infection affect HDAC activities, possibly through signal-dependent post-translational modification. The KSHV protein vGPCR has been reported to induce signaling pathways that converge on HDACs, among other targets [62]. vGPCR induces expression of the ORF50 promoter, which produces the protein RTA (replication and transcription activator) that, in itself, is sufficient for lytic reactivation of KSHV [62,63]. vGPCR activates PKC and PKD signaling pathways associated with regulation of ORF50 expression [62]. These kinases are well-established regulators of nuclear export of class IIa HDACs [51,64], indicating that HDAC phosphorylation during infection may be an important strategy for virus-mediated control of HDAC activity and complex formation. vGPCR signaling was reported to reduce the activity of deacetylases, as shown for both HDACs and sirtuins [62]. HDACs 1, 5 and 7 were shown to associate with the ORF50 promoter during KSHV latency, and the acetylation status of the latency-associated nuclear antigen (LANA) was dependent on HDAC activity [2,44]. The KSHV LANA protein can also interact with the HDAC co-repressor complex mSin3 during EBV infection [65]. Given the importance of temporal coordination of viral gene programs, cell cycle-dependent kinase cascades could provide an additional level of regulation of gene expression during infection. Interestingly, ORF50 is also capable of repressing p53 transcriptional activity through an interaction with the CREB binding protein, CBP [66,67]. As p53 activity is regulated by acetylation, it is tempting to speculate that p53-associated responses to viral infection are, in part, due to misregulation of deacetylase complexes [68,69].

Altogether, these studies have demonstrated that gamma-herpesviruses EBV and KSHV co-opt HDAC complexes to repress viral gene expression. These mechanisms likely allow for maintenance of the viral genome in a latent state until conditions are advantageous for viral replication. Viral infection further alters HDAC activity through activation of phosphorylation signaling cascades, thereby modulating the phosphorylation states and activities of individual HDAC enzymes.

3. Host Employment of HDACs and Acetylation in Defense against Herpesviruses

Comprehensive acetylome studies have revealed that histone and non-histone protein acetylation is comparable in frequency to phosphorylation [12,13]. One study alone identified over 3,500 acetylations across three human cell types using immunoaffinity isolation of acetylated substrates coupled with mass spectrometry analysis [13]. Interestingly, acetylations within several important effectors of innate immunity—RIG-I, IRAK4, OAS2, TRIM25 [13] and, most recently, IFI16 [70]—have been identified, suggesting that acetylation provides dynamic control of important mammalian innate immune functions. Indeed, increasing evidence suggests that HDACs are regulators of inflammatory response, immune signaling and myeloid differentiation [71–74].

3.1. IFI16 Acetylation and Host Detection of Viral DNA

In mammals, induction of host innate immunity in response to viral infection begins with the detection of pathogen-associated molecular patterns (PAMPs) or danger-associated molecular patterns (DAMPs) by intracellular pattern recognition receptors (PRRs). Several classes of PRRs have been characterized, including AIM2-like receptors (ALRs), retinoic acid-inducible gene I-like receptors (RLRs), nucleotide oligomerization domain-like receptors (NLRs), Toll-like receptors (TLRs) and an assorted array of cytoplasmic DNA receptors [75]. These PRRs are predominantly localized to the cytosol, plasma membrane and endosome to sense and respond to a wide range of invading pathogens. Surprisingly, recent studies have extended the range of host immuno-surveillance to the nucleus, where the DNA sensor IFI16 selectively detects the double-stranded DNA genome of herpesviruses during infection [70] (Figure 2).

As an ALR family member, IFI16 senses nuclear and cytoplasmic herpesvirus DNA, inducing pro-inflammatory and interferon responses via distinct pathways to limit viral replication and spread (Figure 2) [70,75–80]. In the cytoplasm, IFI16 associates with the signaling adapter protein STING (stimulator of interferon genes) upon binding of viral DNA, subsequently activating IRF3 and NF-κB transcription factors, which then translocate to the nucleus and induce robust interferon-β (IFN-β) expression [75,80]. However, DNA sensing is not restricted to the cytoplasm, as IFI16 has also been demonstrated to bind herpesvirus DNA in the nucleus during early stages of infection to induce IFN-β expression [70]. Intriguingly, following detection of viral DNA, IFI16 and the additional ALR AIM2 form oligomeric, multi-protein complexes known as inflammasomes [76,78,79,81,82]. In the cytoplasm, these inflammasomes recruit and activate caspase-1, which, in turn, processes the pro-inflammatory cytokines pro-IL-1β and pro-IL-18 to their secreted, biologically active forms. Until recently, the underlying mechanisms regulating these localization-dependent innate immune functions of IFI16 were not well-understood. Li *et al.* identified two acetylations within IFI16 that regulate its sub-cellular distribution [70]. Partly mediated by the HAT p300, acetylation of Lys99 and Lys128 within the nuclear localization signal (NLS) promotes cytoplasmic retention of IFI16, whereas HDAC activity promotes its nuclear import. Nuclear localization of IFI16 was shown to be essential for recognition of nuclear herpesviral DNA during infection [70,76,77], indicating that HDACs may play a critical role in IFI16-mediated DNA sensing. Thus, modification by acetylation provides a means for expanding the range of IFI16-mediated immuno-surveillance of double-stranded DNA viruses and may function as a toggle for additional localization-dependent functions (Figure 2). Observations of the multiple patterns of IFI16 behavior during viral infection suggest that this protein may have varied functions in immune response. While acetylation of IFI16 is critical for positioning this DNA sensor in the appropriate cellular compartment prior to infection, the roles of IFI16 acetylation and associated HDAC functions during infection require further investigation.

IFI16 is not the only PRR known to be acetylated. RIG-I, a sensor of viral double-stranded RNA that acts through the MAVS adapter protein to induce IFN signaling [83], is acetylated at Lys858 within its *C*-terminal repression domain [13]. While Lys858 acetylation has yet to be tested for modulation of RIG-I activity, acetylation of PRRs and HDAC modulation of PRR activities may be a more prominent regulatory feature of the innate immune system than currently appreciated.

Figure 2. Host response to viral DNA is mediated by IFI16. Acetylation-dependent localization of IFI16 allows dual-compartment sensing of viral DNA, promoting pro-inflammatory response and innate immune signaling during herpesvirus infection. (**A**) IFI16 senses HSV-1 DNA within the nucleus. (**B**) IFI16 senses cytoplasmic DNA resulting from transient transfection or viral capsid degradation.

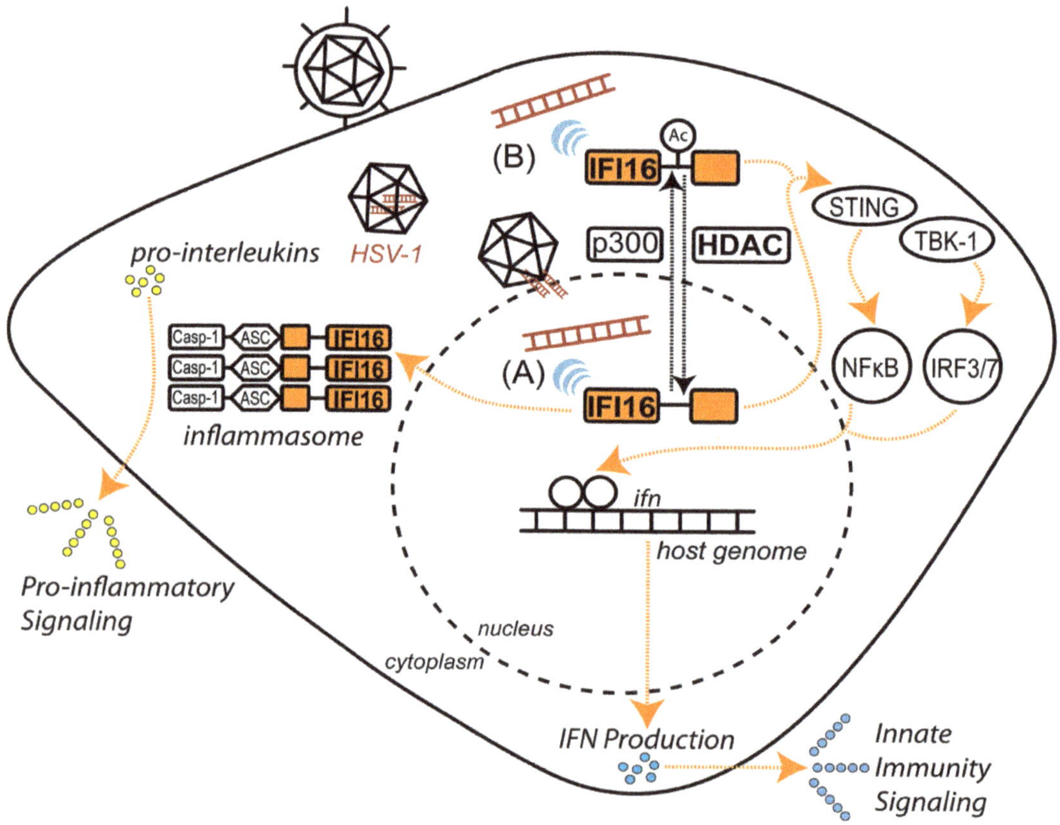

Once PRRs bind their pathogen-derived ligands, innate immune signals are transmitted to neighboring cells via cytokine production and secretion. HDACs have indirectly been implicated in these processes. Animals treated with valproic acid (VPA), a broad-acting HDAC inhibitor, exhibit increased susceptibility to infection by bacterial and fungal pathogens, while being protected from septic shock [73]. In agreement with these observations, VPA-treated macrophages in the presence *E. coli* and *S. aureus* exhibit reduced phagocytosis and subsequent cytokine bursts [74]. Several reports have described attenuated expression of cytokines important in innate immunity signaling (e.g., IFN-β and IFN-γ), pro-inflammatory responses (e.g., TNF-α, IL-6, IL-1β and IL-18) and leukocyte invasion and activation (e.g., MCP-1, G-CSF and CXCL10) following treatment with the pan-HDAC inhibitor, TSA [73,74]. However, dampened cytokine expression does not necessarily correlate with repressive chromatin modifications, as histone H4 acetylation at *Tnf* and *IL6* promoters has been shown to increase following TSA treatment [73]. Thus, it is likely that a significant subset of the immunosuppressive, anti-inflammatory effects of HDAC inhibitors occur at a non-histone level.

3.2. HDAC Association with PML/ND10 Bodies during Herpesvirus Infection

Associated with viral DNA after its nuclear deposition, PML bodies are composed of a set of interferon-inducible proteins that play important roles in host anti-viral defense during herpesvirus infection [84,85]. During HCMV infection, HDACs are recruited to the viral MIEP promoters by Daxx, a component of PML bodies, to repress viral gene expression at early stages of infection [47]. However, this intrinsic immune defense mechanism is counteracted by the activity of viral proteins. Specifically, the HCMV protein pp71 promotes degradation of Daxx, and the interaction of the immediate early viral proteins, IE1 and IE2, with HDAC3 relieves repression of viral transcription [46,47]. This mechanism of evading HDAC-mediated anti-viral response appears to be conserved across species, as the mouse CMV protein mIE1 is also reported to bind mHDAC2, which is recruited to ND10 structures via PML and Daxx [86]. Consistent with a model in which HDAC activity represses viral gene transcription through association with the HCMV MIEP, HDAC inhibition has been demonstrated to rescue IE gene expression [87]. During HSV-1 infection, disruption of ND10 structures is necessary for productive viral replication and is accomplished by ICP0 [88]. Moreover, ICP0 promotes the disruption of HDAC1-CoREST to enhance viral gene expression and replication [31,34]. An *N*-terminal domain of ICP0 shares homology with and binds to a *C*-terminal domain of CoREST immediately adjacent to the HDAC1 binding site [34]. Increased viral gene expression allows the growing population of ICP0 to outcompete HDAC1 in the binding of CoREST. Through this mechanism, ICP0 promotes inhibition of CoREST-associated gene repression by abolishing its interaction with HDAC1. Another viral protein, ICP8, also accumulates adjacent to ND10 structures, where it could function to preferentially bind DNA [28,35]. ICP0-mediated inhibition of HDAC activity is also proposed to facilitate the transition from the expression of viral α genes to β genes [32]. Thus, it is likely that viral protein associations with HDACs and HDAC-containing complexes are temporally regulated during the course of infection to coordinate gene expression for productive viral replication.

3.3. HDAC Non-Histone Substrates in Host Defense

Host response to viral infection is known to be regulated by multiple transcription factors, whose downstream targets include genes associated with apoptotic, immune and pro-inflammatory responses. Several of these transcription factors with critical roles in activation of anti-viral gene programs are known to be regulated by acetylation. For example, the interferon-α receptor (IFNAR) is acetylated at Lys399 following IFN-α binding, directly recruiting interferon regulatory factor 9 (IRF9), along with the signal transducer and activator of transcription 1 (STAT1) and STAT2 [89]. IRF9, STAT1 and STAT2 are all acetylated within their DNA-binding domains, and modification is thought to promote transcriptional activation at interferon-inducible promoters. Similarly, STAT3 dimerization is modulated by the p300-mediated acetylation at Lys685, which promotes nuclear accumulation of STAT3 and transcriptional activation following cytokine-induced signaling [90]. These results suggest that acetylation may be able to positively regulate innate immune signaling pathways, which is in apparent disagreement with global HDAC inhibition studies outlined above. However, recent evidence suggests that the acetylation of STAT1 serves to terminate IFN-α-induced signaling and that deacetylation of STAT1 by HDAC3 promotes its re-association with IFNAR [91]. Thus, HDAC-dependent reinstatement of the STAT1-IFNAR interaction may account for the discrepancy in models for acetylation-dependent regulation of innate immune signaling. As HDACs are effectors of innate immunity signaling, it is not surprising that multiple virus types would develop strategies to promote the disruption of HDAC activities during infection.

Multiple subunits of NF-κB are also regulated by site-specific acetylation (reviewed in [92]). The functional consequences of post-translational modification of NF-κB include modulation of κB-DNA binding by NF-κB, transcriptional activation of NF-κB and association of NF-κB with its negative regulator, IκBα [93]. Specifically, Lys122 and Lys123 of the p65/RelA subunit of NF-κB were shown to be modified by p300/PKAF and HDAC3 [94]. Further analysis revealed that acetylation of NF-κB p65/RelA negatively regulates its binding to κB-DNA and facilitates its nuclear export. In contrast, NF-κB deacetylation has been linked to its activation. Interestingly, several studies have also demonstrated that deacetylation of p65/RelA by SIRT1 and SIRT2 limits NF-κB activity. This is achieved through either direct inhibition of NF-κB transcriptional activity or promotion of its association with IκBα, ultimately leading to diminished secretion of pro-inflammatory cytokines [95–98]. Thus, the association of NF-κB with different deacetylases may be an important determinant of its activity.

These NF-κB functions are carefully regulated during herpesvirus infection in order to redirect NF-κB activity for increased viral gene expression [99,100]. HSV-1 interferes with NF-κB association with the promoter of IκBα and, instead, recruits NF-κB to the ICP0 promoter to facilitate expression of this viral protein [99]. It is conceivable that the altered activity of NF-κB results, at least in part, from changes in its acetylation status, suggesting a possible mechanism by which NF-κB regulation can be exploited in the design of disease treatments. A novel cancer treatment method has recently been proposed, in which treatment of HSV-1 infected cells with TSA induces acetylation and nuclear accumulation of NF-κB, promoting virus production and decreasing the viability of tumor cells [101]. Emerging evidence suggests that NF-κB acetylation may be involved in host immune responses to multiple viruses [102], further highlighting the importance of understanding the regulation of NF-κB and the activity of the enzymes responsible for modulating its acetylation status.

Another critical non-histone HDAC substrate with roles in immune defense during herpesvirus infection is the tumor suppressor, p53. The pro-apoptotic functions of p53, as well as its ability to transactivate IFN-inducible genes during vesicular stomatitis virus (VSV) infection, are dependent on the acetylation state of Lys379, which is negatively regulated by SIRT1 [103]. Interestingly, during HCMV infection, the viral protein IE2 can downregulate p53 function through inhibition of the acetyltransferase p300/CBP [104]. Sequestration of p300/CBP and the transcription factor IRF-3 by ICP0 has also been observed during HSV-1 infection, resulting in attenuated immune response [105]. It has been proposed that HDAC-1, -2 and -3 can downregulate p53 transcriptional activity through deacetylation of residues within its *C*-terminus [106]. In view of these observations, further investigation of the regulatory functions of HDACs with respect to p53 activity during infection is necessary.

3.4. Roles for Additional Acetylation-Modulating Enzymes during Infection: SIRTs and HATs

Further highlighting the significance of protein acetylation during viral infection, recent studies have started to uncover roles for other acetylation-modulating enzymes. While not the focus of this review, it is worth mentioning that the NAD^+-dependent deacetylases, sirtuins (SIRTs) and histone acetyltransferases (HATs) seem to be intimately linked to viral replication. Studies examining the functions of the seven mammalian sirtuins during the progression of viral infection are still limited. However, SIRT1 has been implicated in the progression of human immunodeficiency virus 1 (HIV-1) [102,107–109], human papillomavirus (HPV) [110] and vesicular stomatitis virus (VSV) [111] infection. SIRT1 has also been proposed to control the reactivation of latent varicella zoster virus (VZV) in neurons through the reduction of intracellular NAD^+ levels [112]. Additionally, canine coronavirus (CCoV-II) infection has been shown to induce the expression of SIRT1, SIRT3 and SIRT4 [113], suggesting that the regulation of individual sirtuins is virus specific. Sirtuins possess diverse cellular functions, including modulation of gene expression, DNA repair and apoptosis. Such pathways are commonly exploited by herpesviruses in order to promote viral replication. Therefore, it is tempting to speculate that sirtuins, like the Zn^{2+}-dependent HDACs, have roles in modulation of herpesvirus lifecycles through protein complex associations and regulation of substrate activities within essential pathways.

The modulation of HAT complexes and HAT activities during infection has proven to be an equally interesting subject for investigation. While this review focuses on the modulation of HDAC complexes during herpesvirus infection and the roles of HDACs in host defense mechanisms, it is worthwhile to briefly highlight several examples of roles for HATs during infection. During HSV-1 infection, the circadian HAT CLOCK has been shown to be recruited to ND10 bodies and viral replication compartments, where it associates with the viral proteins, ICP4, ICP27 and ICP22, and the transcription factor, TFIID [114,115]. CLOCK activity promotes the expression of α-genes [114] and, along with its regulator and substrate, BMAL1, remodels viral chromatin [115]. Like their deacetylase counterparts, HAT activities are also modulated by phosphorylation, and, indeed, phosphorylation of TIP60 by a conserved serine/threonine kinase encoded by HSV-1, HCMV, EBV and KSHV has been shown to activate TIP60 during herpesvirus infection and to induce DNA damage responses and chromatin remodeling [116]. TIP60 activity is proposed to have a negative effect on establishment of viral latency, instead promoting active lytic replication [116]. During bovine herpesvirus 1 infection, bICP0 interacts with p300 and may serve to inhibit p300-mediated interferon response to viral stress [117]. Altogether, the dynamic changes in the composition and activity of HAT complexes induced by interactions with viral proteins indicate that these enzymes, like HDACs, have critical roles during herpesvirus infection.

In summary, multiple important regulators of host response to viral infection are dynamically regulated by acetylation and deacetylation, indicating that HDACs are essential upstream modulators of host anti-viral responses. Further analysis of HDAC substrates during viral infection will help define acetylation-dependent mechanisms involved in host response to pathogens, providing additional targets for the development of anti-viral therapeutics.

4. Perspective: "Omic" Approaches in Characterizing HDAC Functions in Virus Infection

As changes in the proteome, metabolome and lipidome of infected cells have started to be established as critical markers for infection, mass spectrometry-based techniques have become an invaluable resource for the field of infectious disease research. Integration of such "omic" methodologies promotes development of a systems biology view of viral infection, which offers a multi-dimensional understanding of the diverse virus-mediated changes in intracellular processes. The impact of such approaches is particularly apparent when considering the diverse functions of HDACs. Omic-based studies can provide insights into the molecular mechanisms underlying HDAC functions during viral infection, including elucidation of their histone and non-histone substrates, their participation in protein complexes and their impact on downstream transcriptional targets (Figure 3).

Figure 3. Assessing HDAC functions during infection through integrative omic approaches. A combination of multi-disciplinary approaches, including metabolomics, proteomics and chemoproteomics, can provide information for comprehensive characterization of the roles that HDACs play during herpesvirus infection.

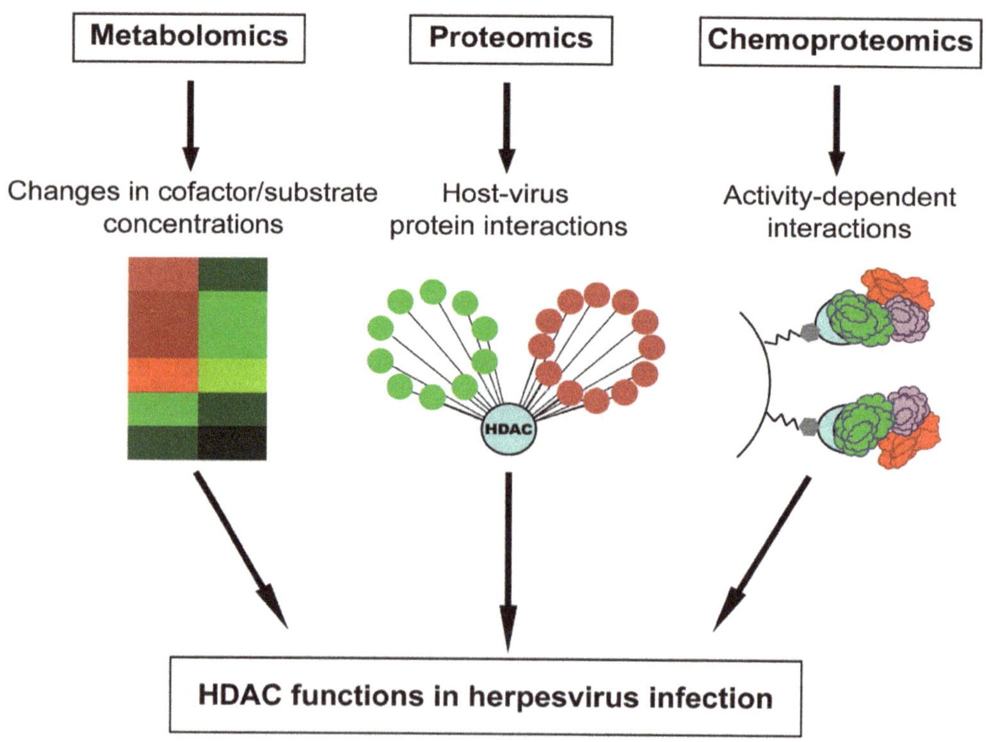

Developments in mass spectrometry and bioinformatics have provided powerful tools for quantifying protein levels and defining interactions and post-translational modifications. Quantitative mass spectrometry incorporating metabolic labeling has been successfully used to assess changes in protein expression levels during pseudorabies virus (PRV) infection, identifying alterations in expression patterns for proteins involved in intracellular transport, translation and host stress response [118]. Similarly, identification of dynamic host-virus protein interactions during infection has contributed significantly to the understanding of both virus-mediated effects on host cell functions and of host defense mechanisms in response to infection (e.g., [38,119–126]). The use of affinity purification coupled with mass spectrometry (AP-MS) has proven effective for both targeted and global protein interaction studies [127]. Furthermore, fluorescent affinity-tags have allowed integration of knowledge regarding protein interactions and localizations, thereby providing a spatial-temporal view of infection [119,128]. Construction of networks incorporating host-virus and virus-virus protein interactions readily illustrates the functional relationships among individual proteins and protein complexes during infection. Application of these methods has advanced the current understanding of virus-host protein interactions during HCMV [38,121,123] and PRV [126] infections. As discussed earlier in this review, proteomic approaches have helped establish the roles of HDACs during HCMV infection, as exemplified by the finding that the HDAC1-containing NuRD complex is recruited by viral proteins during infection [38,39].

On a larger scale, several recent AP-MS studies have examined global host-virus protein interactions, generating comprehensive interaction networks that further highlight the benefit of applying proteomic approaches to investigating viral infection [120,124,125,129]. Moreover, the resulting large-scale protein interaction networks are useful in the development and optimization of statistical methods for characterizing protein associations, including the SAINT algorithm for determining specificity of protein interactions [130]. Curated protein databases, including the HIV-1 Human Protein Interactions Database and VirusMINT, further integrate knowledge of viral protein interactions [131–134]. The expansion of these databases to include proteomic analyses for other viruses will be invaluable for future studies.

In addition to the identification of protein interactions, proteomic approaches allow for identification of post-translational modifications of both viral and host proteins. For example, a recent proteomic study of HSV-1-infected cells led to the identification of multiple phosphorylation and ubiquitination sites within viral proteins [135]. Future investigation and functional characterization of post-translational modifications, including HDAC-regulated acetylations, will expand the current understanding of mechanisms involved in the regulation of viral gene expression and replication.

Alongside advances in AP-MS methodologies, chemoproteomics approaches have emerged as effective techniques for profiling changes in enzymatic activities and for studying activity-dependent protein interactions during infection. Activity-based protein profiling (ABPP) has been applied to the examination of ubiquitin proteases during herpesvirus infection [136]. Chemoproteomic approaches have also been used to resolve the composition of HDAC complexes and to assess the ability of small molecules to inhibit specific HDACs [26]. The development of probes allowing for site-directed capture of HDACs has enabled comprehensive characterization of HDAC substrates and of additional activity-dependent interactions [137,138]. Application of this method for the quantitative study of HDAC activity-dependent interactions during herpesvirus infection will further elucidate the molecular roles of HDACs during infection.

In conjunction with monitoring proteomic changes during infection, examination of alterations in metabolite stability can provide important insight into specific metabolic pathways employed during viral replication cycles. Developments in mass spectrometry-based techniques have allowed quantification of changes in cellular metabolism with increased accuracy [139,140]. Metabolomics studies following either HCMV or HSV-1 infection have revealed variations in host cell metabolic patterns that correlate with viral growth kinetics [139,141–144]. These studies demonstrated that herpesviruses can impact metabolic flux through individual pathways [144]. Specifically, HCMV infection induces glycolytic flux to fuel fatty acid biosynthesis, whereas HSV-1 preferentially stimulates production of components required for pyrimidine nucleotide biosynthesis. Interestingly, HSV-1 infection triggers a significant decrease in intracellular NAD^+ levels that is not observed during HCMV infection, suggesting that NAD^+-dependent deacetylases, SIRTs, may be differentially regulated in the presence of these viruses. Similarly, with developments in mass spectrometry-based lipidome studies [145], virus-induced changes in cellular lipids are becoming more apparent following infection with various types of viruses [146–148], including herpesviruses [149,150]. Overall, the identification of distinct cellular pathways and pathway components necessary for the replication and spread of individual viruses will allow for increased target specificity and selectivity in the design of anti-viral therapeutics [151].

As methodologies for proteomic, metabolomic and lipidomic studies, as well as necessary bioinformatics approaches, are constantly being adapted and improved, it is expected that these "omic" technologies will play an increasingly important role in infectious disease research.

Acknowledgments

We are grateful for funding from NIH/NIDA grant DP1DA026192, NIH grant R21AI102187 and HFSPO award RGY0079/2009-C to IMC and NSF graduate fellowships to AJG and HGB.

References

1. Meier, J.L. Reactivation of the human cytomegalovirus major immediate-early regulatory region and viral replication in embryonal NTera2 cells: Role of trichostatin a, retinoic acid, and deletion of the 21-base-pair repeats and modulator. *J. Virol.* **2001**, *75*, 1581–1593.
2. Lu, F.; Zhou, J.; Wiedmer, A.; Madden, K.; Yuan, Y.; Lieberman, P.M. Chromatin remodeling of the Kaposi's sarcoma-associated herpesvirus ORF50 promoter correlates with reactivation from latency. *J. Virol.* **2003**, *77*, 11425–11435.
3. Danaher, R.J.; Jacob, R.J.; Steiner, M.R.; Allen, W.R.; Hill, J.M.; Miller, C.S. Histone deacetylase inhibitors induce reactivation of herpes simplex virus type 1 in a latency-associated transcript-independent manner in neuronal cells. *J. Neurovirol.* **2005**, *11*, 306–317.
4. Sinclair, J.; Sissons, P. Latency and reactivation of human cytomegalovirus. *J. Gen. Virol.* **2006**, *87*, 1763–1779.
5. Deshmane, S.L.; Fraser, N.W. During latency, herpes-simplex virus type-1 DNA is associated with nucleosomes in a chromatin structure. *J. Virol.* **1989**, *63*, 943–947.

6. Kent, J.R.; Zeng, P.Y.; Atanasiu, D.; Gardner, J.; Fraser, N.W.; Berger, S.L. During lytic infection herpes simplex virus type 1 is associated with histones bearing modifications that correlate with active transcription. *J. Virol.* **2004**, *78*, 10178–10186.

7. Jenkins, P.J.; Binne, U.K.; Farrell, P.J. Histone acetylation and reactivation of Epstein-Barr virus from latency. *J. Virol.* **2000**, *74*, 710–720.

8. Murphy, J.C.; Fischle, W.; Verdin, E.; Sinclair, J.H. Control of cytomegalovirus lytic gene expression by histone acetylation. *EMBO J.* **2002**, *21*, 1112–1120.

9. Kubat, N.J.; Tran, R.K.; McAnany, P.; Bloom, D.C. Specific histone tail modification and not DNA methylation is a determinant of herpes simplex virus type 1 latent gene expression. *J. Virol.* **2004**, *78*, 1139–1149.

10. Cuevas-Bennett, C.; Shenk, T. Dynamic histone H3 acetylation and methylation at human cytomegalovirus promoters during replication in fibroblasts. *J. Virol.* **2008**, *82*, 9525–9536.

11. Toth, Z.; Maglinte, D.T.; Lee, S.H.; Lee, H.-R.; Wong, L.-Y.; Brulois, K.F.; Lee, S.; Buckley, J.D.; Laird, P.W.; Marquez, V.E.; *et al.* Epigenetic analysis of KSHV latent and lytic genomes. *PLoS Pathog.* **2010**, *6*, doi:10.1371/journal.ppat.1001013.

12. Kim, S.C.; Sprung, R.; Chen, Y.; Xu, Y.; Ball, H.; Pei, J.; Cheng, T.; Kho, Y.; Xiao, H.; Xiao, L.; *et al.* Substrate and functional diversity of lysine acetylation revealed by a proteomics survey. *Mol. Cell* **2006**, *23*, 607–618.

13. Choudhary, C.; Kumar, C.; Gnad, F.; Nielsen, M.L.; Rehman, M.; Walther, T.C.; Olsen, J.V.; Mann, M. Lysine acetylation targets protein complexes and co-regulates major cellular functions. *Science* **2009**, *325*, 834–840.

14. Inoue, A.; Fujimoto, D. Enzymatic deacetylation of histone. *Biochem. Biophys. Res. Commun.* **1969**, *36*, 146–150.

15. Berger, S.L. The complex language of chromatin regulation during transcription. *Nature* **2007**, *447*, 407–412.

16. Yang, X.-J.; Seto, E. The Rpd3/Hda1 family of lysine deacetylases: From bacteria and yeast to mice and men. *Nat. Rev. Mol. Cell Biol.* **2008**, *9*, 206–218.

17. Gregoretti, I.V.; Lee, Y.M.; Goodson, H.V. Molecular evolution of the histone deacetylase family: Functional implications of phylogenetic analysis. *J. Mol. Biol.* **2004**, *338*, 17–31.

18. Herbein, G.; Wendling, D. Histone deacetylases in viral infections. *Clin. Epigenetics* **2010**, *1*, 13–24.

19. Hassig, C.A.; Fleischer, T.C.; Billin, A.N.; Schreiber, S.L.; Ayer, D.E. Histone deacetylase activity is required for full transcriptional repression by mSin3A. *Cell* **1997**, *89*, 341–347.

20. Wade, P.A.; Jones, P.L.; Vermaak, D.; Wolffe, A.P. A multiple subunit Mi-2 histone deacetylase from Xenopus laevis cofractionates with an associated Snf2 superfamily ATPase. *Curr. Biol.* **1998**, *8*, 843–846.

21. Zhang, Y.; LeRoy, G.; Seelig, H.P.; Lane, W.S.; Reinberg, D. The dermatomyositis-specific autoantigen Mi2 is a component of a complex containing histone deacetylase and nucleosome remodeling activities. *Cell* **1998**, *95*, 279–289.

22. Tong, J.K.; Hassig, C.A.; Schnitzler, G.R.; Kingston, R.E.; Schreiber, S.L. Chromatin deacetylation by an ATP-dependent nucleosome remodelling complex. *Nature* **1998**, *395*, 917–921.
23. Guenther, M.G.; Lane, W.S.; Fischle, W.; Verdin, E.; Lazar, M.A.; Shiekhattar, R. A core SMRT corepressor complex containing HDAC3 and TBL1, a WD40-repeat protein linked to deafness. *Genes Dev.* **2000**, *14*, 1048–1057.
24. Li, J.W.; Wang, J.; Wang, J.X.; Nawaz, Z.; Liu, J.M.; Qin, J.; Wong, J.M. Both corepressor proteins SMRT and N-CoR exist in large protein complexes containing HDAC3. *EMBO J.* **2000**, *19*, 4342–4350.
25. You, A.; Tong, J.K.; Grozinger, C.M.; Schreiber, S.L. CoREST is an integral component of the CoREST-human histone deacetylase complex. *Proc. Natl. Acad. Sci. USA* **2001**, *98*, 1454–1458.
26. Bantscheff, M.; Hopf, C.; Savitski, M.M.; Dittmann, A.; Grandi, P.; Michon, A.-M.; Schlegl, J.; Abraham, Y.; Becher, I.; Bergamini, G.; *et al.* Chemoproteomics profiling of HDAC inhibitors reveals selective targeting of HDAC complexes. *Nat. Biotechnol.* **2011**, *29*, 255–265.
27. Joshi, P.; Greco, T.M.; Guise, A.J.; Luo, Y.; Yu, F.; Nesvizhskii, A.I.; Cristea, I.M. The functional interactome landscape of the human histone deacetylase family. *Mol. Syst. Biol.* **2013**, *9*, doi:10.1038/msb.2013.26.
28. Gu, H.; Roizman, B. Engagement of the lysine-specific demethylase/HDAC1/CoREST/REST complex by herpes simplex virus 1. *J. Virol.* **2009**, *83*, 4376–4385.
29. Shi, Y.; Lan, F.; Matson, C.; Mulligan, P.; Whetstine, J.R.; Cole, P.A.; Casero, R.A. Histone demethylation mediated by the nuclear amine oxidase homolog LSD1. *Cell* **2004**, *119*, 941–953.
30. Shi, Y.J.; Matson, C.; Lan, F.; Iwase, S.; Baba, T.; Shi, Y. Regulation of LSD1 histone demethylase activity by its associated factors. *Mol. Cell* **2005**, *19*, 857–864.
31. Gu, H.D.; Liang, Y.; Mandel, G.; Roizman, B. Components of the REST/CoREST/histone deacetylase repressor complex are disrupted, modified, and translocated in HSV-1-infected cells. *Proc. Natl. Acad. Sci. USA* **2005**, *102*, 7571–7576.
32. Poon, A.P.W.; Gu, H.; Roizman, B. ICP0 and the U(S)3 protein kinase of herpes simplex virus 1 independently block histone deacetylation to enable gene expression. *Proc. Natl. Acad. Sci. USA* **2006**, *103*, 9993–9998.
33. Zhang, Y.G.; Jones, C. The bovine herpesvirus 1 immediate-early protein (bICP0) associates with histone deacetylase 1 to activate transcription. *J. Virol.* **2001**, *75*, 9571–9578.
34. Gu, H.; Roizman, B. Herpes simplex virus-infected cell protein 0 blocks the silencing of viral DNA by dissociating histone deacetylases from the CoREST-REST complex. *Proc. Natl. Acad. Sci. USA* **2007**, *104*, 17134–17139.
35. Kalamvoki, M.; Roizman, B. Nuclear retention of ICP0 in cells exposed to HDAC inhibitor or transfected with DNA before infection with herpes simplex virus 1. *Proc. Natl. Acad. Sci. USA* **2008**, *105*, 20488–20493.
36. Poon, A.P.W.; Liang, Y.; Roizman, B. Herpes simplex virus 1 gene expression is accelerated by inhibitors of histone deacetylases in rabbit skin cells infected with a mutant carrying a cDNA copy of the infected-cell protein No. 0. *J. Virol.* **2003**, *77*, 12671–12678.

37. Walters, M.S.; Kinchington, P.R.; Banfield, B.W.; Silverstein, S. Hyperphosphorylation of histone deacetylase 2 by alphaherpesvirus US3 kinases. *J. Virol.* **2010**, *84*, 9666–9676.
38. Moorman, N.J.; Cristea, I.M.; Terhune, S.S.; Rout, M.P.; Chait, B.T.; Shenk, T. Human cytomegalovirus protein UL38 inhibits host cell stress responses by antagonizing the tuberous sclerosis protein complex. *Cell Host Microbe* **2008**, *3*, 253–262.
39. Terhune, S.S.; Moorman, N.J.; Cristea, I.M.; Savaryn, J.P.; Cuevas-Bennett, C.; Rout, M.P.; Chait, B.T.; Shenk, T. Human cytomegalovirus UL29/28 protein interacts with components of the NuRD complex which promote accumulation of immediate-early RNA. *PLoS Pathog.* **2010**, *6*, doi:10.1371/journal.ppat.1000965.
40. Reeves, M.; Murphy, J.; Greaves, R.; Fairley, J.; Brehm, A.; Sinclair, J. Autorepression of the human cytomegalovirus major immediate-early promoter/enhancer at late times of infection is mediated by the recruitment of chromatin remodelina enzymes by IE86. *J. Virol.* **2006**, *80*, 9998–10009.
41. Radkov, S.A.; Touitou, R.; Brehm, A.; Rowe, M.; West, M.; Kouzarides, T.; Allday, M.J. Epstein-Barr virus nuclear antigen 3C interacts with histone deacetylase to repress transcription. *J. Virol.* **1999**, *73*, 5688–5697.
42. Knight, J.S.; Lan, K.; Subramanian, C.; Robertson, E.S. Epstein-Barr virus nuclear antigen 3C recruits histone deacetylase activity and associates with the corepressors mSin3A and NCoR in human B-cell lines. *J. Virol.* **2003**, *77*, 4261–4272.
43. Zhou, J.; Snyder, A.R.; Lieberman, P.M. Epstein-barr virus episome stability is coupled to a delay in replication timing. *J. Virol.* **2009**, *83*, 2154–2162.
44. Lu, F.; Day, L.; Gao, S.J.; Lieberman, P.M. Acetylation of the latency-associated nuclear antigen regulates repression of Kaposi's sarcoma-associated herpesvirus lytic transcription. *J. Virol.* **2006**, *80*, 5273–5282.
45. Park, J.J.; Kim, Y.E.; Pham, H.T.; Kim, E.T.; Chung, Y.H.; Ahn, J.H. Functional interaction of the human cytomegalovirus IE2 protein with histone deacetylase 2 in infected human fibroblasts. *J. Gen. Virol.* **2007**, *88*, 3214–3223.
46. Nevels, M.; Paulus, C.; Shenk, T. Human cytomegalovirus immediate-early 1 protein facilitates viral replication by antagonizing histone deacetylation. *Proc. Natl. Acad. Sci. USA* **2004**, *101*, 17234–17239.
47. Saffert, R.T.; Kalejta, R.F. Inactivating a cellular intrinsic immune defense mediated by Daxx is the mechanism through which the human cytomegalovirus pp71 protein stimulates viral immediate-early gene expression. *J. Virol.* **2006**, *80*, 3863–3871.
48. Lomonte, P.; Thomas, J.; Texier, P.; Caron, C.; Khochbin, S.; Epstein, A.L. Functional interaction between class II histone deacetylases and ICPO of herpes simplex virus type 1. *J. Virol.* **2004**, *78*, 6744–6757.
49. Pflum, M.K.H.; Tong, J.K.; Lane, W.S.; Schreiber, S.L. Histone deacetylase I phosphorylation promotes enzymatic activity and complex formation. *J. Biol. Chem.* **2001**, *276*, 47733–47741.
50. Tsai, S.C.; Seto, E. Regulation of histone deacetylase 2 by protein kinase CK2. *J. Biol. Chem.* **2002**, *277*, 31826–31833.

51. Grozinger, C.M.; Schreiber, S.L. Regulation of histone deacetylase 4 and 5 and transcriptional activity by 14-3-3-dependent cellular localization. *Proc. Natl. Acad. Sci. USA* **2000**, *97*, 7835–7840.

52. Wang, A.H.; Kruhlak, M.J.; Wu, J.; Bertos, N.R.; Vezmar, M.; Posner, B.I.; Bazett-Jones, D.P.; Yang, X.J. Regulation of histone deacetylase 4 by binding of 14-3-3 proteins. *Mol. Cell. Biol.* **2000**, *20*, 6904–6912.

53. Kao, H.Y.; Verdel, A.; Tsai, C.C.; Simon, C.; Juguilon, H.; Khochbin, S. Mechanism for nucleocytoplasmic shuttling of histone deacetylase 7. *J. Biol. Chem.* **2001**, *276*, 47496–47507.

54. Greco, T.M.; Yu, F.; Guise, A.J.; Cristea, I.M. Nuclear import of histone deacetylase 5 by requisite nuclear localization signal phosphorylation. *Mol. Cell. Proteomics* **2011**, *10*, doi:10.1074/mcp.M110.004317.

55. Guise, A.J.; Greco, T.M.; Zhang, I.Y.; Yu, F.; Cristea, I.M. Aurora B-dependent regulation of Class IIa histone deacetylases by mitotic nuclear localization signal phosphorylation. *Mol. Cell. Proteomics* **2012**, *11*, 1220–1229.

56. Ahn, J.H.; Brignole, E.J.; Hayward, G.S. Disruption of PML subnuclear domains by the acidic IE1 protein of human cytomegalovirus is mediated through interaction with PML and may modulate a RING finger-dependent cryptic transactivator function of PML. *Mol. Cell. Biol.* **1998**, *18*, 4899–4913.

57. Wu, W.S.; Vallian, S.; Seto, E.; Yang, W.M.; Edmondson, D.; Roth, S.; Chang, K.S. The growth suppressor PML represses transcription by functionally and physically interacting with histone deacetylases. *Mol. Cell. Biol.* **2001**, *21*, 2259–2268.

58. Kao, H.Y.; Ordentlich, P.; Koyano-Nakagawa, N.; Tang, Z.; Downes, M.; Kintner, C.R.; Evans, R.M.; Kadesch, T. A histone deacetylase corepressor complex regulates the Notch signal transduction pathway. *Genes Dev.* **1998**, *12*, 2269–2277.

59. Fischle, W.; Dequiedt, F.; Hendzel, M.J.; Guenther, M.G.; Lazar, M.A.; Voelter, W.; Verdin, E. Enzymatic activity associated with class IIHDACs is dependent on a multiprotein complex containing HDAC3 and SMRT/N-CoR. *Mol. Cell* **2002**, *9*, 45–57.

60. Gruffat, H.; Manet, E.; Sergeant, A. MEF2-mediated recruitment of class 11 HDAC at the EBV immediate early gene BZLF1 links latency and chromatin remodeling. *EMBO Rep.* **2002**, *3*, 141–146.

61. Bryant, H.; Farrell, P.J. Signal transduction and transcription factor modification during reactivation of Epstein-Barr virus from latency. *J. Virol.* **2002**, *76*, 10290–10298.

62. Bottero, V.; Sharma-Walia, N.; Kerur, N.; Paul, A.G.; Sadagopan, S.; Cannon, M.; Chandran, B. Kaposi Sarcoma-associated herpes virus (KSHV) G protein-coupled receptor (vGPCR) activates the ORF50 lytic switch promoter: A potential positive feedback loop for sustained ORF50 gene expression. *Virology* **2009**, *392*, 34–51.

63. Lukac, D.M.; Renne, R.; Kirshner, J.R.; Ganem, D. Reactivation of Kaposi's sarcoma-associated herpesvirus infection from latency by expression of the ORF 50 transactivator, a homolog of the EBV R protein. *Virology* **1998**, *252*, 304–312.

64. Vega, R.B.; Harrison, B.C.; Meadows, E.; Roberts, C.R.; Papst, P.J.; Olson, E.N.; McKinsey, T.A. Protein kinases C and D mediate agonist-dependent cardiac hypertrophy through nuclear export of histone deacetylase 5. *Mol. Cell. Biol.* **2004**, *24*, 8374–8385.
65. Krithivas, A.; Young, D.B.; Liao, G.L.; Greene, D.; Hayward, S.D. Human herpesvirus 8 LANA interacts with proteins of the mSin3 corepressor complex and negatively regulates Epstein-Barr virus gene expression in dually infected PEL cells. *J. Virol.* **2000**, *74*, 9637–9645.
66. Gwack, Y.; Byun, H.; Hwang, S.; Lim, C.; Choe, J. CREB-binding protein and histone deacetylase regulate the transcriptional activity of Kaposi's sarcoma-associated herpesvirus open reading frame 50. *J. Virol.* **2001**, *75*, 1909–1917.
67. Gwack, Y.; Hwang, S.; Byun, H.; Lim, C.; Kim, J.W.; Choi, E.J.; Choe, J. Kaposi's sarcoma-associated herpesvirus open reading frame 50 represses p53-induced transcriptional activity and apoptosis. *J. Virol.* **2001**, *75*, 6245–6248.
68. Gu, W.; Roeder, R.G. Activation of p53 sequence-specific DNA binding by acetylation of the p53 *C*-terminal domain. *Cell* **1997**, *90*, 595–606.
69. Luo, J.Y.; Li, M.Y.; Tang, Y.; Laszkowska, M.; Roeder, R.G.; Gu, W. Acetylation of p53 augments its site-specific DNA binding both *in vitro* and *in vivo*. *Proc. Nat. Acad. Sci. USA* **2004**, *101*, 2259–2264.
70. Li, T.; Diner, B.A.; Chen, J.; Cristea, I.M. Acetylation modulates cellular distribution and DNA sensing ability of interferon-inducible protein IFI16. *Proc. Natl. Acad. Sci. USA* **2012**, *109*, 10558–10563.
71. Nencioni, A.; Beck, J.; Werth, D.; Gruenebach, F.; Patrone, F.; Ballestrero, A.; Brossart, P. Histone deacetylase inhibitors affect dendritic cell differentiation and immunogenicity. *Clin. Cancer Res.* **2007**, *13*, 3933–3941.
72. Halili, M.A.; Andrews, M.R.; Labzin, L.I.; Schroder, K.; Matthias, G.; Cao, C.; Lovelace, E.; Reid, R.C.; Le, G.T.; Hume, D.A.; *et al.* Differential effects of selective HDAC inhibitors on macrophage inflammatory responses to the Toll-like receptor 4 agonist LPS. *J. Leukocyte Biol.* **2010**, *87*, 1103–1114.
73. Roger, T.; Lugrin, J.; le Roy, D.; Goy, G.; Mombelli, M.; Koessler, T.; Ding, X.C.; Chanson, A.L.; Reymond, M.K.; Miconnet, I.; *et al.* Histone deacetylase inhibitors impair innate immune responses to Toll-like receptor agonists and to infection. *Blood* **2011**, *117*, 1205–1217.
74. Mombelli, M.; Lugrin, J.; Rubino, I.; Chanson, A.L.; Giddey, M.; Calandra, T.; Roger, T. Histone deacetylase inhibitors impair antibacterial defenses of macrophages. *J. Infect. Dis.* **2011**, *204*, 1367–1374.
75. Unterholzner, L.; Keating, S.E.; Baran, M.; Horan, K.A.; Jensen, S.B.; Sharma, S.; Sirois, C.M.; Jin, T.; Latz, E.; *et al.* IFI16 is an innate immune sensor for intracellular DNA. *Nat. Immunol.* **2010**, *11*, 997–1004.
76. Kerur, N.; Veettil, M.V.; Sharma-Walia, N.; Bottero, V.; Sadagopan, S.; Otageri, P.; Chandran, B. IFI16 acts as a nuclear pathogen sensor to induce the inflammasome in response to Kaposi Sarcoma-associated herpesvirus infection. *Cell Host Microbe* **2011**, *9*, 363–375.

77. Orzalli, M.H.; DeLuca, N.A.; Knipe, D.M. Nuclear IFI16 induction of IRF-3 signaling during herpesviral infection and degradation of IFI16 by the viral ICP0 protein. *Proc. Natl. Acad. Sci. USA* **2012**, *109*, E3008–E3017.

78. Singh, V.V.; Kerur, N.; Bottero, V.; Dutta, S.; Chakraborty, S.; Ansari, M.A.; Paudel, N.; Chikoti, L.; Chandran, B. Kaposi's sarcoma-associated herpesvirus latency in endothelial and B cells activates interferon gamma-inducible protein 16 (IFI16) mediated inflammasomes. *J. Virol.* **2013**, *87*, 4417–4431.

79. Johnson, K.E.; Chikoti, L.; Chandran, B. HSV-1 infection induces activation and subsequent inhibition of the IFI16 and NLRP3 inflammasomes. *J. Virol.* **2013**, *87*, 5005–5018.

80. Horan, K.A.; Hansen, K.; Jakobsen, M.R.; Holm, C.K.; Soby, S.; Unterholzner, L.; Thompson, M.; West, J.A.; Iversen, M.B.; Rasmussen, S.B.; *et al.* Proteasomal degradation of herpes simplex virus capsids in macrophages releases DNA to the cytosol for recognition by DNA sensors. *J. Immunol.* **2013**, *190*, 2311–2319.

81. Fernandes-Alnemri, T.; Yu, J.W.; Datta, P.; Wu, J.; Alnemri, E.S. AIM2 activates the inflammasome and cell death in response to cytoplasmic DNA. *Nature* **2009**, *458*, 509–513.

82. Rathinam, V.A.; Jiang, Z.; Waggoner, S.N.; Sharma, S.; Cole, L.E.; Waggoner, L.; Vanaja, S.K.; Monks, B.G.; Ganesan, S.; Latz, E.; *et al.* The AIM2 inflammasome is essential for host defense against cytosolic bacteria and DNA viruses. *Nat. Immunol.* **2009**, *11*, 395–402.

83. Yoneyama, M.; Kikuchi, M.; Natsukawa, T.; Shinobu, N.; Imaizumi, T.; Miyagishi, M.; Taira, K.; Akira, S.; Fujita, T. The RNA helicase RIG-I has an essential function in double-stranded RNA-induced innate antiviral responses. *Nat. Immunol.* **2004**, *5*, 730–737.

84. Maul, G.G.; Ishov, A.M.; Everett, R.D. Nuclear domain 10 as preexisting potential replication start sites of herpes simplex virus type-1. *Virology* **1996**, *217*, 67–75.

85. Tavalai, N.; Papior, P.; Rechter, S.; Leis, M.; Stamminger, T. Evidence for a role of the cellular ND10 protein PML in mediating intrinsic immunity against human cytomegalovirus infections. *J. Virol.* **2006**, *80*, 8006–8018.

86. Tang, Q.Y.; Maul, G.G. Mouse cytomegalovirus immediate-early protein 1 binds with host cell repressors to relieve suppressive effects on viral transcription and replication during lytic infection. *J. Virol.* **2003**, *77*, 1357–1367.

87. Groves, I.J.; Reeves, M.B.; Sinclair, J.H. Lytic infection of permissive cells with human cytomegalovirus is regulated by an intrinsic "pre-immediate-early" repression of viral gene expression mediated by histone post-translational modification. *J. Gen. Virol.* **2009**, *90*, 2364–2374.

88. Burkham, J.; Coen, D.M.; Hwang, C.B.C.; Weller, S.K. Interactions of herpes simplex virus type 1 with ND10 and recruitment of PML to replication compartments. *J. Virol.* **2001**, *75*, 2353–2367.

89. Tang, X.; Gao, J.S.; Guan, Y.J.; McLane, K.E.; Yuan, Z.L.; Ramratnam, B.; Chin, Y.E. Acetylation-dependent signal transduction for type I interferon receptor. *Cell* **2007**, *131*, 93–105.

90. Yuan, Z.L.; Guan, Y.J.; Chatterjee, D.; Chin, Y.E. Stat3 dimerization regulated by reversible acetylation of a single lysine residue. *Science* **2005**, *307*, 269–273.

91. Kramer, O.H.; Knauer, S.K.; Greiner, G.; Jandt, E.; Reichardt, S.; Guhrs, K.H.; Stauber, R.H.; Bohmer, F.D.; Heinzel, T. A phosphorylation-acetylation switch regulates STAT1 signaling. *Genes Dev.* **2009**, *23*, 223–235.

92. Chen, L.F.; Greene, W.C. Regulation of distinct biological activities of the NF-kappaB transcription factor complex by acetylation. *J. Mol. Med.* **2003**, *81*, 549–557.

93. Quivy, V.; van Lint, C. Regulation at multiple levels of NF-kappaB-mediated transactivation by protein acetylation. *Biochem. Pharmacol.* **2004**, *68*, 1221–1229.

94. Kiernan, R.; Bres, V.; Ng, R.W.; Coudart, M.P.; el Messaoudi, S.; Sardet, C.; Jin, D.Y.; Emiliani, S.; Benkirane, M. Post-activation turn-off of NF-kappa B-dependent transcription is regulated by acetylation of p65. *J. Biol. Chem.* **2003**, *278*, 2758–2766.

95. Chen, L.; Fischle, W.; Verdin, E.; Greene, W.C. Duration of nuclear NF-kappaB action regulated by reversible acetylation. *Science* **2001**, *293*, 1653–1657.

96. Yeung, F.; Hoberg, J.E.; Ramsey, C.S.; Keller, M.D.; Jones, D.R.; Frye, R.A.; Mayo, M.W. Modulation of NF-kappaB-dependent transcription and cell survival by the SIRT1 deacetylase. *EMBO J.* **2004**, *23*, 2369–2380.

97. Rothgiesser, K.M.; Erener, S.; Waibel, S.; Luscher, B.; Hottiger, M.O. SIRT2 regulates NF-kappaB dependent gene expression through deacetylation of p65 Lys310. *J. Cell Sci.* **2010**, *123*, 4251–4258.

98. Yang, H.; Zhang, W.; Pan, H.; Feldser, H.G.; Lainez, E.; Miller, C.; Leung, S.; Zhong, Z.; Zhao, H.; Sweitzer, S.; *et al.* SIRT1 activators suppress inflammatory responses through promotion of p65 deacetylation and inhibition of NF-kappaB activity. *PLoS One* **2012**, 7, e46364.

99. Amici, C.; Rossi, A.; Costanzo, A.; Ciafre, S.; Marinari, B.; Balsamo, M.; Levrero, M.; Santoro, M.G. Herpes simplex virus disrupts NF-kappaB regulation by blocking its recruitment on the IkappaBalpha promoter and directing the factor on viral genes. *J. Biol. Chem.* **2006**, *281*, 7110–7117.

100. El Mjiyad, N.; Bontems, S.; Gloire, G.; Horion, J.; Vandevenne, P.; Dejardin, E.; Piette, J.; Sadzot-Delvaux, C. Varicella-zoster virus modulates NF-kappaB recruitment on selected cellular promoters. *J. Virol.* **2007**, *81*, 13092–13104.

101. Katsura, T.; Iwai, S.; Ota, Y.; Shimizu, H.; Ikuta, K.; Yura, Y. The effects of trichostatin A on the oncolytic ability of herpes simplex virus for oral squamous cell carcinoma cells. *Canc. Gene Ther.* **2009**, *16*, 237–245.

102. Kwon, H.S.; Brent, M.M.; Getachew, R.; Jayakumar, P.; Chen, L.F.; Schnolzer, M.; McBurney, M.W.; Marmorstein, R.; Greene, W.C.; Ott, M. Human immunodeficiency virus type 1 Tat protein inhibits the SIRT1 deacetylase and induces T cell hyperactivation. *Cell Host Microbe* **2008**, *3*, 158–167.

103. Munoz-Fontela, C.; Gonzalez, D.; Marcos-Villar, L.; Campagna, M.; Gallego, P.; Gonzalez-Santamaria, J.; Herranz, D.; Gu, W.; Serrano, M.; Aaronson, S.A.; *et al.* Acetylation is indispensable for p53 antiviral activity. *Cell Cycle* **2011**, *10*, 3701–3705.

104. Hsu, C.H.; Chang, M.D.; Tai, K.Y.; Yang, Y.T.; Wang, P.S.; Chen, C.J.; Wang, Y.H.; Lee, S.C.; Wu, C.W.; Juan, L.J. HCMV IE2-mediated inhibition of HAT activity downregulates p53 function. *EMBO J.* **2004**, *23*, 2269–2280.
105. Melroe, G.T.; Silva, L.; Schaffer, P.A.; Knipe, D.M. Recruitment of activated IRF-3 and CBP/p300 to herpes simplex virus ICP0 nuclear foci: Potential role in blocking IFN-beta induction. *Virology* **2007**, *360*, 305–321.
106. Juan, L.J.; Shia, W.J.; Chen, M.H.; Yang, W.M.; Seto, E.; Lin, Y.S.; Wu, C.W. Histone deacetylases specifically down-regulate p53-dependent gene activation. *J. Biol. Chem.* **2000**, *275*, 20436–20443.
107. Pagans, S.; Pedal, A.; North, B.J.; Kaehlcke, K.; Marshall, B.L.; Dorr, A.; Hetzer-Egger, C.; Henklein, P.; Frye, R.; McBurney, M.W.; *et al.* SIRT1 regulates HIV transcription via Tat deacetylation. *PLoS Biol.* **2005**, *3*, 210–220.
108. Zhang, H.-S.; Zhou, Y.; Wu, M.-R.; Zhou, H.-S.; Xu, F. Resveratrol inhibited Tat-induced HIV-1 LTR transactivation via NAD(+)-dependent SIRT1 activity. *Life Sci.* **2009**, *85*, 484–489.
109. Thakur, B.K.; Chandra, A.; Dittrich, T.; Welte, K.; Chandra, P. Inhibition of SIRT1 by HIV-1 viral protein Tat results in activation of p53 pathway. *Biochem. Biophys. Res. Commun.* **2012**, *424*, 245–250.
110. Allison, S.J.; Jiang, M.; Milner, J. Oncogenic viral protein HPV E7 up-regulates the SIRT1 longevity protein in human cervical cancer cells. *Aging* **2009**, *1*, 316–327.
111. Campagna, M.; Herranz, D.; Garcia, M.A.; Marcos-Villar, L.; Gonzalez-Santamaria, J.; Gallego, P.; Gutierrez, S.; Collado, M.; Serrano, M.; Esteban, M.; *et al.* SIRT1 stabilizes PML promoting its sumoylation. *Cell Death Differ.* **2011**, *18*, 72–79.
112. Picchione, K.E.; Bhattacharjee, A. Viral genome silencing by neuronal sirtuin 1. *J. Neurovirol.* **2011**, *17*, 184–188.
113. Marfc, G.; Tafani, M.; Fiorito, F.; Pagnini, U.; Iovane, G.; De Martino, L. Involvement of FOXO transcription factors, TRAIL-FasL/Fas, and sirtuin proteins family in canine coronavirus type II-Induced apoptosis. *PLoS One* **2011**, *6*, e27313.
114. Kalamvoki, M.; Roizman, B. Circadian CLOCK histone acetyl transferase localizes at ND10 nuclear bodies and enables herpes simplex virus gene expression. *Proc. Natl. Acad. Sci. USA* **2010**, *107*, 17721–17726.
115. Kalamvoki, M.; Roizman, B. The histone acetyltransferase CLOCK is an essential component of the herpes simplex virus 1 transcriptome that includes TFIID, ICP4, ICP27, and ICP22. *J. Virol.* **2011**, *85*, 9472–9477.
116. Li, R.; Zhu, J.; Xie, Z.; Liao, G.; Liu, J.; Chen, M.-R.; Hu, S.; Woodard, C.; Lin, J.; Taverna, S.D.; *et al.* Conserved herpesvirus kinases target the DNA damage response pathway and TIP60 histone acetyltransferase to promote virus replication. *Cell Host Microbe* **2011**, *10*, 390–400.
117. Zhang, Y.G.; Jiang, Y.Q.; Geiser, V.; Zhou, J.; Jones, C. Bovine herpesvirus 1 immediate-early protein (bICP0) interacts with the histone acetyltransferase p300, which stimulates productive infection and gC promoter activity. *J. Gen. Virol.* **2006**, *87*, 1843–1851.

118. Skiba, M.; Mettenleiter, T.C.; Karger, A. Quantitative whole-cell proteome analysis of pseudorabies virus-infected cells. *J. Virol.* **2008**, *82*, 9689–9699.
119. Cristea, I.M.; Carroll, J.-W.N.; Rout, M.P.; Rice, C.M.; Chait, B.T.; MacDonald, M.R. Tracking and elucidating Alphavirus-host protein interactions. *J. Biol. Chem.* **2006**, *281*, 30269–30278.
120. Calderwood, M.A.; Venkatesan, K.; Xing, L.; Chase, M.R.; Vazquez, A.; Holthaus, A.M.; Ewence, A.E.; Li, N.; Hirozane-Kishikawa, T.; Hill, D.E.; *et al.* Epstein-Barr virus and virus human protein interaction maps. *Proc. Natl. Acad. Sci. USA* **2007**, *104*, 7606–7611.
121. Moorman, N.J.; Sharon-Friling, R.; Shenk, T.; Cristea, I.M. A targeted spatial-temporal proteomics approach implicates multiple cellular trafficking pathways in human cytomegalovirus virion maturation. *Mol. Cell. Proteomics* **2010**, *9*, 851–860.
122. Cristea, I.M.; Rozjabek, H.; Molloy, K.R.; Karki, S.; White, L.L.; Rice, C.M.; Rout, M.P.; Chait, B.T.; MacDonald, M.R. Host factors associated with the sindbis virus RNA-dependent RNA polymerase: Role for G3BP1 and G3BP2 in virus replication. *J. Virol.* **2010**, *84*, 6720–6732.
123. Cristea, I.M.; Moorman, N.J.; Terhune, S.S.; Cuevas, C.D.; O'Keefe, E.S.; Rout, M.P.; Chait, B.T.; Shenk, T. Human cytomegalovirus pUL83 stimulates activity of the viral immediate-early promoter through its interaction with the cellular IFI16 protein. *J. Virol.* **2010**, *84*, 7803–7814.
124. Doolittle, J.M.; Gomez, S.M. Mapping protein interactions between Dengue virus and its human and insect hosts. *PLoS Negl. Trop. Dis.* **2011**, *5*, e954.
125. Jager, S.; Cimermancic, P.; Gulbahce, N.; Johnson, J.R.; McGovern, K.E.; Clarke, S.C.; Shales, M.; Mercenne, G.; Pache, L.; Li, K.; *et al.* Global landscape of HIV-human protein complexes. *Nature* **2012**, *481*, 365–370.
126. Kramer, T.; Greco, T.M.; Taylor, M.P.; Ambrosini, A.E.; Cristea, I.M.; Enquist, L.W. Kinesin-3 mediates axonal sorting and directional transport of alphaherpesvirus particles in neurons. *Cell Host Microbe* **2012**, *12*, 806–814.
127. Miteva, Y.V.; Budayeva, H.G.; Cristea, I.M. Proteomics-based methods for discovery, quantification, and validation of protein-protein interactions. *Anal. Chem.* **2013**, *85*, 749–768.
128. Cristea, I.M.; Williams, R.; Chait, B.T.; Rout, M.P. Fluorescent proteins as proteomic probes. *Mol. Cell. Proteomics* **2005**, *4*, 1933–1941.
129. Kaczkowski, B.; Rossing, M.; Andersen, D.K.; Dreher, A.; Morevati, M.; Visser, M.A.; Winther, O.; Nielsen, F.C.; Norrild, B. Integrative analyses reveal novel strategies in HPV11,-16 and -45 early infection. *Sci. Rep.* **2012**, *2*, 515.
130. Choi, H.; Larsen, B.; Lin, Z.-Y.; Breitkreutz, A.; Mellacheruvu, D.; Fermin, D.; Qin, Z.S.; Tyers, M.; Gingras, A.-C.; Nesvizhskii, A.I. SAINT: Probabilistic scoring of affinity purification-mass spectrometry data. *Nat. Methods* **2011**, *8*, 70–73.
131. Ptak, R.G.; Fu, W.; Sanders-Beer, B.E.; Dickerson, J.E.; Pinney, J.W.; Robertson, D.L.; Rozanov, M.N.; Katz, K.S.; Maglott, D.R.; Pruitt, K.D.; *et al.* Cataloguing the HIV type 1 human protein interaction network. *AIDS Res. Hum. Retroviruses* **2008**, *24*, 1497–1502.
132. Fu, W.; Sanders-Beer, B.E.; Katz, K.S.; Maglott, D.R.; Pruitt, K.D.; Ptak, R.G. Human immunodeficiency virus type 1, human protein interaction database at NCBI. *Nucleic Acids Res.* **2009**, *37*, D417–D422.

133. Chatr-aryamontri, A.; Ceol, A.; Peluso, D.; Nardozza, A.; Panni, S.; Sacco, F.; Tinti, M.; Smolyar, A.; Castagnoli, L.; Vidal, M.; *et al.* VirusMINT: A viral protein interaction database. *Nucleic Acids Res.* **2009**, *37*, D669–D673.
134. Pinney, J.W.; Dickerson, J.E.; Fu, W.; Sanders-Beer, B.E.; Ptak, R.G.; Robertson, D.L. HIV-host interactions: A map of viral perturbation of the host system. *AIDS* **2009**, *23*, 549–554.
135. Bell, C.; Desjardins, M.; Thibault, P.; Radtke, K. Proteomics analysis of herpes simplex virus type 1-infected cells reveals dynamic changes of viral protein expression, ubiquitylation, and phosphorylation. *J. Proteome Res.* **2013**, *12*, 1820–1829.
136. Gredmark, S.; Schlieker, C.; Quesada, V.; Spooner, E.; Ploegh, H.L. A functional ubiquitin-specific protease embedded in the large tegument protein (ORF64) of murine gammaherpesvirus 68 is active during the course of infection. *J. Virol.* **2007**, *81*, 10300–10309.
137. Salisbury, C.M.; Cravatt, B.F. Activity-based probes for proteomic profiling of histone deacetylase complexes. *Proc. Natl. Acad. Sci. USA* **2007**, *104*, 1171–1176.
138. Salisbury, C.M.; Cravatt, B.F. Optimization of activity-based probes for proteomic profiling of histone deacetylase complexes. *J. Am. Chem. Soc.* **2008**, *130*, 2184–2194.
139. Munger, J.; Bajad, S.U.; Coller, H.A.; Shenk, T.; Rabinowitz, J.D. Dynamics of the cellular metabolome during human cytomegalovirus infection. *PLoS Pathog.* **2006**, *2*, e132.
140. Milne, S.B.; Mathews, T.P.; Myers, D.S.; Ivanova, P.T.; Brown, H.A. Sum of the parts: Mass spectrometry-based metabolomics. *Biochemistry* **2013**, *52*, 3829–3840.
141. Munger, J.; Bennett, B.D.; Parikh, A.; Feng, X.J.; McArdle, J.; Rabitz, H.A.; Shenk, T.; Rabinowitz, J.D. Systems-level metabolic flux profiling identifies fatty acid synthesis as a target for antiviral therapy. *Nat. Biotechnol.* **2008**, *26*, 1179–1186.
142. Chambers, J.W.; Maguire, T.G.; Alwine, J.C. Glutamine metabolism is essential for human cytomegalovirus infection. *J. Virol.* **2010**, *84*, 1867–1873.
143. Yu, Y.; Clippinger, A.J.; Alwine, J.C. Viral effects on metabolism: Changes in glucose and glutamine utilization during human cytomegalovirus infection. *Trends Microbiol.* **2011**, *19*, 360–367.
144. Vastag, L.; Koyuncu, E.; Grady, S.L.; Shenk, T.E.; Rabinowitz, J.D. Divergent effects of human cytomegalovirus and herpes simplex virus-1 on cellular metabolism. *PLoS Pathog.* **2011**, *7*, e1002124.
145. Ivanova, P.T.; Milne, S.B.; Myers, D.S.; Brown, H.A., Lipidomics: A mass spectrometry based systems level analysis of cellular lipids. *Curr. Opin. Chem. Biol.* **2009**, *13*, 526–531.
146. Brugger, B.; Glass, B.; Haberkant, P.; Leibrecht, I.; Wieland, F.T.; Krausslich, H.G. The HIV lipidome: A raft with an unusual composition. *Proc. Natl. Acad. Sci. USA* **2006**, *103*, 2641–2646.
147. Bruegger, B.; Krautkraemer, E.; Tibroni, N.; Munte, C.E.; Rauch, S.; Leibrecht, I.; Glass, B.; Breuer, S.; Geyer, M.; Kraeusslich, H.-G.; *et al.* Human immunodeficiency virus type 1 nef protein modulates the lipid composition of virions and host cell membrane microdomains. *Retrovirology* **2007**, *4*, doi:10.1186/1742-4690-4-70.
148. Diamond, D.L.; Syder, A.J.; Jacobs, J.M.; Sorensen, C.M.; Walters, K.-A.; Proll, S.C.; McDermott, J.E.; Gritsenko, M.A.; Zhang, Q.; Zhao, R.; *et al.* Temporal proteome and lipidome profiles reveal hepatitis C virus-associated reprogramming of hepatocellular metabolism and bioenergetics. *PLoS Pathog.* **2010**, *6*, e1000719.

149. Liu, S.T.H.; Sharon-Friling, R.; Ivanova, P.; Milne, S.B.; Myers, D.S.; Rabinowitz, J.D.; Brown, H.A.; Shenk, T., Synaptic vesicle-like lipidome of human cytomegalovirus virions reveals a role for SNARE machinery in virion egress. *Proc. Natl. Acad. Sci. USA* **2011**, *108*, 12869–12874.
150. Gudleski-O'Regan, N.; Greco, T.M.; Cristea, I.M.; Shenk, T. Increased expression of LDL receptor-related protein 1 during human cytomegalovirus infection reduces virion cholesterol and infectivity. *Cell Host Microbe* **2012**, *12*, 86–96.
151. Rabinowitz, J.D.; Purdy, J.G.; Vastag, L.; Shenk, T.; Koyuncu, E. Metabolomics in drug target discovery. *Cold Spring Harb. Symp. Quant. Biol.* **2011**, *76*, 235–246.

4

Chromatin, Non-Coding RNAs, and the Expression of HIV

Jessica N. Groen [1] and Kevin V. Morris [1,2,*]

1 School of Biotechnology and Biomolecular Sciences, The University of New South Wales, Sydney, NSW 2052, Australia; E-Mail: jessica.n.groen@gmail.com

2 Department of Molecular and Experimental Medicine, The Scripps Research Institute, La Jolla, CA 92037, USA

* Author to whom correspondence should be addressed; E-Mail: kmorris@unsw.edu.au;

Abstract: HIV is a chronic viral infection affecting an estimated 34 million people worldwide. Current therapies employ the use of a cocktail of antiretroviral medications to reduce the spread and effects of HIV, however complete eradication from an individual currently remains unattainable. Viral latency and regulation of gene expression is a key consideration when developing effective treatments. While our understanding of these processes remains incomplete new developments suggest that non-coding RNA (ncRNA) mediated regulation may provide an avenue to controlling both viral expression and latency. Here we discuss the importance of known regulatory mechanisms and suggest directions for further study, in particular the use ncRNAs in controlling HIV expression.

Keywords: HIV; non-coding RNA; chromatin remodeling; latency; reactivation

1. Introduction

Upon entering a cell, HIV integrates into the genome of the host and essentially functions as an endogenous gene. The ability of HIV to remain dormant, in a relatively quiescent state in the infected cell remains the major barrier in providing an effective cure. Highly active antiretroviral therapy (HAART) is the current standard of care, and although viral load may be reduced to extremely low if not undetectable levels, it is unable to deplete viral reservoirs, and thus the HIV infection remains a lifelong infection. The HIV-1 provirus employs numerous mechanisms to regulate its patterns of gene expression that are vital to the maintenance of latency in cells and therefore its survival. Currently, most of the literature surrounding HIV gene regulation focuses on the role of the long terminal repeat (LTR), and the interactions between of Tat and TAR. This view may be incomplete as new insights suggest a role for long non-coding RNAs (lncRNAs) in the regulation of gene expression patterns in many organisms however their role in HIV is still yet to be elucidated. These ncRNAs have the potential to impact viral lifecycles and pathogenesis in cells and therefore a more holistic understanding of the mechanisms of HIV viral latency and reactivation are paramount if therapeutics are to be developed to eradicate HIV.

2. Regulation of HIV-1 Chromatin and Latency

2.1. The HIV LTR

HIV-1 gene expression is regulated primarily at a transcriptional level by a series of *cis*-acting elements and *trans*-regulatory components located within the LTR at both the 5' and 3' ends of the provirus. The HIV-1 5' LTR comprises of three distinct regions, U3, R and U5, each with different elements involved in transcriptional regulation. The U3 region contains three functional domains, which regulate HIV-1 positive sense transcription: a core promoter region, core enhancer region and a modulatory region (Reviewed in [1]). The promoter region contains numerous transcription factor-binding sites, most notably, a TATA box and three Sp1 binding sites as well as an initiator element [2–4]. Following the promoter region is the core enhancer domain, which contains two NF-κB sites. Interaction between the Sp1 and NF-κB proteins is essential for positive regulation of HIV-1 transcription as the binding of NF-κB alone to the enhancer region is not sufficient for transcriptional activation [5] (Figure 1).

Figure 1. The LTR promoter of HIV. The genomic organization of HIV-1 is shown with lines emphasizing/delineating the 5' LTR/promoter. The transcription factor AP1, NFAT-1, IL-2RE, NF-kB, Sp1 and LBP-1 binding sites, TATA box, upstream weak transcriptional start TAGAA, Tat activating region (TAR), and the AAUAA poly-adenylation sites downstream of TAR in the LTR are shown. Note not all transcription factor binding sites are shown.

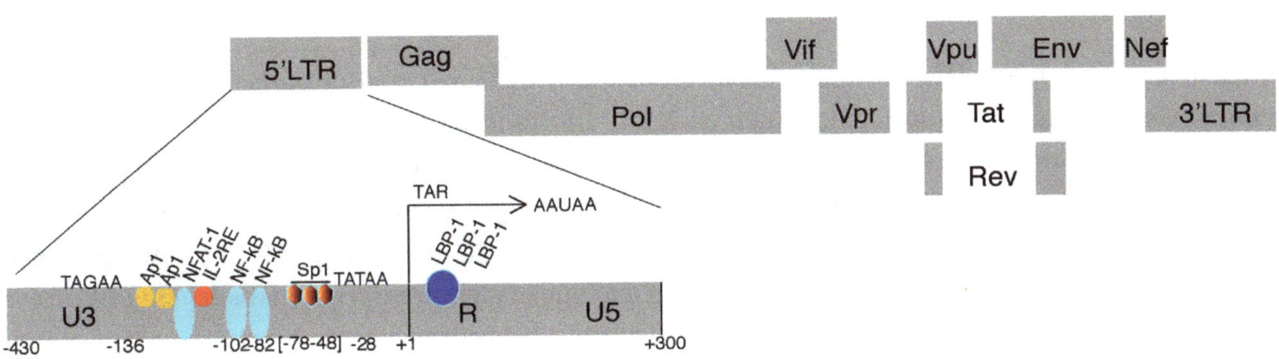

Many other cellular proteins have also been suggested to have sequence-specific interactions with the modulatory region, contributing to both positive and negative regulation of HIV-1 transcription (Reviewed in [1]). The R region, downstream of the U3 region, contains the transactivation response element (TAR); a viral stem-loop RNA structure which has been well documented to recruit and bind the Tat protein for efficient transcriptional elongation ([6,7], reviewed in [8]). CBP and p300 are coactivating proteins, which acetylate Tat, permitting its association with TAR RNA [9–12]. The Tat/TAR association synergistically enhances transcriptional efficiency of proviral RNA. The U5 region has also been shown to contain important motifs, which are involved in transactivation of the HIV-1 provirus [13,14]. The capacity of the HIV-1 LTR to mediate complex DNA-protein interactions, which positively and negatively regulate transcription, reveals its importance in the HIV viral lifecycle.

2.2. HIV Chromatin Regulation

Post-integration into the host genome, the provirus undergoes packaging into chromatin. Histones are highly conserved proteins, which form the foundation of chromatin structure. Histone proteins associate with DNA to form highly organised and compact structures. This structural unit is termed the nucleosome; and its tight arrangement will act as a barrier for DNA-binding factors such as transcription factors. Limited access to specific proviral sequences impacts the ability of the virus to express genes. Although histones have historically been thought of only as structural elements of the chromatin fibres, it has become evident that they are crucial players in the regulation of gene transcription and have the ability to alter the course of transcription regulation machinery through their histone code [15]. Covalent chemical modifications of the N-terminus of histone tails form the basis of their regulatory capacity and the histone code. These epigenetic modifications such as acetylation, phosphorylation, methylation, ubiquitination and ribosylation are key markers on the protruding histone tails, which may alter chromatin structure and regulation of gene expression (Reviewed in [16]).

The remodeling and modification of chromatin architecture has since been suggested to be an important factor in the transcriptional regulation of HIV-1 [17,18]. Upon HIV-1 integration into the host genome, the deposition of two nucleosomes, nuc-1 and nuc-0 occurs at two defined regions of the proviral LTR [19]. The deposition of nuc-1 plays an integral role in the suppression of HIV-1 gene expression, ultimately implicating chromatin modification as a key aspect of viral gene repression and latency [20].

Histone deacetylases (HDACs) have been associated with HIV-1 transcriptional silencing and viral latency. Cellular transcription factors, such as YY1, LSF and more recently c-Myc, Sp1 and AP-4, have been shown to be involved in the recruitment of HDAC1 to the viral LTR, repressing the HIV-1 promoter and maintaining viral latency [21–23]. These changes result in an impaired ability of RNA polymerase II to localise to the HIV-1 promoter and initiate transcription [24]. Following HDAC1 recruitment to the LTR, nucleosome deacetylation and subsequent transcriptional silencing of proviral transcriptional expression have been observed [25].

Another epigenetic modification, DNA methylation, has also been identified as a contributing mechanism for viral latency. HIV DNA may become methylated within the viral LTR, which has been associated with transcriptional silencing and the inhibition of the methylation has been shown to result in the reactivation of previously latent HIV [26–28]. DNA methylation however, does not seem to be the main silencing mechanism as the effect appears to be reversible and partially methylated promoters may still be reactivated [26].

Likewise, other epigenetic modifications to nucleosomes may play a role in transcriptional activation of HIV-1. It has been shown that the acetylation of histones is correlated with transcriptional activation of the HIV-1 promoter [20]. Acetylation primarily occurs at the lysine residues of the histone tails, which reduces the positive charge of the tails, lowering their affinity for DNA and ultimately causing partial or full disassociation with the DNA [29]. Histone acetyltransferases (HATs) have an opposite action to HDACs and have been known to interact with and be recruited to the viral promoter by the viral protein Tat [9,30,31]. Acetylation of the H3 and H4 histones has been shown to play a strikingly significant role in the onset of viral mRNA transcription in HIV-1 infected cells. In conditions under which the HIV-1 viral promoter is transcriptionally inactive, its activation by Tat correlates with acetylation of H3 and H4 on nuc-0 prior to the onset of viral mRNA production [32]. Furthermore, HAT activity at the promoter sites of genes has been shown to enhance gene transcription although alone it is not able to induce expression of viral expression (Reviewed in [33,34]).

Essentially, the ability of HIV-1 to alter chromatin structure and epigenetic modifications through cellular and viral transcriptional regulation mechanisms ultimately determines the path of transcriptional activation or viral latency in HIV.

3. NcRNAs and Their Role in Genetic Regulation

It has long been accepted that the genome is regulated by a series of aforementioned epigenetic modifications known as the histone code and HIV also appears to be under this mode of gene regulation. The mystery about the concise choreography and execution of the histone code continues to be enigmatic as we delve further into the nuances of the genome. Previous estimates suggested that up to ninety eight per cent of the genome was 'junk', however recent observations suggest that this is not the case. It turns out that these so-called 'junk regions' of the genome are active and may in fact be assiduous writers of the histone code controlling transcriptional and epigenetic states, among other things. The association of these ncRNAs with chromatin remodeling complexes shapes the future of their bound genes.

3.1. LncRNAs, Xist and PTENpg1

In humans, lncRNAs have been found to play a substantial role in chromatin remodeling and gene silencing in both normal cellular function as well as the development of diseases. The most eloquent example of this is the inactivation of the entire X chromosome during cell development. In mammalian females, one copy of the X chromosome is transcriptionally silent for the life of the cell. This is to ensure that the correct 'dosage' of expression of the chromosome is achieved with respect to males, who only possess one copy [35]. The silencing of the entire chromosome is mediated by a sophisticated long intergenic noncoding RNA (lincRNA) known as Xist, which is a multiexonic, spliced RNA that possesses its own 5' cap and polyA tail [35–38]. PRC2 is a large complex with histone methyltransferase activity and is required for the extensive formation of the transcriptionally silent heterochromatin by trimethylation of histone H3 on lysine 27 (Reviewed in [39,40]). The PRC2 complex has been shown to bind RepA; and in turn is bound with Xist to target PRC2 histone methyltransferase activity on the future silent X chromosome [41]. This is the most well recognized example of how a lncRNA can facilitate extensive and essential changes to chromatin and dramatically alter gene expression.

Non-coding RNAs are not only vital for normal development but can also play a role in the development of human diseases such as cancer, Alzheimer's disease and α-thalassemia [42,43]. The tumor suppressor gene, PTEN, is post-transcriptionally regulated by a lncRNA termed PTEN pseudogene 1 (PTENpg1) [44]. PTENpg1 in turn is modulated by a PTENpg1 encoded asRNA, which exists as one of two isoforms, α and β [45]. The α isoform has been shown to epigenetically silence PTEN transcription while the β isoform interacts with the sense pseudogene to alter the stability and localization of the transcript [45]. The sophistication of directive regulation by lncRNAs allows them to exert substantial control over gene expression and that the equilibrium by which they exist is fundamental for normal cellular functioning.

3.2. MicroRNAs (miRNAs) and Small Interfering RNAs (siRNAs); The Role of Dicer and Drosha

LncRNAs are not the only ncRNAs that have a regulatory effect on the genome. MiRNAs and siRNAs are the workhorses of RNA-directed RNA-processing. The action they exert on processing machinery is termed RNA interference (RNAi). miRNAs are small sequences of about 20–24 nucleotides which regulate gene expression by binding specific cellular mRNA transcripts and directing them to degradation (Reviewed in [46]). The nuclear enzyme, Drosha, and the cytoplasmic enzyme, Dicer are responsible for the maturation of miRNAs in a multistep process (Reviewed in [47]). After the maturation of the miRNA, other components of the RNA induced silencing complex (RISC) are recruited, most of these being nucleases, and degrade target RNA (Reviewed in [48]). The suggested method of targeting particular transcripts comes from the miRNA sequence homology with the mRNA that is to targeted and ultimately degraded [49]. MiRNAs have been found in many species of plants, animals and even in a number of viruses, including the Epstein-Barr Virus (EBV) [50–58]. Since viral genomes are extremely compact, utilization of both the positive and negative sense strands seems to be the ideal way to capitalize on their limited regulatory and coding capacity space.

3.3. Mechanisms of RNA-Directed Epigenetic Modification

It is thought that the main mechanism for ncRNA directed epigenetic modifications occurs both in *cis* and in *trans* through specific RNA:DNA and likely RNA:RNA interactions (in the case of *trans*).

Cis-acting RNAs are localised to their point of transcription and act directly on surrounding genes on the same chromosome. Acting in *cis*, it is likely that ncRNAs are transcribed with a histone-modifying protein-binding site, such as the histone methyltransferase PRC2. The PRC2 protein is recruited to the lncRNA while the RNA is still tethered to its transcription site by RNA polymerase II. Transcription factors such as YY1 are then recruited which clamp the hanging protein:ncRNA complex to the chromatin (Reviewed in [59]). The chromatin-modifying protein is then free to induce epigenetic changes such as histone methylation. It has been shown that up to 20% of lincRNAs associate with the histone methyltransferase PRC2 [60].

Trans-acting RNAs differ to this as they are not tethered to their site of synthesis but rather are able to move freely and act on genes that are on different chromosomes, some distance away [45]. The ncRNAs are able to recruit histone-modifying proteins and act as a scaffold by which these proteins can associate and form complexes [61]. The mechanism by which *trans*-acting ncRNAs target certain genetic regions to be epigenetically altered is debatable. While there are examples of targeting through sequence homology, whereby the ncRNA forms a DNA:RNA hybrid with the complementary target gene, this may not always be the case. The lncRNA HOTAIR has been shown to interact with up to 850 genome wide target [62] suggesting it is not sequence-specific but that the RNA itself has a structural role in the scaffold. Another potential hypothesis is that the lncRNA interacts with an RNA intermediate at the gene target site. These promoter associated RNAs, named such as they are derived from the promoter of the target gene, have been shown to be mechanistically relevant in antisense RNA (asRNA) directed transcriptional gene silencing [63] and thus have been included as a potential mechanism for lncRNA-directed epigenetic modification. The precise mechanism or combination of mechanisms for *trans*-regulation of epigenetic modification is still yet to be elucidated and may be multifactorial. For a more detailed review on the mechanism of ncRNA-directed epigenetic silencing see Beisel and Paro, 2011 [64].

4. HIV and Non-Coding RNAs

It is important to recognize the multiplicity of complex regulatory mechanisms surrounding HIV-1 transcriptional and translational control in order for us to decipher the puzzle of HIV viral latency and reactivation. In addition to chromatin remodeling complexes and the direction of the LTR, other regulatory means are present to control HIV-1 viral expression.

4.1. HIV and asRNAs

Gene expression of retroviruses usually occurs by the transcription of a single transcript, which may be differentiated through splicing events. Transcription is initiated from the 5' end in the LTR, where there are many of the necessary binding sites for transcription factors and regulators of gene expression (Figure 1). With the discovery of new antisense transcripts generated in the HTLV-1 retrovirus [65–67], the long-held belief that retroviruses transcribe their genome in a single direction has become redundant and naturally it has been speculated that a similar antisense transcript may exist in other retroviruses such as HIV-1. The possible existence of an antisense protein (ASP) was first proposed by Miller using computational models and analysis of highly conserved regions of HIV-1 proviral DNA [68]. Since then, an asRNA coding for a putative ASP have been characterized [69], however the existence of an actual ASP protein has not yet been determined [70]. Furthermore, it was shown that the regulation this asRNA exerts over the proviral genome may not be due to the ASP, but rather the asRNA itself [71]. Therefore although the existence of the ASP is debatable, there is a growing evidence suggesting a role for the HIV expressed asRNA in controlling HIV-1 expression [72–74]. Supporting this notion a recent study by Kobayashi-Ishihara *et al.* has demonstrated that asRNAs may have a regulatory role in HIV-1 viral replication, in particular, regulation of positive sense transcription [75]. These data suggest that the aforementioned asRNA may actually be reclassified as a lncRNA due to its functions in gene regulation, however further studies will be required to elucidate the true function of this HIV expressed asRNA in regulating HIV.

Chromatin remodeling has already been described as an important mechanism for the regulation of viral latency in HIV. Chromatin remodeling in humans is facilitated, at least in part, by lncRNAs that have the ability to form RNA-protein complexes with histone modifying proteins and direct them to the target region (Reviewed in [76–78]). Although no lncRNAs have yet been discovered in HIV, their presence in a wide variety of organisms and their role in chromatin remodeling and gene expression would suggest that this is an area of potential interest when considering a possible driving mechanism in HIV latency.

4.2. HIV and miRNAs

In addition to the long asRNAs being utilized by viruses, miRNAs have also been found to be produced by viruses such as EBV and HSV-1. These miRNAs appear to be involved in the post-transcription regulation of viral mRNA transcripts and also modulating host cell gene expression, essentially with the virus hijacking host miRNA pathways for its own benefit and survival ([55], and reviewed in [79]). MiRNAs are generated from imperfect stem-loop precursors by the enzymes Drosha and Dicer. HIV-1 contains two of these such structures, TAR and RRE [80] so it seems reasonable to extrapolate that it may be able to act in the same way as other viruses, using host machinery to process its own miRNAs. A study by Benasser *et al.* hypothesized, using computational analysis that HIV was also capable of generating up to ten viable viral miRNAs (vmiRNAs) [81]. Further studies have demonstrated that the HIV TAR element is bound by and processed by host-derived Dicer to yield a vmiRNA [82–84]. This vmiRNA, processed from the HIV-1 TAR element, was found to inhibit LTR-driven gene expression, potentially through sequence homology to the TAR element and transcriptional gene silencing [82]. It has also been suggested that HIV may produce vmiRNAs as a part of its pathogenic mechanism. Findings indicate that the HIV-1 proviral genome may have the capacity to produce inhibitory vmiRNAs that interfere with host immunity [85]. These vmiRNAs have been found to theoretically have the ability to block translation of factors such as CD28, CD4 and some interleukins [85]. Supporting this model, HIV-1 has also been shown through deep sequencing analysis, to produce viral small interfering RNAs (vsiRNAs) to further modulate both cellular and viral gene expression [86,87].

5. Final Remarks and Future Work

HIV-1 is a complex retrovirus with many regulatory mechanisms in place to control latency, reactivation and gene expression. Although these mechanisms are not yet fully understood, there has been a trend toward widening the scope of the search. Chromatin remodeling complexes and the mechanisms in which they are directed is under particularly intense study due to the increasing amounts of data implicating them as important factors in gene expression. Among the masses of data, lncRNAs seem to be particularly well represented as regulators of chromatin complexes. Further investigation into this area may see the emergence of previously unknown ncRNAs, be they miRNAs, or lncRNAs, in the epigenetic regulation of viral expression and host-virus interactions.

Acknowledgments

The project was supported by NIAID R56 AI096861-01, and PO1 AI099783-01 to KVM.

References

1. Pereira, L.A.; Bentley, K.; Peeters, A.; Churchill, M.J.; Deacon, N.J. A compilation of cellular transcription factor interactions with the HIV-1 LTR promoter. *Nucleic Acids Res.* **2000**, *28*, 663–668.
2. Jones, K.A.; Peterlin, B.M. Control of RNA initiation and elongation at the HIV-1 promoter. *Annu. Rev. Biochem.* **1994**, *63*, 717–743.
3. Jones, K.A.; Kadonaga, J.T.; Luciw, P.A.; Tjian, R. Activation of the AIDS retrovirus promoter by the cellular transcription factor, Sp1. *Science* **1986**, *232*, 755–759.
4. Rittner, K.; Churcher, M.J.; Gait, M.J.; Karn, J. The human immunodeficiency virus long terminal repeat includes a specialised initiator element which is required for Tat-responsive transcription. *J. Mol. Biol.* **1995**, *248*, 562–580.
5. Majello, B.; de Luca, P.; Hagen, G.; Suske, G.; Lania, L. Different members of the Sp1 multigene family exert opposite transcriptional regulation of the long terminal repeat of HIV-1. *Nucleic Acids Res.* **1994**, *22*, 4914–4921.
6. Graeble, M.A.; Churcher, M.J.; Lowe, A.D.; Gait, M.J.; Karn, J. Human immunodeficiency virus type 1 transactivator protein, Tat, stimulates transcriptional read-through of distal terminator sequences *in vitro*. *Proc. Natl. Acad. Sci. USA* **1993**, *90*, 6184–6188.

7. Wei, P.; Garber, M.E.; Fang, S.-M.; Fischer, W.H.; Jones, K.A. A Novel CDK9-Associated C-Type Cyclin Interacts Directly with HIV-1 Tat and Mediates Its High-Affinity, Loop-Specific Binding to TAR RNA. *Cell* **1998**, *92*, 451–462.
8. Brigati, C.; Giacca, M.; Noonan, D.M.; Albini, A. HIV Tat, its TARgets and the control of viral gene expression. *FEMS Microbiol. Lett.* **2003**, *220*, 57–65.
9. Col, E.; Caron, C.; Seigneurin-Berny, D.; Gracia, J.; Favier, A.; Khochbin, S. The histone acetyltransferase, hGCN5, interacts with and acetylates the HIV transactivator, Tat. *J. Biol. Chem.* **2001**, *276*, 28179–28184.
10. Deng, L.; de la Fuente, C.; Fu, P.; Wang, L.; Donnelly, R.; Wade, J.D.; Lambert, P.; Li, H.; Lee, C.G.; Kashanchi, F. Acetylation of HIV-1 Tat by CBP/P300 increases transcription of integrated HIV-1 genome and enhances binding to core histones. *Virology* **2000**, *277*, 278–295.
11. Kiernan, R.E.; Vanhulle, C.; Schiltz, L.; Adam, E.; Xiao, H.; Maudoux, F.; Calomme, C.; Burny, A.; Nakatani, Y.; Jeang, K.T.; *et al.* HIV-1 tat transcriptional activity is regulated by acetylation. *EMBO J.* **1999**, *18*, 6106–6118.
12. Ott, M.; Schnolzer, M.; Garnica, J.; Fischle, W.; Emiliani, S.; Rackwitz, H.R.; Verdin, E. Acetylation of the HIV-1 Tat protein by p300 is important for its transcriptional activity. *Curr. Biol.* **1999**, *9*, 1489–1492.
13. Rabbi, M.F.; Saifuddin, M.; Gu, D.S.; Kagnoff, M.F.; Roebuck, K.A. U5 region of the human immunodeficiency virus type 1 long terminal repeat contains TRE-like cAMP-responsive elements that bind both AP-1 and CREB/ATF proteins. *Virology* **1997**, *233*, 235–245.
14. Roebuck, K.A.; Gu, D.S.; Kagnoff, M.F. Activating protein-1 cooperates with phorbol ester activation signals to increase HIV-1 expression. *AIDS* **1996**, *10*, 819–826.
15. Luger, K.; Richmond, T.J. The histone tails of the nucleosome. *Curr. Opin. Genet. Dev.* **1998**, *8*, 140–146.
16. Strahl, B.D.; Allis, C.D. The language of covalent histone modifications. *Nature* **2000**, *403*, 41–45.
17. He, G.; Ylisastigui, L.; Margolis, D.M. The regulation of HIV-1 gene expression: The emerging role of chromatin. *DNA Cell Biol.* **2002**, *21*, 697–705.
18. Pumfery, A.; Deng, L.; Maddukuri, A.; de la Fuente, C.; Li, H.; Wade, J.D.; Lambert, P.; Kumar, A.; Kashanchi, F. Chromatin remodeling and modification during HIV-1 Tat-activated transcription. *Curr. HIV Res.* **2003**, *1*, 343–362.
19. Verdin, E. DNase I-hypersensitive sites are associated with both long terminal repeats and with the intragenic enhancer of integrated human immunodeficiency virus type 1. *J. Virol.* **1991**, *65*, 6790–6799.
20. Van Lint, C.; Emiliani, S.; Ott, M.; Verdin, E. Transcriptional activation and chromatin remodeling of the HIV-1 promoter in response to histone acetylation. *EMBO J.* **1996**, *15*, 1112–1120.
21. Coull, J.J.; Romerio, F.; Sun, J.M.; Volker, J.L.; Galvin, K.M.; Davie, J.R.; Shi, Y.; Hansen, U.; Margolis, D.M. The human factors YY1 and LSF repress the human immunodeficiency virus type 1 long terminal repeat via recruitment of histone deacetylase 1. *J. Virol.* **2000**, *74*, 6790–6799.

22. Jiang, G.; Espeseth, A.; Hazuda, D.J.; Margolis, D.M. c-Myc and Sp1 contribute to proviral latency by recruiting histone deacetylase 1 to the human immunodeficiency virus type 1 promoter. *J. Virol.* **2007**, *81*, 10914–10923.
23. Imai, K.; Okamoto, T. Transcriptional repression of human immunodeficiency virus type 1 by AP-4. *J. Biol. Chem.* **2006**, *281*, 12495–12505.
24. Williams, S.A.; Chen, L.F.; Kwon, H.; Ruiz-Jarabo, C.M.; Verdin, E.; Greene, W.C. NF-kappaB p50 promotes HIV latency through HDAC recruitment and repression of transcriptional initiation. *EMBO J.* **2006**, *25*, 139–149.
25. Coull, J.J.; He, G.; Melander, C.; Rucker, V.C.; Dervan, P.B.; Margolis, D.M. Targeted derepression of the Human Immunodeficiency Virus type 1 long terminal repeat by pyrrole-imidazole polyamides. *J. Virol.* **2002**, *76*, 12349–12354.
26. Kauder, S.E.; Bosque, A.; Lindqvist, A.; Planelles, V.; Verdin, E. Epigenetic regulation of HIV-1 latency by cytosine methylation. *PLoS Pathog.* **2009**, *5*, e1000495.
27. Bednarik, D.P.; Cook, J.A.; Pitha, P.M. Inactivation of the HIV LTR by DNA CpG methylation: Evidence for a role in latency. *EMBO J.* **1990**, *9*, 1157–1164.
28. Bednarik, D.P.; Duckett, C.; Kim, S.U.; Perez, V.L.; Griffis, K.; Guenthner, P.C.; Folks, T.M. DNA CpG methylation inhibits binding of NF-kappa B proteins to the HIV-1 long terminal repeat cognate DNA motifs. *New Biol.* **1991**, *3*, 969–976.
29. Hong, L.; Schroth, G.P.; Matthews, H.R.; Yau, P.; Bradbury, E.M. Studies of the DNA binding properties of histone H4 amino terminus. Thermal denaturation studies reveal that acetylation markedly reduces the binding constant of the H4 "tail" to DNA. *J. Biol. Chem.* **1993**, *268*, 305–314.
30. Marzio, G.; Tyagi, M.; Gutierrez, M.I.; Giacca, M. HIV-1 tat transactivator recruits p300 and CREB-binding protein histone acetyltransferases to the viral promoter. *Proc. Natl. Acad. Sci. USA* **1998**, *95*, 13519–13524.
31. Hottiger, M.O.; Nabel, G.J. Interaction of human immunodeficiency virus type 1 Tat with the transcriptional coactivators p300 and CREB binding protein. *J. Virol.* **1998**, *72*, 8252–8256.
32. Lusic, M.; Marcello, A.; Cereseto, A.; Giacca, M. Regulation of HIV-1 gene expression by histone acetylation and factor recruitment at the LTR promoter. *EMBO J.* **2003**, *22*, 6550–6561.
33. Narlikar, G.J.; Fan, H.Y.; Kingston, R.E. Cooperation between complexes that regulate chromatin structure and transcription. *Cell* **2002**, *108*, 475–487.
34. Cosma, M.P. Ordered recruitment: Gene-specific mechanism of transcription activation. *Mol. Cell* **2002**, *10*, 227–236.
35. Panning, B.; Dausman, J.; Jaenisch, R. X chromosome inactivation is mediated by Xist RNA stabilization. *Cell* **1997**, *90*, 907–916.
36. Gartler, S.M.; Goldman, M.A. X-Chromosome inactivation. In *eLS*; John Wiley & Sons, Ltd.: New York, NY, USA, 2001.
37. Brown, C.J.; Ballabio, A.; Rupert, J.L.; Lafreniere, R.G.; Grompe, M.; Tonlorenzi, R.; Willard, H.F. A gene from the region of the Human X inactivation centre is expressed exclusively from the inactive X chromosome. *Nature* **1991**, *349*, 38–44.

38. Penny, G.D.; Kay, G.F.; Sheardown, S.A.; Rastan, S.; Brockdorff, N. Requirement for Xist in X chromosome inactivation. *Nature* **1996**, *379*, 131–137.
39. Simon, J.A.; Kingston, R.E. Mechanisms of Polycomb gene silencing: Knowns and unknowns. *Nat. Rev. Mol. Cell Biol.* **2009**, *10*, 697–708.
40. Plath, K.; Fang, J.; Mlynarczyk-Evans, S.K.; Cao, R.; Worringer, K.A.; Wang, H.; de la Cruz, C.C.; Otte, A.P.; Panning, B.; Zhang, Y. Role of histone H3 lysine 27 methylation in X inactivation. *Science* **2003**, *300*, 131–135.
41. Zhao, J.; Sun, B.K.; Erwin, J.A.; Song, J.J.; Lee, J.T. Polycomb proteins targeted by a short repeat RNA to the mouse X chromosome. *Science* **2008**, *322*, 750–756.
42. Faghihi, M.A.; Modarresi, F.; Khalil, A.M.; Wood, D.E.; Sahagan, B.G.; Morgan, T.E.; Finch, C.E.; St Laurent, G., 3rd; Kenny, P.J.; Wahlestedt, C. Expression of a noncoding RNA is elevated in Alzheimer's disease and drives rapid feed-forward regulation of beta-secretase. *Nat. Med.* **2008**, *14*, 723–730.
43. Tufarelli, C.; Stanley, J.A.; Garrick, D.; Sharpe, J.A.; Ayyub, H.; Wood, W.G.; Higgs, D.R. Transcription of antisense RNA leading to gene silencing and methylation as a novel cause of human genetic disease. *Nat. Genet.* **2003**, *34*, 157–165.
44. Poliseno, L.; Salmena, L.; Zhang, J.; Carver, B.; Haveman, W.J.; Pandolfi, P.P. A coding-independent function of gene and pseudogene mRNAs regulates tumour biology. *Nature* **2010**, *465*, 1033–1038.
45. Johnsson, P.; Ackley, A.; Vidarsdottir, L.; Lui, W.; Corcoran, M.; Grandér, D.; Morris, K.V. A pseudogene long non-coding RNA network regulates PTEN transcription and translation in human cells. *Nat. Struct. Mol. Biol.* **2013**, in press.
46. Kawasaki, H.; Wadhwa, R.; Taira, K. World of small RNAs: From ribozymes to siRNA and miRNA. *Differentiation* **2004**, *72*, 58–64.
47. Lee, Y.; Ahn, C.; Han, J.; Choi, H.; Kim, J.; Yim, J.; Lee, J.; Provost, P.; Radmark, O.; Kim, S.; *et al*. The nuclear RNase III Drosha initiates microRNA processing. *Nature* **2003**, *425*, 415–419.
48. Sontheimer, E.J. Assembly and function of RNA silencing complexes. *Nat. Rev. Mol. Cell Biol.* **2005**, *6*, 127–138.
49. Conrad, R.; Barrier, M.; Ford, L.P. Role of miRNA and miRNA processing factors in development and disease. *Birth Defects Res. C Embryo Today* **2006**, *78*, 107–117.
50. Reinhart, B.J.; Slack, F.J.; Basson, M.; Pasquinelli, A.E.; Bettinger, J.C.; Rougvie, A.E.; Horvitz, H.R.; Ruvkun, G. The 21-nucleotide let-7 RNA regulates developmental timing in Caenorhabditis elegans. *Nature* **2000**, *403*, 901–906.
51. Lagos-Quintana, M.; Rauhut, R.; Lendeckel, W.; Tuschl, T. Identification of Novel genes coding for small expressed RNAs. *Science* **2001**, *294*, 853–857.
52. Lau, N.C.; Lim, L.P.; Weinstein, E.G.; Bartel, D.P. An abundant class of tine RNAs with probable regulatory roles in Caenorhabditis elegans. *Science* **2001**, *294*, 858–862.
53. Mourelatos, Z.; Dostie, J.; Paushkin, S.; Sharma, A.; Charroux, B.; Abel, L.; Rappsilber, J.; Mann, M.; Dreyfuss, G. miRNPs: A novel class of ribonucleoproteins containing numerous microRNAs. *Genes Dev.* **2002**, *16*, 720–728.

54. Lagos-Quintana, M.; Rauhut, R.; Yalcin, A.; Meyer, J.; Lendeckel, W.; Tuschl, T. Identification of tissue-specific microRNAs from mouse. *Curr. Biol.* **2002**, *12*, 735–739.
55. Pfeffer, S.; Zavolan, M.; Grasser, F.A.; Chien, M.; Russo, J.J.; Ju, J.; John, B.; Enright, A.J.; Marks, D.; Sander, C.; *et al.* Identification of virus-encoded microRNAs. *Science* **2004**, *304*, 734–736.
56. Umbach, J.L.; Kramer, M.F.; Jurak, I.; Karnowski, H.W.; Coen, D.M.; Cullen, B.R. MicroRNAs expressed by herpes simplex virus 1 during latent infection regulate viral mRNAs. *Nature* **2008**, *454*, 780–783.
57. Sullivan, C.S.; Sung, C.K.; Pack, C.D.; Grundhoff, A.; Lukacher, A.E.; Benjamin, T.L.; Ganem, D. Murine Polyomavirus encodes a microRNA that cleaves early RNA transcripts but is not essential for experimental infection. *Virology* **2009**, *387*, 157–167.
58. Singh, J.; Singh, C.P.; Bhavani, A.; Nagaraju, J. Discovering microRNAs from Bombyx mori nucleopolyhedrosis virus. *Virology* **2010**, *407*, 120–128.
59. Lee, J.T. Epigenetic regulation by long noncoding RNAs. *Science* **2012**, *338*, 1435–1439.
60. Khalil, A.M.; Guttman, M.; Huarte, M.; Garber, M.; Raj, A.; Rivea Morales, D.; Thomas, K.; Presser, A.; Bernstein, B.E.; van Oudenaarden, A.; *et al.* Many human large intergenic noncoding RNAs associate with chromatin-modifying complexes and affect gene expression. *Proc. Natl. Acad. Sci. USA* **2009**, *106*, 11667–11672.
61. Tsai, M.C.; Manor, O.; Wan, Y.; Mosammaparast, N.; Wang, J.K.; Lan, F.; Shi, Y.; Segal, E.; Chang, H.Y. Long noncoding RNA as modular scaffold of histone modification complexes. *Science* **2010**, *329*, 689–693.
62. Gupta, R.A.; Shah, N.; Wang, K.C.; Kim, J.; Horlings, H.M.; Wong, D.J.; Tsai, M.C.; Hung, T.; Argani, P.; Rinn, J.L.; *et al.* Long non-coding RNA HOTAIR reprograms chromatin state to promote cancer metastasis. *Nature* **2010**, *464*, 1071–1076.
63. Han, J.; Kim, D.; Morris, K.V. Promoter-associated RNA is required for RNA-directed transcriptional gene silencing in human cells. *Proc. Natl. Acad. Sci. USA* **2007**, *104*, 12422–12427.
64. Beisel, C.; Paro, R. Silencing chromatin: Comparing modes and mechanisms. *Nat. Rev. Genet.* **2011**, *12*, 123–135.
65. Mesnard, J.M.; Barbeau, B.; Devaux, C. HBZ, a new important player in the mystery of adult T-cell leukemia. *Blood* **2006**, *108*, 3979–3982.
66. Gaudray, G.; Gachon, F.; Basbous, J.; Biard-Piechaczyk, M.; Devaux, C.; Mesnard, J.M. The complementary strand of the human T-cell leukemia virus type 1 RNA genome encodes a bZIP transcription factor that down-regulates viral transcription. *J. Virol.* **2002**, *76*, 12813–12822.
67. Larocca, D.; Chao, L.A.; Seto, M.H.; Brunck, T.K. Human T-cell leukemia virus minus strand transcription in infected T-cells. *Biochem. Biophys. Res. Commun.* **1989**, *163*, 1006–1013.
68. Miller, R.H. Human immunodeficiency virus may encode a novel protein on the genomic DNA plus strand. *Science* **1988**, *239*, 1420–1422.

69. Michael, N.L.; Vahey, M.T.; d'Arcy, L.; Ehrenberg, P.K.; Mosca, J.D.; Rappaport, J.; Redfield, R.R. Negative-strand RNA transcripts are produced in human immunodeficiency virus type 1-infected cells and patients by a novel promoter downregulated by Tat. *J. Virol.* **1994**, *68*, 979–987.
70. Torresilla, C.; Larocque, E.; Landry, S.; Halin, M.; Coulombe, Y.; Masson, J.Y.; Mesnard, J.M.; Barbeau, B. Detection of the HIV-1 minus strand-encoded Antisense Protein and its association with autophagy. *J. Virol.* **2013**, *87*, 5089–5105.
71. Tagieva, N.E.; Vaquero, C. Expression of naturally occurring antisense RNA inhibits human immunodeficiency virus type 1 heterologous strain replication. *J. Gen. Virol.* **1997**, *78*, 2503–2511.
72. Landry, S.; Halin, M.; Lefort, S.; Audet, B.; Vaquero, C.; Mesnard, J.M.; Barbeau, B. Detection, characterization and regulation of antisense transcripts in HIV-1. *Retrovirology* **2007**, *4*, 71.
73. Bentley, K.; Deacon, N.; Sonza, S.; Zeichner, S.; Churchill, M. Mutational analysis of the HIV-1 LTR as a promoter of negative sense transcription. *Arch. Virol.* **2004**, *149*, 2277–2294.
74. Peeters, A.; Lambert, P.F.; Deacon, N.J. A fourth Sp1 site in the human immunodeficiency virus type 1 long terminal repeat is essential for negative-sense transcription. *J. Virol.* **1996**, *70*, 6665–6672.
75. Kobayashi-Ishihara, M.; Yamagishi, M.; Hara, T.; Matsuda, Y.; Takahashi, R.; Miyake, A.; Nakano, K.; Yamochi, T.; Ishida, T.; Watanabe, T. HIV-1-encoded antisense RNA suppresses viral replication for a prolonged period. *Retrovirology* **2012**, *9*, 38.
76. Grewal, S.I.; Moazed, D. Heterochromatin and epigenetic control of gene expression. *Science* **2003**, *301*, 798–802.
77. Hsieh, J.; Fire, A. Recognition and silencing of repeated DNA. *Annu. Rev. Genet.* **2000**, *34*, 187–204.
78. Morris, K.V. The emerging role of RNA in the regulation of gene transcription in human cells. *Semin. Cell Dev. Biol.* **2011**, *22*, 351–358.
79. Narayanan, A.; Kehn-Hall, K.; Bailey, C.; Kashanchi, F. Analysis of the roles of HIV-derived microRNAs. *Expert Opin. Biol. Ther.* **2011**, *11*, 17–29.
80. Jeang, K.T.; Chang, Y.; Berkhout, B.; Hammarskjold, M.L.; Rekosh, D. Regulation of HIV expression: Mechanisms of action of Tat and Rev. *AIDS* **1991**, *5*, S3–S14.
81. Bennasser, Y.; Le, S.Y.; Yeung, M.L.; Jeang, K.T. HIV-1 encoded candidate micro-RNAs and their cellular targets. *Retrovirology* **2004**, *1*, 43.
82. Klase, Z.; Kale, P.; Winograd, R.; Gupta, M.V.; Heydarian, M.; Berro, R.; McCaffrey, T.; Kashanchi, F. HIV-1 TAR element is processed by Dicer to yield a viral micro-RNA involved in chromatin remodeling of the viral LTR. *BMC Mol. Biol.* **2007**, *8*, 63.
83. Bennasser, Y.; Yeung, M.L.; Jeang, K.T. HIV-1 TAR RNA subverts RNA interference in transfected cells through sequestration of TAR RNA-binding protein, TRBP. *J. Biol. Chem.* **2006**, *281*, 27674–27678.
84. Purzycka, K.J.; Adamiak, R.W. The HIV-2 TAR RNA domain as a potential source of viral-encoded miRNA. A reconnaissance study. *Nucleic Acids Symp. Ser. (Oxf.)* **2008**, doi:10.1093/nass/nrn259.
85. Couturier, J.P.; Root-Bernstein, R.S. HIV may produce inhibitory microRNAs (miRNAs) that block production of CD28, CD4 and some interleukins. *J. Theor. Biol.* **2005**, *235*, 169–184.

86. Schopman, N.C.; Willemsen, M.; Liu, Y.P.; Bradley, T.; van Kampen, A.; Baas, F.; Berkhout, B.; Haasnoot, J. Deep sequencing of virus-infected cells reveals HIV-encoded small RNAs. *Nucleic Acids Res.* **2012**, *40*, 414–427.
87. Bennasser, Y.; Le, S.Y.; Benkirane, M.; Jeang, K.T. Evidence that HIV-1 encodes an siRNA and a suppressor of RNA silencing. *Immunity* **2005**, *22*, 607–619.

5

Biochemical and Functional Interactions of Human Papillomavirus Proteins with Polycomb Group Proteins

Margaret E. McLaughlin-Drubin * and Karl Munger *

Division of Infectious Diseases, Brigham and Women's Hospital and Department of Medicine, Harvard Medical School, 181 Longwood Avenue, MCP 861, Boston, MA 02115, USA

* Authors to whom correspondence should be addressed;
E-Mails: mdrubin@rics.bwh.harvard.edu (M.E.M.-D.); kmunger@rics.bwh.harvard.edu (K.M.);

Abstract: The role of enzymes involved in polycomb repression of gene transcription has been studied extensively in human cancer. Polycomb repressive complexes mediate oncogene-induced senescence, a principal innate cell-intrinsic tumor suppressor pathway that thwarts expansion of cells that have suffered oncogenic hits. Infections with human cancer viruses including human papillomaviruses (HPVs) and Epstein-Barr virus can trigger oncogene-induced senescence, and the viruses have evolved strategies to abrogate this response in order to establish an infection and reprogram their host cells to establish a long-term persistent infection. As a consequence of inhibiting polycomb repression and evading oncogene induced-senescence, HPV infected cells have an altered epigenetic program as evidenced by aberrant homeobox gene expression. Similar alterations are frequently observed in non-virus associated human cancers and may be harnessed for diagnosis and therapy.

Keywords: cervical cancer; biomarker; histone methylation; tumor suppressor

---

1. Introduction

1.1. Human Papillomaviruses

Human papillomaviruses (HPVs) are members of the *Papillomaviridae,* a large family of viruses that infect epithelial cells. Papillomaviruses consist of approximately 8 kb double stranded circular DNA genomes packaged into 55 nm icosahedral capsids. Only one of the two strands is transcribed and encodes five to six "early" (E) open reading frames (ORFs) that encode non-structural regulatory proteins and two "late" (L) ORFs, L1 and L2, from which the major and minor capsid proteins, respectively, are translated. Papillomaviruses exhibit exquisite species specificity, and as a consequence there are no heterologous animal systems to model the natural course of HPV infections.

Almost 200 HPV genotypes have been identified, and they are categorized by the degree of sequence similarity into specific papillomavirus genera [1]. The alpha HPVs have received considerable experimental attention, since they are classified as "high-risk" and "low-risk" based on the propensity for malignant progression of the lesions that they cause. Low-risk HPVs such as HPV6 and HPV11 cause generally benign warts of the genital or oral mucosa whereas infections with "high-risk" HPVs cause lesions of these same target tissues that can undergo malignant progression [2]. Almost 100% of human cervical cancers as well as a large fraction of other anogenital tract and oral carcinomas are caused by high-risk alpha HPV infections [3]. Even though highly efficacious prophylactic vaccines—that prevent infection with the most highly abundant low-risk HPVs (HPV6 and HPV11) and high-risk HPVs (HPV16 and HPV18)—are on the market, the acceptance of these vaccines in the US population has been low [4]. Moreover, because of their cost, these vaccines are not universally available to populations in low-income countries, where cervical carcinoma remains one of the leading causes of cancer death in women [5]. In addition, cervical carcinoma generally develop years or decades after the initial infection and since the prophylactic vaccines do not protect from pre-existing infections or prevent malignant progression, it will be decades before these vaccines will have a noticeable impact on the incidence of HPV-associated cancers [6]. Hence, infections with high-risk alpha HPVs will continue to be one of the most common sexually transmitted diseases and a major cause of morbidity and mortality for decades to come.

Like other viruses, HPVs are obligatory intracellular parasites that need to reprogram the infected host cell to establish an infection and complete their life cycles and produce viral progeny. In the case of HPVs that is a particularly challenging endeavor. First of all, despite extensive splicing due to their limited coding potential, HPVs can only produce a limited number of non-structural proteins. Only two of these, E1 and E2, are mechanistically involved in viral genome replication. E1 has ATPase and DNA helicase activity, and in complex with E2, it binds the viral origin of replication, where it assembles into a hexameric complex that forms a scaffold for binding cellular replication proteins [7]. HPVs do not encode any other proteins that are rate-limiting for replication such as nucleotide biosynthesis enzymes or a DNA polymerase, and these viruses are acutely dependent on the availability of the cellular DNA synthesis machinery to replicate their genomes. Moreover, the productive HPV life cycle is coupled to the differentiation status of the infected squamous epithelial cell [8]. The squamous epithelium is the largest organ of the human body and is in a constant state of self-renewal. Within this tissue, basal epithelial cells are the only cells that undergo cell division and are the targets of HPV infection. To maintain the integrity of the multilayer epithelial structure, basal epithelial cells divide asymmetrically. One daughter cell retains undifferentiated, DNA synthesis-competent basal cell characteristics, whereas the other daughter cell is poised to undergo cell cycle withdrawal and terminal differentiation, while it is pushed towards the surface of the epithelium and is eventually sloughed off. When the epithelium is injured, however, some basal cells can also undergo symmetrical division to replenish the population of basal cells and close the wound (Figure 1). Since the productive HPV life cycle including production of viral progeny only occurs in terminally differentiated cells, the virus needs to encode proteins that uncouple cell cycle withdrawal from the differentiation program to allow differentiating cells to remain DNA synthesis competent so as to permit viral genome replication. The viral E6 and E7 proteins, which in high-risk HPVs have potent oncogenic activities, are the major drivers of this process. A second and equally important aspect of the viral life cycle is the ability of high-risk HPVs to establish a long-term persistent infection of undifferentiated, basal epithelial cells [8]. One attractive model is that during persistent infection, cells harboring HPV genomes either undergo division only infrequently or that they preferentially undergo symmetrical cell division, yielding two equal basal like cells where the genome is maintained but no infectious progeny is produced. This model has not been tested experimentally, mostly because there are no adequate experimental systems that allow long-term study of a squamous epithelium *in vitro*.

Figure 1. Cell division in a squamous epithelium. (**A**) Asymmetric cell division of a basal epithelial cell yields two unequal daughter cells. One remains an undifferentiated, DNA synthesis competent basal epithelial cell whereas the other daughter is a differentiating epithelial cell that will terminally withdraw from the cell division cycle. Human papillomaviruses (HPV) genomes segregated into such cells will retain these cells in a DNA replication competent state and complete their full replicative life cycle including viral progeny synthesis. (**B**) Symmetric cell division will yield two basal like cells. This mode of cell division is to replenish basal epithelial cell during wound healing. After the initial infection, HPVs establish a long-term persistent infection of these cells where the viral genome is maintained at a low copy number. The viral genome undergoes replication every time the cell replicates its genome. See text for details.

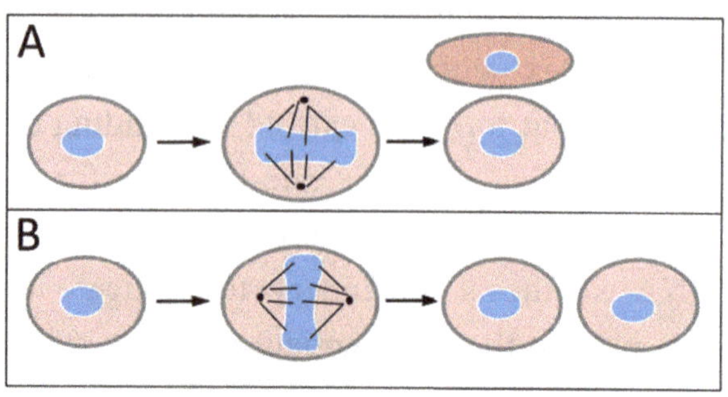

In high-risk HPV-associated cancers the viral genome frequently integrates during malignant progression and only two viral genes, E6 and E7 are consistently expressed in cervical carcinoma cells [9,10]. E6 and E7 each have potent transforming activities and can immortalize primary human epithelial cells and induce genomic instability that drives development of fully transformed, carcinogenic cells [11]. Expression of E6 and E7 in transgenic mice from a keratin K14 promoter that drives their expression in basal epithelial cells in combination with low dose estrogen treatment causes cervical carcinoma development [12]. Cervical carcinoma cells are "addicted" to E6/E7 expression and undergo cell cycle arrest, senescence or cell death when E6/E7 expression is extinguished [13–15]. Hence, HPV E6/E7-mediated cellular reprogramming for the purpose of establishing and maintaining a long-term persistent infection and to generate viral progeny is a risky proposition for the infected host cell as well as the virus, as it can lead to cancer formation and the ultimate demise of the host and the viral genome that is trapped within that host.

In addition to targeting specific transcriptional programs, HPV E6 and E7 proteins are known to affect epigenetic control mechanisms to more globally perturb the transcriptional competence of the infected host cells. Not surprisingly, high-risk HPV E6 and E7 proteins have been reported to biochemically interact with and/or functionally alter a variety of epigenetic enzymes including DNA methylases and histone modifying enzymes. This article focuses on interactions of the HPV E7 protein with components and regulators of Polycomb group (PcG) proteins.

1.2. Polycomb Group Proteins and Homeobox Genes

PcG genes were discovered in *Drosophila melanogaster* and named to denote a mutant phenotype that, in addition to segmentation defects, displays formation of aberrant sex combs on the legs of male flies. PcG proteins form macromolecular repressor complexes, polycomb repressive complexes (PRCs), that globally regulate transcriptional competence of genes that play important roles in cell fate specification and maintenance of stem cell pools [16].

There are two major PRC species, designated PRC1 and PRC2, which play critical roles in epigenetic gene silencing. PRC2 contains the EZH2 enzyme, which places a trimethyl mark on lysine 27 of histone H3 (H3K27me3). This repressive mark causes chromatin compaction and gene silencing. PRC1 occupies H3K27me3 marked chromatin and further silences the chromatin by mono-ubiquitination of lysine 119 on histone H2A (H2AK119Ub) (Figure 2). Some PRC1 complexes can also silence gene expression in the absence of repressive H3K27me3 marks since H2AK119Ub marked chromatin is a binding site for the L3MBTL2 protein, which then establish repressive structures [17] that are particularly important in pluripotent stem cells [18].

There is compelling evidence that PRCs regulate epithelial cell differentiation as well as expansion of basal cell pools during wound healing [19–21]. As described in more detail above, HPVs may need to target both of these processes to allow for viral progeny synthesis and establishment of long-term persistent infection, respectively. Hence, PRC components and molecules that regulate their activity are attractive targets for HPV proteins.

Figure 2. Polycomb mediated silencing of gene expression. The polycomb repressive complex 2 (PRC2) silences chromatin by trimethylating lysine residue 27 (K27me3) of histone H3, causing chromatin compaction. H3K27me3 marked chromatin is bound by PRC1, which further silences gene expression by monoubiquitinating lysine residue 119 (K119Ub) of histone H2A.

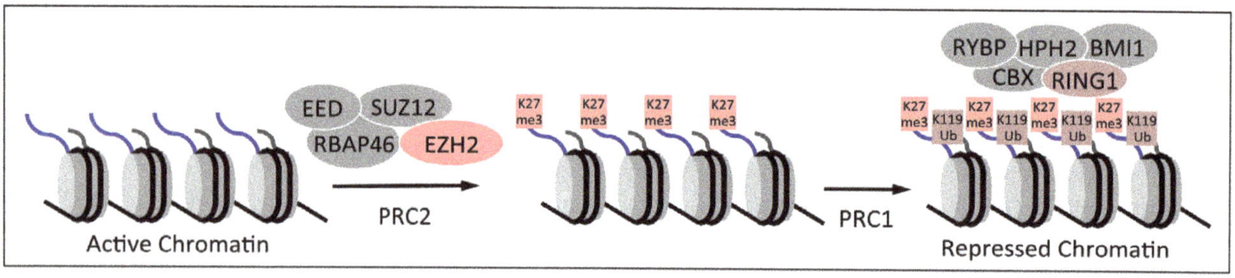

The best-known transcriptional targets of PRCs are the homeobox (*HOX*) genes, which encode a family of related transcription factors that contain a homeodomain. *HOX* family members are frequently dysregulated during carcinogenesis [22,23] and germline *HOXB13* mutations have been linked to an increased risk for the development of prostate cancer [24]. HOX proteins are not only downstream transcriptional targets of PRCs, but they also mediate PRC repressor activities on some of their target genes [25].

2. Dysregulation of Homeobox Gene Expression in Cervical Cancers

Not surprisingly, dysregulated HOX gene expression has also been reported during cervical carcinogenesis. In an early study, *HOX* gene expression was analyzed in a series of cervical carcinoma lines and compared to expression in normal cervical epithelium. These studies documented aberrant expression of *HOXA1*, *B2*, *B4*, *C5*, *C10* and *D13* in some of the cancer lines but there was no evidence for coding mutations in *HOX* genes [26]. Differential *HOXC5* expression was also observed in a study where *HOX* gene expression in normal keratinocytes was compared to the HPV16 positive SiHa cervical carcinoma line. This study also provided evidence for increased expression of *HOXC8* in SiHa cells [27], and another study provided additional evidence for *HOXB4* overexpression in cervical carcinomas [28]. Collectively, however, these results are difficult to interpret and may simply reflect the differences in differentiation states of the normal keratinocytes and the cervical carcinoma lines that were analyzed.

The most compelling evidence for aberrant *HOX* gene expression in cervical carcinoma was provided by a study performed with clinical specimens. Gene expression analysis of normal cervix, high-grade premalignant lesions and frank cancers provided strong evidence for upregulation of *HOXC10* expression during cervical cancer progression. Using cell culture based experiments the authors were able to link *HOXC10* expression to the acquisition of the invasive phenotype during cervical carcinogenesis [29].

3. Association of HPV16 E7 with Polycomb Group Proteins

3.1. HPV16 E7

The HPV16 E7 ORF encodes a low-molecular size, 98 amino acid protein that lacks intrinsic enzymatic and specific DNA binding activities. E7 is consistently expressed in cervical cancer even after integration of the viral genome into a host chromosome. It exerts its biological activities through associating with and functionally reprogramming host protein complexes that play critical roles in signal transduction. The best-studied cellular target of HPV16 E7 is pRB, the protein encoded by the retinoblastoma susceptibility gene (RB1), and the related p107 (RBL1) and p130 (RBL2) proteins [11]. However, additional important cellular targets of HPV16 E7 exist, and with the development of proteomic methods, identification of putative transformation targets for the HPV E7 protein has been a mainstay of HPV research [30].

3.2. Association of HPV16 E7 with E2F6 Containing Polycomb Repressive Complexes

One of the first proteomic studies with twin-epitope tagged HPV16 E7 ectopically expressed in HeLa cells, led to the identification of multiple previously unappreciated cellular HPV16 E7 targets, including the E2F6 transcriptional repressor [31,32]. E2F6 is a non-canonical member of the E2F family of transcription factors as it lacks the C-terminal binding site for pRB family member, and hence its transcriptional activity is not modulated by pRB binding. Like other E2F family members, E2F6 associates with a dimerization partner (DP1 or DP2) to form a transcriptionally active DNA binding complex. The E2F6/DP1 or DP2 heterodimer functions as a transcriptional repressor that is expressed in late S-phase, presumably to down-regulate E2F transcriptional target genes and stimulate S-phase exit [33,34]. HPV16 E7 associates with the C-terminal repressor domain of E2F6 and abrogates its repressive activity on E2F6 target genes. The ability to target E2F6 is shared with low-risk HPV E7 proteins, and the simian vacuolating virus 40 large tumor antigen (SV40 TAg) and the adenovirus (Ad) E1A protein also share the ability to inhibit E2F6 repression [32].

E2F6 is also a component of PRCs and several, apparently distinct, E2F6 containing PRCs have been described [35–38]. Examination of E7 associated proteins revealed evidence for the presence multiple additional PRC components, including BMI1, PCGF2 (MEL-18), CBX4 (hPC2), RING1, MGA and L3MBTL2 [32]. Many of these proteins have been specifically described as components of E2F6-associated PRCs, and hence it is likely that HPV16 E7 can associate with and potentially modify activities of E2F6 containing PRCs. It has not been investigated whether low-risk HPV E7 proteins, SV40 TAg or Ad E1A can also associate with E2F6 containing PRCs.

Detection of E2F6 containing nuclear dots, presumably representing E2F6 containing PRCs were diminished in HPV16 E7 expressing cells, and an HPV16 E7 mutant that does not associate with E2F6 had no effect on the number of detectable E2F6 nuclear dots [32]. This finding is consistent with the model that E7 binding may alter the composition of E2F6 containing PRCs. This model, however, has not yet been tested experimentally.

3.3. Decreased Trimethylation of Lysine 27 of Histone H3 in HPV16 E7 Expressing Cells

Analysis of H3K27me3 levels in HPV16 E7 expressing primary human keratinocytes revealed a dramatic decrease in the H3K27me3 mark compared to donor and passage matched control vector expressing keratinocytes. Interestingly, there was no comparable decrease in the H3K27me2 and H3K27me1 marks [39]. Similar decreases in the H3K27me3 mark were also detected in clinical specimens of HPV16 positive high-grade premalignant squamous intraepithelial lesions (SILs) of the cervix [39,40]. Studies with a U2OS human osteosarcoma cell line with tetracycline-inducible E7 expression showed that the observed decrease of the repressive H3K27me3 mark is a direct and immediate effect of HPV16 E7 expression [39]. H3K27 staining diminishes within 72 hours of E7 induction and is restored when E7 expression is switched off. These results may provide an alternative explanation for the observed loss of detection of E2F6 containing PRCs in HPV16 E7 expressing cells.

4. Modulation of Polycomb Group Protein Expression by HPV16 Oncoproteins

4.1. Increased EZH2 Expression in HPV E7 Expressing Cells

The enzymatic PRC2 component, the H3K27 methyltransferase EZH2, is a bona fide human oncogene that is overexpressed and amplified in human tumors [41–43]. EZH2 transcription is regulated by E2F transcription factors [41]. HPV16 E7 targets pRB, p107 and p130 for proteasomal degradation and associates with E2F6 and therefore interferes with E2F transcriptional repressor activities, causing deregulated and increased expression of E2F transcriptional targets. Consistent with this model, HPV16 E7 transcriptionally activates EZH2 through its E2F sites and EZH2 is highly overexpressed in cervical lesions and tumors [44]. Interestingly, cervical carcinoma cells appear addicted to EZH2; depletion caused G1 cell cycle arrest and a low level of apoptosis.

High levels of EZH2 expression in HPV-positive cervical carcinomas and HPV E7 expressing cell lines and their apparent addiction to EZH2 is particularly remarkable since the H3K27me3 mark is decreased, not increased, in such cell lines. Different potential mechanistic explanations have been proposed to account for this apparently paradoxical finding. There is evidence that the enzymatic activity of EZH2 in PRC2 complexes is negatively regulated by AKT mediated phosphorylation at serine residue (S) 21 [45]. Since HPV16 E6 and E7 have both been reported to cause AKT activation [46,47] it is conceivable that PRC2 complex-associated EZH2 enzymatic activity may be low despite high-level overexpression in HPV16 positive lesions and cancers. A recent exciting study has shown that EZH2 phosphorylation on S21 acts as a functional switch that promotes EZH2 association with an androgen receptor containing transcription factor complex and in this context EZH2 acts as a polycomb independent activator of gene expression [48]. This study also provided compelling evidence that the oncogenic activity of EZH2 in castration-resistant prostate cancer cells is based on this polycomb independent activity of EZH2 [48]. EZH2 has also been detected in PRC complexes that catalyze H1K26 methylation [49]. It will be important to determine the posttranslational modifications of EZH2 and the biochemical composition of EZH2 complexes in HPV16 E7 expressing cells.

4.2. Modulation of BMI1 Expression by HPV E6 and E7

Expression of other PcG proteins in HPV16 E6/E7 expressing cells has also been studied. Levels of the PRC1 components SUZ12 and EED were reported to be unchanged but the levels of BMI1 were dramatically reduced in HPV16 E6/E7 expressing cells [40]. These results were somewhat surprising since BMI1 is a well-known oncogene that is frequently overexpressed in human tumors including cervical carcinomas [50–53], and it has even been suggested that BMI1 autoantibodies may be useful as a biomarker of cervical carcinomas [54].

In another study, HPV16 E6 was shown to increase BMI1 expression in primary human keratinocytes, and levels remained high in HPV E6/E7 immortalized keratinocyte lines. Most intriguingly, BMI1 could substitute for E6 and cooperate with E7 to cause keratinocyte immortalization [55]. This result is consistent with an earlier study that showed that BMI1 depletion in the HPV18 positive HeLa cervical carcinoma line caused S-phase depletion and G1 growth arrest [56].

5. Modulation of PRC Regulators by HPV16 E7

5.1. Upregulation of the H3K27 Demethylases KDM6A and KDM6B

H3K27 trimethylation is a dynamic process that is reversed by two demethylases, KDM6A (UTX) and KDM6B (JMJD3) (Figure 3). A mechanistic explanation for the dramatically decreased H3K27me3 levels in HPV16 positive cervical lesions and cancers was provided by the finding that KDM6A and KDM6B are expressed at markedly higher levels in these cells [39].

Figure 3. PRC2 mediated gene silencing is reversible. The EZH2 histone methyl transferase in PRC2 silences gene expression by adding the trimethyl mark on lysine residue 27 of histone H3, and this mark can be removed by one of the two H3K27 specific demethylases, KDM6A or KDM6B. See text for details.

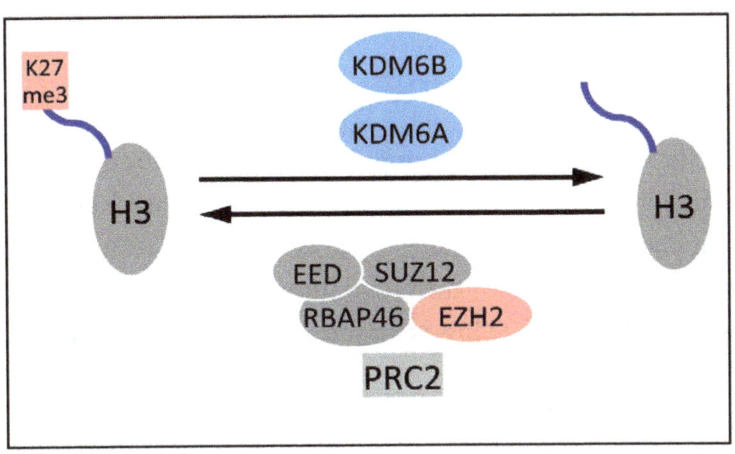

Even though KDM6A and KDM6B have identical catalytic activities and substrate specificities, they have different chromatin targets. KDM6A is encoded on the X-chromosome but escapes X-inactivation [57]. A related gene, UTY, is encoded on the Y chromosome but the UTY protein appears to lack histone demethylase enzymatic activity [58].

The fact that KDM6A and KDM6B have non-overlapping and non-redundant biological activities and that KDM6A may have biological activities that are independent of enzymatic activities have been impressively validated in genetically engineered mouse models (GEMMs). Studies with KDM6A$^{-/-}$ GEMMs revealed that KDM6A plays an important role in activating cardiac differentiation [59]. KDM6A$^{-/-}$ female mice died at E12.5 with defects in neural tube, yolk sac, and cardiac development, whereas approximately 20% of KDM6A$^{-/-}$ male mice survived. These animals are fertile, but are smaller and have a reduced life span [58,60,61]. Studies with embryonic stem (ES) cells derived from these GEMMs and GEMMs expressing enzymatically inactive KDM6A, revealed that KDM6A regulated embryonic development may be independent of its enzymatic activity [61].

KDM6B$^{-/-}$ GEMMs show perinatal lethality due to respiratory failure, which is caused by a developmental defect of the respiratory neuronal network [62]. KDM6B may also have biological activities that may not dependent on H3K27 demethylation. In macrophages KDM6B is induced by NF-kB in response to inflammatory stimuli and modulates expression of PRC silenced genes [63]. This KDM6B activity also does not appear to primarily depend on H3K27 demethylation [64].

The observed non-redundant activities of KDM6A and KDM6B may reflect incorporation of the two proteins into different multiprotein complexes. KDM6A is associated with H3K4 methyl transferase activity containing Mixed-Lineage-Leukemia (MLL)2/3 complexes [65,66]. KDM6A containing MLL2/3 complexes might link H3K27 demethylation to H3K4 methylation, and KDM6A/MLL2/3 complexes can convert transcriptionally silenced chromatin to a transcriptionally competent state. KDM6A mutations have been detected in some tumors [67], whereas KDM6B is upregulated in some cancers, particularly metastatic prostate carcinomas [68].

HPV16 E7 upregulates expression of KDM6A and KDM6B, at least in part at the level of transcription. The exact mechanisms of transcriptional induction of KDM6A and KDM6B expression remain to be determined. Upregulation of KDM6B, however, is clearly independent of HPV16 E7-mediated pRB degradation and activation of canonical E2F transcription factors [39].

5.2. KDM6B Controls Epithelial Differentiation

Genes that are specifically expressed during skin differentiation frequently carry H3K27me3 repressive marks in undifferentiated basal epithelial cells and are subject to PRC transcriptional regulation. Differentiation causes removal of these marks and relief from PCG repression. Even though KDM6B levels remain unchanged during differentiation, the removal of the repressive H3K27me3 mark is mostly mediated by KDM6B. This is based on the observation that KDM6B depletion in keratinocytes inhibited differentiation whereas ectopic expression accelerated differentiation. KDM6B enzymatic activity was required for acceleration of epithelial differentiation [69]. These results predict that HPV16 E7 expression not only changes *HOX* gene expression but also induces expression of genes that are normally only expressed in differentiating epithelial cells (Figure 4). This might play an important role in the viral life cycle as the switch from early to late viral gene expression is mediated by differentiation cues.

Figure 4. HPV16 E7 causes increased KDM6A and KDM6B expression. E7 mediated KDM6A and KDM6B induction affects multiple transcriptional programs, including keratinocyte differentiation and cell identity. KDM6B induction represents a cellular defense response to E7 oncogene expression that is to trigger cell cycle arrest and senescence. HPV16 E7 short-circuits this response by targeting the retinoblastoma tumor suppressor for degradation. Several other viruses including EBV have developed strategies to subvert such cellular defense responses. See text for details.

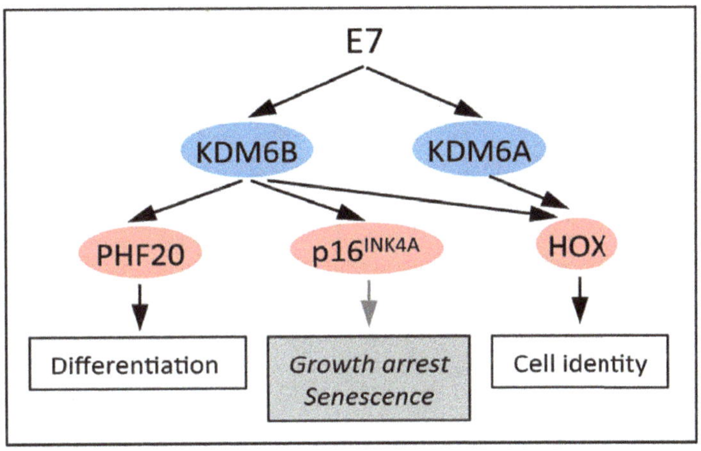

5.3. KDM6B Mediates the Oncogene-Induced Senescence (OIS) Response to RAS/RAF

Oncogene induced senescence (OIS) is one of the cell intrinsic tumor suppressor responses that has evolved to eliminate aberrantly proliferating and therefore potentially tumorigenic cells from the proliferative pool. OIS was initially discovered with the *RAS* oncogene and is signaled through transcriptional upregulation of the $p16^{INK4A}$ tumor suppressor [70] (Figure 5). In some cell types, particularly in mouse cells, the partially overlapping gene encoding $p14^{ARF}$ (or $p19^{ARF}$ in mouse cells) is also induced and causes activation of the p53 tumor suppressor by inhibiting ubiquitination by MDM2 [71]. The $p16^{INK4A}$ protein is a component of the retinoblastoma tumor suppressor pathway and inhibits CDK4/6-cyclin D mediated pRB phosphorylation and S-phase entry (Figure 5). It is frequently mutated, deleted or transcriptionally silenced in human tumors and tumor cell lines, supporting the notion that overcoming the OIS response is a major bottleneck in human cancer development.

Expression of $p16^{INK4A}$ in normal human cells is generally low because the gene is silenced by H3K27 trimethylation and PRCs. In response to RAS/RAF stimulation, KDM6B expression is transcriptionally activated, potentially through AP1, causing removal of the H3K27me3 mark and enhanced $p16^{INK4A}$ expression. This then signals G1 arrest and senescence through activation of the pRB tumor suppressor. Notably, however, RAS/RAF stimulation does not induce KDM6A expression nor does it consistently cause de-silencing of the $p14^{ARF}$ promoter [71,72].

Figure 5. Induction and abrogation of the Oncogene Induced Senescence (OIS) tumor suppressor response by HPV16 E7. (**A**) The retinoblastoma tumor suppressor (pRB) pathway regulates S-phase cell cycle entry. Activity of pRB is regulated by phosphorylation by cyclin dependent kinase 4 or 6 (CDK4/6). CDK4/6 activity is activated by association with a D-type cyclin (CCND) and negatively regulated by association with one of several small molecule inhibitors ($p16^{INK4A}$, $p18^{INK4C}$ and $p19^{INK4D}$), which are induced in response to different growth suppressive stimuli. CDK4/6 phosphorylation of pRB at the G1/S boundary inactivates the transcriptional repressor activity of the pRB/E2F complex and signals S-phase entry. (**B**) Oncogenic stimuli such as RAS/RAF signaling or HPV16 E7 expression causes KDM6B expression and de-repression of $p16^{INK4A}$ expression, which inhibits CDK4/6 activity and pRB phosphorylation, causing G1 cell cycle arrest and senescence (OIS). (**C**) HPV16 E7 has evolved to evade OIS by targeting pRB for ubiquitin mediated proteasomal degradation.

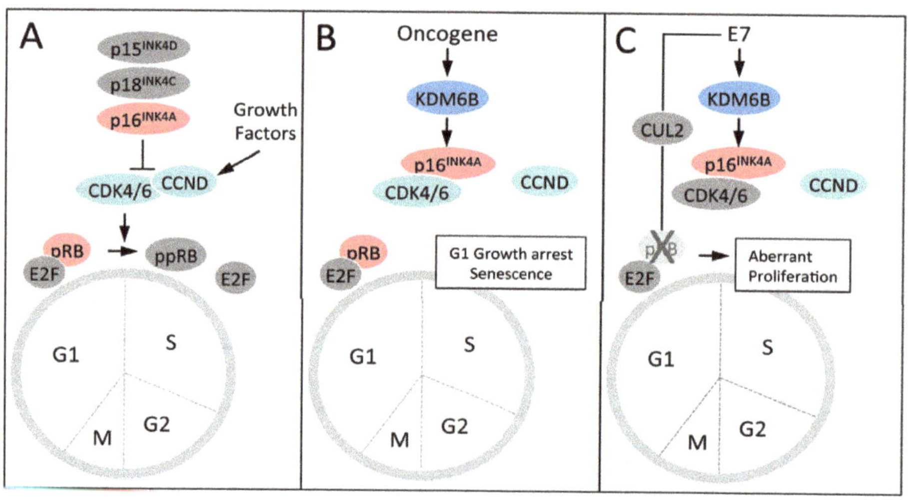

5.4. HPV16 E7 Induces the Cervical Cancer Biomarker $p16^{INK4A}$ through KDM6B

The $p16^{INK4A}$ tumor suppressor is an important biomarker for high-risk HPV-associated lesions and cancers and is induced by E7 [73,74]. It was initially thought that E7 induced $p16^{INK4A}$ through E2F activation [75], but there are no E2F response elements in the $p16^{INK4A}$ promoter and a pRB binding/degradation deficient HPV16 E7 mutant that does not activate E2F transcription, induces $p16^{INK4A}$ expression as efficiently as wild-type HPV16 E7 [39]. More recent studies have clearly shown that high level $p16^{INK4A}$ expression in cervical lesions and cancer represents a readout of an E7 induced OIS response [39]. How E7 triggers the response and how it is signaled to the KDM6B promoter is unclear, but E7 proteins also blunts OIS signaling by targeting pRB for ubiquitin dependent proteasomal degradation. Indeed, earlier studies have shown that pRB degradation, not merely binding, is necessary to fully inhibit pRB induced senescence [76]. Notably, $p14^{ARF}$ expression is also increased in E7 expressing cells but in contrast to $p16^{INK4A}$, depletion of KDM6B does not decrease $p14^{ARF}$ levels or the H3K27me3 mark at the $p14^{ARF}$ promoter [39].

Abrogation of the p16^{INK4A} OIS block in primary lymphocytes also represents a major roadblock to transformation by Epstein-Barr virus (EBV) [77]. The EBV proteins EBNA3A and EBNA3C cooperate to epigenetically silence the p16^{INK4A} promoter through a mechanism that involves the transcriptional repressor C-terminal binding protein (CtBP) [78,79]. Transcriptional silencing of other PRC controlled genes, such as the apoptosis regulator BIM, likely also contribute to EBV transformation [80]. Similarly, the hepatitis B virus (HBV) X protein downregulates the PRC2 protein SUZ12, which is essential for placing the H3K27me3 mark [81].

It is interesting to note that high-level p16^{INK4A} expression has also been detected in a number of other cancer types, including lung, prostate, breast and ovarian cancers [82–85]. In most cases, high level p16^{INK4A} expression is linked to pRB mutations [86], and it will be important to determine whether p16^{INK4A} expression is also mediated by KDM6B in such tumors. As mentioned previously, KDM6B upregulation has been reported in metastatic prostate carcinomas [68].

Cervical carcinoma cells are "addicted" to HPV E6/E7 oncogene expression and undergo growth arrest, senescence and cell death when expression of the viral oncoproteins is silenced [13–15]. Loss of HPV E6 or E7 expression can each individually induce senescence through re-activation of the p53 and pRB pathways, respectively [87–89]. It will be interesting to determine whether epigenetic mechanisms in general and PcG group proteins in particular are involved in signaling induction of senescence responses in these cases.

5.5. Dysregulated Homeobox Gene Expression in HPV16 E7 Expressing Cells

In contrast to RAF/RAS stimulation, HPV16 E7 also causes increased expression of the H3K27-specific demethylase KDM6A [39,40]. It is not clear whether KDM6A expression also represents a cellular tumor suppressive defense response, how E7 triggers it and what the transcriptional consequences of KDM6A expression may be. The fact that KDM6A has been classified as a putative tumor suppressor [67] may support the model that KDM6A may also be induced as a consequence of E7 triggering a cell intrinsic tumor suppressive defense response. Therefore it will be important to determine the mechanisms of E7 mediated KDM6A induction, the transcriptional consequences of KDM6A expression and the mechanisms by which E7 subverts KDM6A tumor suppressor activity.

It is known that KDM6A controls expression of *HOX* genes and indeed, *HOX* gene expression is dysregulated in HPV16 E7 expressing cells [39]. As pointed out in a previous section, *HOX* gene expression is frequently dysregulated in human cancers, including cervical carcinomas, and some *HOX* genes have been shown to contribute to cancer formation. Aberrant *HOX* gene expression in E7 expressing cells suggests that *HOX* gene dysregulation observed in cervical carcinoma cells is caused by HPV E7 expression and suggests that HPV infection causes reprogramming of the epigenetic make up of epithelial cells.

5.6. KDM6A and KDM6B are Essential in Cervical Carcinoma Cells

It is not intuitively obvious that KDM6A and/or KDM6B upregulation by HPV16 E7 would contribute to E7 transformation, since abrogation of downstream transcriptional consequences, such as $p16^{INK4A}$ mediated OIS signaling, is critical for HPV, EBV and possibly HBV cell transformation. Hence, it was surprising that KDM6A as well as KDM6B depletion dramatically inhibited viability of the HPV16 positive CaSki cervical carcinoma line [39]. This finding suggests that survival of HPV E7 expressing cells is critically dependent on KDM6A and KDM6B targets. Even though it cannot be ruled out that these enzymes may have substrates other than methylated H3K27, it is likely that these represent transcriptional targets. The full delineation of KDM6A and KDM6B targets represents a major effort, but it is feasible by determining the full spectrum of human genes that have altered H3K27me3 marks in response to KDM6A or KDM6B using chromatin immunoprecipitation followed by DNA sequencing (ChIPSeq) in combination with expression profiling.

6. Concluding Remarks

Dysregulation of the histone code and activation of transcriptional programs in the “wrong” cell type is a hallmark of carcinogenesis. The REST transcriptional repressor, for example, is responsible for silencing neuronal-specific gene expression in non-neuronal cells. REST is a major tumor suppressor in colon, lung and breast cancers [90–92] and may be key to the neuro-endocrine character of some of these tumors. Similarly, PcG group proteins have been implicated in human carcinogenesis and some, including *BMI1* and *EZH2* are bona fide oncogenes that are overexpressed in many tumor types. The H3K27 demethylases KDM6A and KDM6B have also been implicated in carcinogenesis and the finding that KDM6B is the major mediator of OIS further supports the involvement of these enzymes in cancer formation.

One of the most exciting possibilities is that, unlike genetic mutations, epigenetic alterations may be reversed by inhibiting the enzymes that cause them. Even though some functions of KDM6A and KDM6B appear to be independent of their enzymatic activities, a recently developed KDM6 selective inhibitor was show to affect proinflammatory signaling in macrophages [93], even though previous studies suggested that KDM6B modulation of expression of PRC silenced genes in response to inflammatory stimuli [63] may not primarily depend on H3K27 demethylation [64]. Given the result that KDM6A as well as KDM6B expression is essential for viability to cervical carcinoma cells, KDM6 inhibition should be evaluated as a therapeutic modality for some human cancers.

Acknowledgments

Research on epigenetic alterations caused by HPV infections in the authors’ laboratories is supported by PHS grants R01 CA066980 (KM) and K01 CA143010 (MEM-D) from the National Cancer Institute.

References

1. Bernard, H.U.; Burk, R.D.; Chen, Z.; van Doorslaer, K.; Hausen, H.; de Villiers, E.M. Classification of papillomaviruses (PVs) based on 189 PV types and proposal of taxonomic amendments. *Virology* **2010**, *401*, 70–79.
2. Moody, C.A.; Laimins, L.A. Human papillomavirus oncoproteins: Pathways to transformation. *Nat. Rev. Cancer* **2010**, *10*, 550–560.
3. Munoz, N.; Bosch, F.X.; de Sanjose, S.; Herrero, R.; Castellsague, X.; Shah, K.V.; Snijders, P.J.; Meijer, C.J. Epidemiologic classification of human papillomavirus types associated with cervical cancer. *N. Engl. J. Med.* **2003**, *348*, 518–527.
4. Jemal, A.; Simard, E.P.; Dorell, C.; Noone, A.M.; Markowitz, L.E.; Kohler, B.; Eheman, C.; Saraiya, M.; Bandi, P.; Saslow, D.; *et al.* Annual report to the nation on the status of cancer, 1975–2009, Featuring the burden and trends in human papillomavirus(HPV)-associated cancers and HPV vaccination coverage levels. *J. Nat. Cancer Inst.* **2013**, *105*, 175–201.
5. Kane, M.A.; Serrano, B.; de Sanjose, S.; Wittet, S. Implementation of human papillomavirus immunization in the developing world. *Vaccine* **2012**, *30* (Suppl. 5), F192–F200.
6. Frazer, I.H. Prevention of cervical cancer through papillomavirus vaccination. *Nat. Rev. Immunol.* **2004**, *4*, 46–54.
7. Hebner, C.M.; Laimins, L.A. Human papillomaviruses: Basic mechanisms of pathogenesis and oncogenicity. *Rev. Med. Virol.* **2006**, *16*, 83–97.
8. Bodily, J.; Laimins, L.A. Persistence of human papillomavirus infection: Keys to malignant progression. *Trends Microbiol.* **2011**, *19*, 33–39.
9. Baker, C.C.; Phelps, W.C.; Lindgren, V.; Braun, M.J.; Gonda, M.A.; Howley, P.M. Structural and translational analysis of human papillomavirus type 16 sequences in cervical carcinoma cell lines. *J. Virol.* **1987**, *61*, 962–971.
10. Schwarz, E.; Freese, U.K.; Gissmann, L.; Mayer, W.; Roggenbuck, B.; Stremlau, A.; zur Hausen, H. Structure and transcription of human papillomavirus sequences in cervical carcinoma cells. *Nature* **1985**, *314*, 111–114.
11. McLaughlin-Drubin, M.E.; Munger, K. Oncogenic activities of human papillomaviruses. *Virus Res.* **2009**, *143*, 195–208.
12. Riley, R.R.; Duensing, S.; Brake, T.; Munger, K.; Lambert, P.F.; Arbeit, J.M. Dissection of human papillomavirus E6 and E7 function in transgenic mouse models of cervical carcinogenesis. *Cancer Res.* **2003**, *63*, 4862–4871.
13. Francis, D.A.; Schmid, S.I.; Howley, P.M. Repression of the integrated papillomavirus E6/E7 promoter is required for growth suppression of cervical cancer cells. *J. Virol.* **2000**, *74*, 2679–2686.
14. Goodwin, E.C.; DiMaio, D. Repression of human papillomavirus oncogenes in HeLa cervical carcinoma cells causes the orderly reactivation of dormant tumor suppressor pathways. *Proc. Natl. Acad. Sci. USA* **2000**, *97*, 12513–81251.

15. Thierry, F.; Yaniv, M. The BPV-1 E2 trans-acting protein can be either an activator or repressor of the HPV-18 regulatory region. *EMBO* **1987**, *6*, 3391–3397.

16. Bracken, A.P.; Helin, K. Polycomb group proteins: Navigators of lineage pathways led astray in cancer. *Nat. Rev. Cancer* **2009**, *9*, 773–784.

17. Trojer, P.; Cao, A.R.; Gao, Z.; Li, Y.; Zhang, J.; Xu, X.; Li, G.; Losson, R.; Erdjument-Bromage, H.; Tempst, P.; *et al.* L3MBTL2 protein acts in concert with PcG protein-mediated monoubiquitination of H2A to establish a repressive chromatin structure. *Mol. Cell* **2011**, *42*, 438–450.

18. Qin, J.; Whyte, W.A.; Anderssen, E.; Apostolou, E.; Chen, H.H.; Akbarian, S.; Bronson, R.T.; Hochedlinger, K.; Ramaswamy, S.; Young, R.A.; *et al.* The polycomb group protein L3mbtl2 assembles an atypical PRC1-family complex that is essential in pluripotent stem cells and early development. *Cell Stem Cell* **2012**, *11*, 319–332.

19. Zhang, J.; Bardot, E.; Ezhkova, E. Epigenetic regulation of skin: Focus on the Polycomb complex. *Cell Mol. Life Sci.* **2012**, *69*, 2161–2172.

20. Eckert, R.L.; Adhikary, G.; Rorke, E.A.; Chew, Y.C.; Balasubramanian, S. Polycomb group proteins are key regulators of keratinocyte function. *J. Invest. Dermatol.* **2011**, *131*, 295–301.

21. Shaw, T.; Martin, P. Epigenetic reprogramming during wound healing: Loss of polycomb-mediated silencing may enable upregulation of repair genes. *EMBO Rep.* **2009**, *10*, 881–886.

22. Eklund, E. The role of Hox proteins in leukemogenesis: Insights into key regulatory events in hematopoiesis. *Crit. Rev. Oncog.* **2011**, *16*, 65–76.

23. Kelly, Z.L.; Michael, A.; Butler-Manuel, S.; Pandha, H.S.; Morgan, R.G. HOX genes in ovarian cancer. *J. Ovarian. Res.* **2011**, *4*, e16.

24. Ewing, C.M.; Ray, A.M.; Lange, E.M.; Zuhlke, K.A.; Robbins, C.M.; Tembe, W.D.; Wiley, K.E.; Isaacs, S.D.; Johng, D.; Wang, Y.; *et al.* Germline mutations in HOXB13 and prostate-cancer risk. *N. Engl. J. Med.* **2012**, *366*, 141–149.

25. Martin, N.; Popov, N.; Aguilo, F.; O'Loghlen, A.; Raguz, S.; Snijders, A.P.; Dharmalingam, G.; Li, S.; Thymiakou, E.; Carroll, T.; *et al.* Interplay between homeobox proteins and polycomb repressive complexes in p16 regulation. *EMBO* **2013**, *32*, 982–995

26. Hung, Y.C.; Ueda, M.; Terai, Y.; Kumagai, K.; Ueki, K.; Kanda, K.; Yamaguchi, H.; Akise, D.; Ueki, M. Homeobox gene expression and mutation in cervical carcinoma cells. *Cancer Sci.* **2003**, *94*, 437–441.

27. Alami, Y.; Castronovo, V.; Belotti, D.; Flagiello, D.; Clausse, N. HOXC5 and HOXC8 expression are selectively turned on in human cervical cancer cells compared to normal keratinocytes. *Biochem. Biophys. Res. Commun.* **1999**, *257*, 738–745.

28. Barba-de la Rosa, A.P.; Briones-Cerecero, E.; Lugo-Melchor, O.; de Leon-Rodriguez, A.; Santos, L.; Castelo-Ruelas, J.; Valdivia, A.; Pina, P.; Chagolla-Lopez, A.; Hernandez-Cueto, D.; *et al.* Hox B4 as potential marker of non-differentiated cells in human cervical cancer cells. *J. Cancer Res. Clin. Oncol.* **2012** *138*, 293–300.

29. Zhai, Y.; Kuick, R.; Nan, B.; Ota, I.; Weiss, S.J.; Trimble, C.L.; Fearon, E.R.; Cho, K.R. Gene expression analysis of preinvasive and invasive cervical squamous cell carcinomas identifies HOXC10 as a key mediator of invasion. *Cancer Res.* **2007**, *67*, 10163–10172.
30. White, E.A.; Howley, P.M. Proteomic approaches to the study of papillomavirus-host interactions. *Virology* **2013**, *435*, 57–69.
31. Huh, K.W.; DeMasi, J.; Ogawa, H.; Nakatani, Y.; Howley, P.M.; Munger, K. Association of the human papillomavirus type 16 E7 oncoprotein with the 600-kDa retinoblastoma protein-associated factor, p600. *Proc. Natl. Acad. Sci. USA* **2005**, *102*, 11492–11497.
32. McLaughlin-Drubin, M.E.; Huh, K.W.; Munger, K. Human papillomavirus type 16 E7 oncoprotein associates with E2F6. *J. Virol.* **2008**, *82*, 8695–8705.
33. Cartwright, P.; Muller, H.; Wagener, C.; Holm, K.; Helin, K. E2F-6: A novel member of the E2F family is an inhibitor of E2F-dependent transcription. *Oncogene* **1998**, *17*, 611–623.
34. Gaubatz, S.; Wood, J.G.; Livingston, D.M. Unusual proliferation arrest and transcriptional control properties of a newly discovered E2F family member, E2F-6. *Proc. Natl. Acad. Sci. USA* **1998**, *95*, 9190–9195.
35. Trimarchi, J.M.; Fairchild, B.; Wen, J.; Lees, J.A. The E2F6 transcription factor is a component of the mammalian Bmi1-containing polycomb complex. *Proc. Natl. Acad. Sci. USA* **2001**, *98*, 1519–1524.
36. Ogawa, H.; Ishiguro, K.; Gaubatz, S.; Livingston, D.M.; Nakatani, Y. A complex with chromatin modifiers that occupies E2F- and Myc-responsive genes in G0 cells. *Science* **2002**, *296*, 1132–1136.
37. Attwooll, C.; Oddi, S.; Cartwright, P.; Prosperini, E.; Agger, K.; Steensgaard, P.; Wagener, C.; Sardet, C.; Moroni, M.C.; Helin, K. A novel repressive E2F6 complex containing the polycomb group protein, EPC1, that interacts with EZH2 in a proliferation-specific manner. *J. Biol. Chem.* **2005**, *280*, 1199–1208.
38. Deshpande, A.M.; Akunowicz, J.D.; Reveles, X.T.; Patel, B.B.; Saria, E.A.; Gorlick, R.G.; Naylor, S.L.; Leach, R.J.; Hansen, M.F. PHC3, a component of the hPRC-H complex, associates with E2F6 during G0 and is lost in osteosarcoma tumors. *Oncogene* **2007**, *26*, 1714–1722.
39. McLaughlin-Drubin, M.E.; Crum, C.P.; Munger, K. Human papillomavirus E7 oncoprotein induces KDM6A and KDM6B histone demethylase expression and causes epigenetic reprogramming. *Proc. Natl. Acad. Sci. USA* **2011**, *108*, 2130–2135.
40. Hyland, P.L.; McDade, S.S.; McCloskey, R.; Dickson, G.J.; Arthur, K.; McCance, D.J.; Patel, D. Evidence for alteration of EZH2, BMI1, and KDM6A and epigenetic reprogramming in human papillomavirus type 16 E6/E7-expressing keratinocytes. *J. Virol.* **2011**, *85*, 10999–11006.
41. Bracken, A.P.; Pasini, D.; Capra, M.; Prosperini, E.; Colli, E.; Helin, K. EZH2 is downstream of the pRB-E2F pathway, Essential for proliferation and amplified in cancer. *EMBO J.* **2003**, *22*, 5323–5335.
42. Morin, R.D.; Johnson, N.A.; Severson, T.M.; Mungall, A.J.; An, J.; Goya, R.; Paul, J.E.; Boyle, M.; Woolcock, B.W.; Kuchenbauer, F.; *et al.* Somatic mutations altering EZH2 (Tyr641) in follicular and diffuse large B-cell lymphomas of germinal-center origin. *Nat. Genet.* **2010**, *42*, 181–185.
43. Chase, A.; Cross, N.C. Aberrations of EZH2 in cancer. *Clin. Cancer Res.* **2011**, *17*, 2613–2618.
44. Holland, D.; Hoppe-Seyler, K.; Schuller, B.; Lohrey, C.; Maroldt, J.; Durst, M.; Hoppe-Seyler, F.

Activation of the enhancer of zeste homologue 2 gene by the human papillomavirus E7 oncoprotein. *Cancer Res.* **2008**, *68*, 9964–9972.

45. Cha, T.L.; Zhou, B.P.; Xia, W.; Wu, Y.; Yang, C.C.; Chen, C.T.; Ping, B.; Otte, A.P.; Hung, M.C. Akt-mediated phosphorylation of EZH2 suppresses methylation of lysine 27 in histone H3. *Science* **2005**, *310*, 306–310.
46. Menges, C.W.; Baglia, L.A.; Lapoint, R.; McCance, D.J. Human papillomavirus type 16 E7 up-regulates AKT activity through the retinoblastoma protein. *Cancer Res.* **2006**, *66*, 5555–5559.
47. Spangle, J.M.; Munger, K. The human papillomavirus type 16 E6 oncoprotein activates mTORC1 signaling and increases protein synthesis. *J. Virol.* **2010**, *84*, 9398–9407.
48. Xu, K.; Wu, Z.J.; Groner, A.C.; He, H.H.; Cai, C.; Lis, R.T.; Wu, X.; Stack, E.C.; Loda, M.; Liu, T.; *et al.* EZH2 oncogenic activity in castration-resistant prostate cancer cells is Polycomb-independent. *Science* **2012**, *338*, 1465–1469.
49. Kuzmichev, A.; Margueron, R.; Vaquero, A.; Preissner, T.S.; Scher, M.; Kirmizis, A.; Ouyang, X.; Brockdorff, N.; Abate-Shen, C.; Farnham, P.; *et al.* Composition and histone substrates of polycomb repressive group complexes change during cellular differentiation. *Proc. Natl. Acad. Sci. USA* **2005**, *102*, 1859–1864.
50. Honig, A.; Weidler, C.; Hausler, S.; Krockenberger, M.; Buchholz, S.; Koster, F.; Segerer, S.E.; Dietl, J.; Engel, J.B. Overexpression of polycomb protein BMI-1 in human specimens of breast, Ovarian, endometrial and cervical cancer. *Anticancer Res.* **2010**, *30*, 1559–1564.
51. Min, L.; Dong-Xiang, S.; Xiao-Tong, G.; Ting, G.; Xiao-Dong, C. Clinicopathological and prognostic significance of Bmi-1 expression in human cervical cancer. *Acta Obstet. Gynecol. Scand.* **2011**, *90*, 737–745.
52. Zhang, X.; Wang, C.X.; Zhu, C.B.; Zhang, J.; Kan, S.F.; Du, L.T.; Li, W.; Wang, L.L.; Wang, S. Overexpression of Bmi-1 in uterine cervical cancer: Correlation with clinicopathology and prognosis. *Int. J. Gynecol. Cancer* **2010**, *20*, 1597–1603.
53. Zhang, X.; Wang, C.; Wang, L.; Du, L.; Wang, S.; Zheng, G.; Li, W.; Zhuang, X.; Dong, Z. Detection of circulating Bmi-1 mRNA in plasma and its potential diagnostic and prognostic value for uterine cervical cancer. *Int. J. Cancer* **2012**, *131*, 165–172.
54. Tong, Y.Q.; Liu, B.; Zheng, H.Y.; He, Y.J.; Gu, J.; Li, F.; Li, Y. BMI-1 autoantibody as a new potential biomarker for cervical carcinoma. *PLoS One* **2011**, *6*, e27804.
55. Miller, J.; Dakic, A.; Chen, R.; Palechor-Ceron, N.; Dai, Y.; Kallakury, B.; Schlegel, R.; Liu, X. HPV16 E7 Protein and hTERT proteins defective for telomere maintenance cooperate to immortalize human keratinocytes. *PLoS Pathog.* **2013**, *9*, e1003284.
56. Chen, F.; Li, Y.; Wang, L.; Hu, L. Knockdown of BMI-1 causes cell-cycle arrest and derepresses p16INK4a, HOXA9 and HOXC13 mRNA expression in HeLa cells. *Med. Oncol.* **2011**, *28*, 1201–1209.
57. Greenfield, A.; Carrel, L.; Pennisi, D.; Philippe, C.; Quaderi, N.; Siggers, P.; Steiner, K.; Tam, P.P.; Monaco, A.P.; Willard, H.F.; *et al.* The UTX gene escapes X inactivation in mice and humans. *Hum. Mol. Genet.* **1998**, *7*, 737–742.

58. Shpargel, K.B.; Sengoku, T.; Yokoyama, S.; Magnuson, T. UTX and UTY demonstrate histone demethylase-independent function in mouse embryonic development. *PLoS Genet.* **2012**, *8*, e1002964.
59. Lee, S.; Lee, J.W.; Lee, S.K. UTX, a histone H3-lysine 27 demethylase, acts as a critical switch to activate the cardiac developmental program. *Dev. Cell* **2012**, *22*, 25–37.
60. Welstead, G.G.; Creyghton, M.P.; Bilodeau, S.; Cheng, A.W.; Markoulaki, S.; Young, R.A.; Jaenisch, R. X-linked H3K27me3 demethylase Utx is required for embryonic development in a sex-specific manner. *Proc. Natl. Acad. Sci. USA* **2012**, *109*, 13004–13009.
61. Wang, C.; Lee, J.E.; Cho, Y.W.; Xiao, Y.; Jin, Q.; Liu, C.; Ge, K. UTX regulates mesoderm differentiation of embryonic stem cells independent of H3K27 demethylase activity. *Proc. Natl. Acad. Sci. USA* **2012**, *109*, 15324–15329.
62. Burgold, T.; Voituron, N.; Caganova, M.; Tripathi, P.P.; Menuet, C.; Tusi, B.K.; Spreafico, F.; Bevengut, M.; Gestreau, C.; Buontempo, S.; *et al*. The H3K27 demethylase JMJD3 is required for maintenance of the embryonic respiratory neuronal network, Neonatal breathing, and survival. *Cell Rep.* **2012**, *2*, 1244–1258.
63. De Santa, F.; Totaro, M.G.; Prosperini, E.; Notarbartolo, S.; Testa, G.; Natoli, G. The histone H3 lysine-27 demethylase Jmjd3 links inflammation to inhibition of polycomb-mediated gene silencing. *Cell* **2007**, *130*, 1083–1094.
64. De Santa, F.; Narang, V.; Yap, Z.H.; Tusi, B.K.; Burgold, T.; Austenaa, L.; Bucci, G.; Caganova, M.; Notarbartolo, S.; Casola, S.; *et al*. Jmjd3 contributes to the control of gene expression in LPS-activated macrophages. *EMBO* **2009**, *28*, 3341–3352.
65. Lee, M.G.; Villa, R.; Trojer, P.; Norman, J.; Yan, K.P.; Reinberg, D.; Di Croce, L.; Shiekhattar, R. Demethylation of H3K27 regulates polycomb recruitment and H2A ubiquitination. *Science* **2007**, *318*, 447–450.
66. Issaeva, I.; Zonis, Y.; Rozovskaia, T.; Orlovsky, K.; Croce, C.M.; Nakamura, T.; Mazo, A.; Eisenbach, L.; Canaani, E. Knockdown of ALR (MLL2) reveals ALR target genes and leads to alterations in cell adhesion and growth. *Mol. Cell Biol.* **2007**, *27*, 1889–1903.
67. van Haaften, G.; Dalgliesh, G.L.; Davies, H.; Chen, L.; Bignell, G.; Greenman, C.; Edkins, S.; Hardy, C.; O'Meara, S.; Teague, J.; *et al*. Somatic mutations of the histone H3K27 demethylase gene UTX in human cancer. *Nat. Genet.* **2009**, *41*, 521–523.
68. Xiang, Y.; Zhu, Z.; Han, G.; Lin, H.; Xu, L.; Chen, C.D. JMJD3 is a histone H3K27 demethylase. *Cell Res.* **2007**, *17*, 850–857.
69. Sen, G.L.; Webster, D.E.; Barragan, D.I.; Chang, H.Y.; Khavari, P.A. Control of differentiation in a self-renewing mammalian tissue by the histone demethylase JMJD3. *Gene. Develop.* **2008**, *22*, 1865–1870.
70. Serrano, M.; Lin, A.W.; McCurrach, M.E.; Beach, D.; Lowe, S.W. Oncogenic ras provokes premature cell senescence associated with accumulation of p53 and p16INK4a. *Cell* **1997**, *88*, 593–602.
71. Barradas, M.; Anderton, E.; Acosta, J.C.; Li, S.; Banito, A.; Rodriguez-Niedenfuhr, M.; Maertens, G.; Banck, M.; Zhou, M.M.; Walsh, M.J.; *et al*. Histone demethylase JMJD3 contributes to epigenetic control of INK4a/ARF by oncogenic RAS. *Gene. Develop.* **2009**, *23*, 1177–1182.

72. Agger, K.; Cloos, P.A.; Rudkjaer, L.; Williams, K.; Andersen, G.; Christensen, J.; Helin, K. The H3K27me3 demethylase JMJD3 contributes to the activation of the INK4A-ARF locus in response to oncogene- and stress-induced senescence. *Gene. Develop.* **2009**, *23*, 1171–1176.
73. Sano, T.; Oyama, T.; Kashiwabara, K.; Fukuda, T.; Nakajima, T. Expression status of p16 protein is associated with human papillomavirus oncogenic potential in cervical and genital lesions. *Amer. J. Pathol.* **1998**, *153*, 1741–1748.
74. Klaes, R.; Friedrich, T.; Spitkovsky, D.; Ridder, R.; Rudy, W.; Petry, U.; Dallenbach-Hellweg, G.; Schmidt, D.; von Knebel Doeberitz, M. Overexpression of p16(INK4A) as a specific marker for dysplastic and neoplastic epithelial cells of the cervix uteri. *Int. J. Cancer* **2001**, *92*, 276–284.
75. Khleif, S.N.; DeGregori, J.; Yee, C.L.; Otterson, G.A.; Kaye, F.J.; Nevins, J.R.; Howley, P.M. Inhibition of cyclin D-CDK4/CDK6 activity is associated with an E2F-mediated induction of cyclin kinase inhibitor activity. *Proc. Natl. Acad. Sci. USA* **1996**, *93*, 4350–4354.
76. Gonzalez, S.L.; Stremlau, M.; He, X.; Basile, J.R.; Münger, K. Degradation of the retinoblastoma tumor suppressor by the human papillomavirus type 16 E7 oncoprotein is important for functional inactivation and is separable from proteasomal degradation of E7. *J. Virol.* **2001**, *75*, 7583–7591.
77. Skalska, L.; White, R.E.; Parker, G.A.; Sinclair, A.J.; Paschos, K.; Allday, M.J. Induction of p16(INK4a) is the major barrier to proliferation when Epstein-Barr Virus (EBV) transforms primary B cells into lymphoblastoid cell lines. *PLoS Pathog.* **2013**, *9*, e1003187.
78. Skalska, L.; White, R.E.; Franz, M.; Ruhmann, M.; Allday, M.J. Epigenetic repression of p16(INK4A) by latent Epstein-Barr virus requires the interaction of EBNA3A and EBNA3C with CtBP. *PLoS Pathog.* **2010**, *6*, e1000951.
79. White, R.E.; Groves, I.J.; Turro, E.; Yee, J.; Kremmer, E.; Allday, M.J. Extensive co-operation between the Epstein-Barr virus EBNA3 proteins in the manipulation of host gene expression and epigenetic chromatin modification. *PLoS One* **2010**, *5*, e13979.
80. Paschos, K.; Parker, G.A.; Watanatanasup, E.; White, R.E.; Allday, M.J. BIM promoter directly targeted by EBNA3C in polycomb-mediated repression by EBV. *Nucleic Acids Res.* **2012**, *40*, 7233–7246.
81. Andrisani, O.M. Deregulation of epigenetic mechanisms by the hepatitis B virus x protein in hepatocarcinogenesis. *Viruses* **2013**, *5*, 858–872.
82. Herschkowitz, J.I.; He, X.; Fan, C.; Perou, C.M. The functional loss of the retinoblastoma tumour suppressor is a common event in basal-like and luminal B breast carcinomas. *Breast Cancer Res.* **2008**, *10*, R75.
83. Jarrard, D.F.; Modder, J.; Fadden, P.; Fu, V.; Sebree, L.; Heisey, D.; Schwarze, S.R.; Friedl, A. Alterations in the p16/pRb cell cycle checkpoint occur commonly in primary and metastatic human prostate cancer. *Cancer Lett.* **2002**, *185*, 191–199.
84. Kommoss, S.; du Bois, A.; Ridder, R.; Trunk, M.J.; Schmidt, D.; Pfisterer, J.; Kommoss, F. Independent prognostic significance of cell cycle regulator proteins p16(INK4a) and pRb in advanced-stage ovarian carcinoma including optimally debulked patients: a translational research subprotocol of a randomised study of the Arbeitsgemeinschaft Gynaekologische Onkologie Ovarian Cancer Study Group. *Br. J. Cancer* **2007**, *96*, 306–313.

85. Andujar, P.; Wang, J.; Descatha, A.; Galateau-Salle, F.; Abd-Alsamad, I.; Billon-Galland, M.A.; Blons, H.; Clin, B.; Danel, C.; Housset, B.; *et al.* p16INK4A inactivation mechanisms in non-small-cell lung cancer patients occupationally exposed to asbestos. *Lung Cancer* **2010**, *67*, 23–30.
86. Malumbres, M.; Barbacid, M. To cycle or not to cycle: a critical decision in cancer. *Nat. Rev. Cancer* **2001**, *1*, 222–231.
87. Horner, S.M.; DeFilippis, R.A.; Manuelidis, L.; DiMaio, D. Repression of the human papillomavirus E6 gene initiates p53-dependent, Telomerase-independent senescence and apoptosis in HeLa cervical carcinoma cells. *J. Virol.* **2004**, *78*, 4063–4073.
88. Psyrri, A.; DeFilippis, R.A.; Edwards, A.P.; Yates, K.E.; Manuelidis, L.; DiMaio, D. Role of the retinoblastoma pathway in senescence triggered by repression of the human papillomavirus E7 protein in cervical carcinoma cells. *Cancer Res.* **2004**, *64*, 3079–3086.
89. DeFilippis, R.A.; Goodwin, E.C.; Wu, L.; DiMaio, D. Endogenous human papillomavirus E6 and E7 proteins differentially regulate proliferation, senescence, and apoptosis in HeLa cervical carcinoma cells. *J. Virol.* **2003**, *77*, 1551–1563.
90. Westbrook, T.F.; Martin, E.S.; Schlabach, M.R.; Leng, Y.; Liang, A.C.; Feng, B.; Zhao, J.J.; Roberts, T.M.; Mandel, G.; Hannon, G.J.; *et al.* A genetic screen for candidate tumor suppressors identifies REST. *Cell* **2005**, *121*, 837–848.
91. Coulson, J.M.; Edgson, J.L.; Woll, P.J.; Quinn, J.P. A splice variant of the neuron-restrictive silencer factor repressor is expressed in small cell lung cancer: A potential role in derepression of neuroendocrine genes and a useful clinical marker. *Cancer Res.* **2000**, *60*, 1840–1844.
92. Westbrook, T.F.; Hu, G.; Ang, X.L.; Mulligan, P.; Pavlova, N.N.; Liang, A.; Leng, Y.; Maehr, R.; Shi, Y.; Harper, J.W.; *et al.* SCFbeta-TRCP controls oncogenic transformation and neural differentiation through REST degradation. *Nature* **2008**, *452*, 370–374.
93. Kruidenier, L.; Chung, C.W.; Cheng, Z.; Liddle, J.; Che, K.; Joberty, G.; Bantscheff, M.; Bountra, C.; Bridges, A.; Diallo, H.; *et al.* A selective jumonji H3K27 demethylase inhibitor modulates the proinflammatory macrophage response. *Nature* **2012**, *488*, 404–408.

6

Bromodomain Proteins in HIV Infection

Daniela Boehm [1,2,†], **Ryan J. Conrad** [1,2,†] **and Melanie Ott** [1,2,*]

[1] Gladstone Institute of Virology and Immunology, San Francisco, CA 94158, USA;
E-Mails: daniela.boehm@gladstone.ucsf.edu (D.B.); Ryan.Conrad@ucsf.edu (R.J.C.)

[2] Department of Medicine, University of California, San Francisco, CA 94158, USA

† These authors contributed equally to this work.

* Author to whom correspondence should be addressed; E-Mail: mott@gladstone.ucsf.edu;

Abstract: Bromodomains are conserved protein modules of ~110 amino acids that bind acetylated lysine residues in histone and non-histone proteins. Bromodomains are present in many chromatin-associated transcriptional regulators and have been linked to diverse aspects of the HIV life cycle, including transcription and integration. Here, we review the role of bromodomain-containing proteins in HIV infection. We begin with a focus on acetylated viral factors, followed by a discussion of structural and biological studies defining the involvement of bromodomain proteins in the HIV life cycle. We end with an overview of promising new studies of bromodomain inhibitory compounds for the treatment of HIV latency.

Keywords: bromodomains; HIV; PCAF; PBAF; p300; CBP; TRIM28; BRD2; BRD4

---

1. The Bromodomain Protein Family

Reversible modifications of nucleosome components are increasingly acknowledged for their regulatory potential [1]. One such modification is acetylation, which involves the transfer of an acetyl group from acetyl-coenzyme A (acetyl-CoA) to the ε-amino group of lysine side chains on histone and non-histone proteins [2,3]. This modification is catalyzed by lysine acetyltransferases (KATs, also known as HATs), whose action is reversed by lysine deacetylases (KDACS, also known as HDACs) or sirtuins (SIRTs). Histone acetylation is a well-studied modification that antagonizes the nucleosomal DNA-protein interaction, promoting chromatin accessibility and transcriptional activation [4]. However, aside from causing physiochemical changes in the nucleosome core, acetylation also generates novel and unique interaction interfaces for the assembly of macromolecular complexes important for a variety of cellular processes.

The bromodomain is a conserved protein module of ~110 amino acids that recognizes and binds ε-*N*-acetylated lysine residues in histone and non-histone proteins [5,6]. Recognition of acetyl-lysine residues by bromodomain-containing proteins is at least partly responsible for the functional consequences linked to protein acetylation. The first reference to a bromodomain can be traced to the Drosophila gene *brahma* (*brm*) [7], and the human bromodomain family to date includes 46 distinct proteins and 61 unique bromodomains (Figure 1A) [8]. Select transcriptional regulators (*i.e.*, BRD4, TAF1, TIF1), chromatin-modifying enzymes (*i.e.*, p300, PCAF, MLL), and nucleosome remodelers (*i.e.*, SMARAC2, PB1, BAZ1B) contain bromodomains [6].

Structurally, bromodomains are comprised of four left-handed α-helices (αZ, αA, αB, and αC) connected by two loops (ZA and BC loops) (Figure 1B) [5]. This structure forms a deep hydrophobic cavity that serves as the acetyl-lysine recognition site [8]. While the helical regions are moderately conserved among different bromodomains, the loop regions are highly variable in both length and sequence composition [8]. This loop variability guides the substrate specificity observed among members of the bromodomain family. Co-crystal structures of bromodomains with various acetylated peptides demonstrate that the neutralized acetyl-lysine residue forms a hydrogen bond with an asparagine residue found in most bromodomains (Figure 1C). Some bromodomains exhibit higher affinity for multiply acetylated substrates, while the affinities of others are regulated by additional post-translational modifications of the ligand, such as phosphorylation [8,9].

2. HIV Infection and Reversible Acetylation

Reversible acetylation of histone and non-histone proteins plays a key role in HIV transcription and is a lead target in preclinical and clinical efforts to reverse HIV latency [10–14]. Upon integration into the human genome, the HIV proviral cDNA is organized into higher-order chromatin and becomes subject to regulation by host chromatin-modifying enzymes, including acetyltransferases and deacetylases [15]. Indeed, it has been shown that following stimulation with phorbol esters, distinct lysines in histone H3 (H3K9 and H3K14) become rapidly acetylated within a single nucleosome (nuc-1) located immediately downstream of the viral transcription start site [16]. However, the HIV provirus differs from cellular genes because it encodes a viral protein called transactivator of transcription (Tat). Tat is essential for HIV replication. It relieves a powerful block to the elongation of HIV transcripts by cooperatively binding to (1) an RNA stem-loop structure called TAR present at the 5' end of all nascent viral transcripts and (2) the positive transcription elongation factor b (P-TEFb), which together with other elongation factors, including PAF1c, forms a "super-elongation complex" [17,18].

Additionally, Tat is known to recruit several acetyltransferases to the HIV LTR, thus enhancing HIV transcription in the context of chromatin. These include KAT3B/EP300/p300 [19], KAT3A/CREBBP/CBP [19], KAT2A/GCN5 [16], and KAT2B/PCAF [16]. Conversely, several HDACs have been shown to bind to the HIV promoter located in the 5' long terminal repeat (LTR) through interactions with cellular transcription factors, including YY1 [20], LSF [20], NF-κB [21], AP-4 [22], CBF-1 [23], c-Myc and Sp1 [24]. HDAC inhibitors, which are known to activate HIV from latency in cell culture models [25], are being clinically tested for their potential to reactivate HIV from transcriptional latency [10].

Figure 1. The human bromodomain family. (**A**) Phylogenetic tree of 57 human bromodomains. Those bromodomain-containing proteins that have been shown to interact with HIV proteins are denoted in red with the corresponding viral factor indicated alongside. Phylogenetic trees were generated using Seaview v4.4.1 with individual bromodomain sequences obtained from [23]. (**B**) Structure of the first bromodomain of BRD4 (purple) in complex with a diacetylated histone peptide (blue). Histone acetyllysine residues are shown in yellow. Structural representations in (B,**C**) were rendered using Chimera (UCSF) with PDB: 3UVW (**C**) Top view of interaction between first bromodomain of BRD4 and a diacetylated histone peptide. The hydrogen bond between the canonical bromodomain asparagine residue (N140 in BRD4) and the histone acetyllysine residue is shown in red with an estimated length of 2.94A.

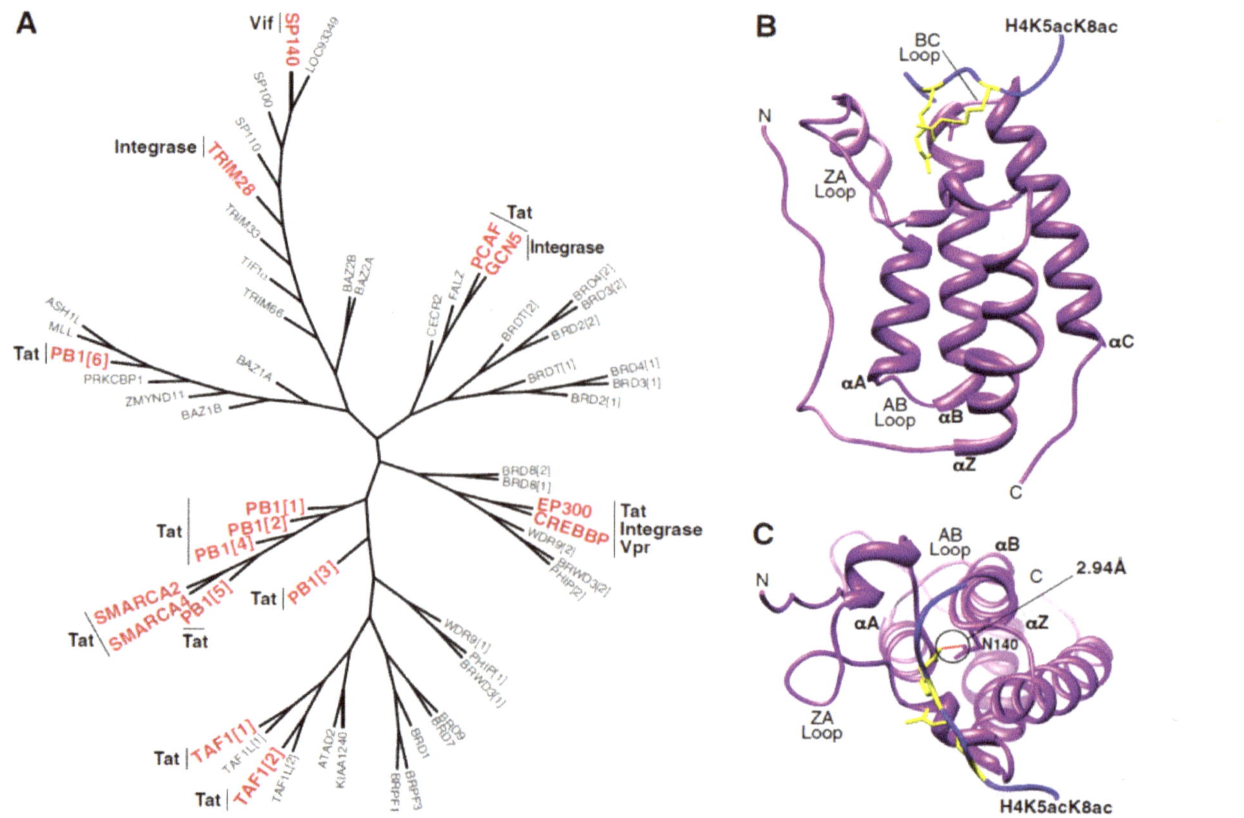

Tat itself is subject to reversible acetylation. Tat is acetylated by KAT2B/PCAF at lysine 28 within a characteristic cysteine-rich region required for its interaction with P-TEFb [26]. Tat is also acetylated by KAT3B/EP300/p300 and the close KAT2B/PCAF homologue KAT2A/GCN5 at lysines 50 and 51 located in its basic RNA-binding domain [26–28]. Both acetylation events positively support Tat's transcriptional activity [29,30] and are reversed by the deacetylase activities of HDAC6 and SIRT1 [31,32]. In addition to Tat, HIV integrase, a DNA-binding protein that catalyzes 3' processing and strand transfer of the viral genome, is acetylated by KAT3B/EP300/p300 at lysines 264, 266 and 273 [33]. These residues are also subject to acetylation by KAT2A/GCN5, in addition to lysine 258 [34]. Integrase acetylation increases the affinity of the enzyme for DNA and also enhances strand-transfer catalysis *in vitro*. Lastly, Vpr, a viral protein implicated in nuclear translocation of the HIV pre-integration complex, HIV-mediated G_2/M arrest, and transcription of viral and cellular promoters, interacts with KAT3B/EP300/p300 [35]. Mutational analysis suggests that the Vpr-p300 interaction occurs independently of the p300 bromodomain [35], and it is unclear whether Vpr is acetylated.

3. Interactions between Bromodomain-Containing Proteins and HIV Proteins

3.1. Acetylation-Dependent Interactions

3.1.1. p300/CBP-Associated Factor (PCAF)

KAT2B/PCAF (p300/CBP-associated factor) is a histone acetyltransferase that contains a *N*-acetyltransferase domain and a *C*-terminal bromodomain. KAT2B/PCAF also participates in the reversible acetylation of various non-histone proteins, including p53, β-catenin, retinoblastoma protein (Rb), and several transcriptional regulators, such as the general transcription factors $TF_{II}E\beta$ and $TF_{II}F$ and the sequence-specific transcription factors E2F1, c-Myc, and MyoD (reviewed in [36]) [37]. In HIV infection, KAT2B/PCAF acetylates Tat at lysine 28 [26,38]. Acetylation of Tat on lysine 28 facilitates recruitment of P-TEFb kinase, resulting in the efficient phosphorylation of the heptad repeats in the carboxyl terminus of cellular RNA polymerase II and thus promoting HIV transcript elongation [26,29,38]. KAT2B/PCAF is recruited to Tat through an acetylation-dependent mechanism (Figure 2). Acetylated K50 in Tat acts as a specific binding partner of the KAT2B/PCAF bromodomain, an interaction that was examined by NMR spectroscopy at the structural level and characteristically involves additional residues in Tat that interact with the KAT2B/PCAF bromodomain in an acetylated K50-dependent manner [39,40]. KAT2B/PCAF binding to Tat positively supports HIV transcription either through enhanced lysine 28 acetylation in Tat, or enhanced local histone acetylation during HIV transcriptional elongation. Consequently, mutations in the KAT2B/PCAF bromodomain that suppress interactions with acetylated Tat or treatment with small molecules that specifically bind the KAT2B/PCAF bromodomain effectively suppress Tat transactivation, supporting the concept that this interaction could serve as a specific target for anti-HIV transcription therapeutics [39,41].

3.1.2. SWItch/Sucrose Non-Fermentable (SWI/SNF)

Members of the SWI/SNF family form evolutionarily conserved chromatin-remodeling complexes that utilize the energy of ATP hydrolysis to induce nucleosome remodeling. Two important and distinct SWI/SNF complexes have been described in humans: BAF and PBAF. These complexes contain either Brg-1 (also known at SMARCA4) or BRM (also known at SMARCA2) as the major catalytic subunit together with several accessory proteins. BAF is distinguished by the presence of the BAF250a/b subunit, while PBAF contains BAF180 (also known as Polybromo or PB1), BAF200, and BRD7 subunits. BAF has been shown to repress HIV transcription by positioning the nuc-1 nucleosome immediately downstream of the transcription start site in a manner that encumbers processive transcription [42]. Such repressive remodeling events may be crucial for the maintenance of HIV latency in the absence of Tat. Conversely, the PBAF complex is required for robust Tat-mediated transactivation of HIV expression [43,44]. Both shared constituents of BAF and PBAF, Brg-1 and BRM, interact with Tat. These interactions are regulated by acetylation of Tat, with K50 acetylation enhancing the Tat-Brg1 interaction [45] and inhibiting the Tat-BRM interaction [46]. The interaction between acetylated Tat and Brg-1 was mapped to the Brg-1 bromodomain, while the Tat-BRM interaction was shown to be bromodomain-independent [46]. Tat displays enhanced interaction with the PBAF-specific constituent BAF200 in a K50/K51-dependent manner [47]. In addition, Tat acetylated at K50/K51 interacts with PBAF through the BAF180 subunit, an interaction that facilitates Tat-mediated transactivation (Figure 2) [42]. It is likely, though not experimentally confirmed, that acetylated Tat interacts with one or more of the six bromodomains present in BAF180. These findings evoke a model in which Tat acetylation at K50/K51 functions to switch the repressive BAF complex with the activating PBAF complex through specific interactions with several bromodomain-containing proteins in the PBAF complex, including Brg-1 and BAF180.

3.1.3. Bromodomain-Containing Protein 4 (BRD4)

BRD4 is a mitotic chromosome-associated protein that serves as an important regulator of post-mitotic transcription by recruiting various transcriptional regulators to acetylated chromatin. BRD4 is also required for maintaining a proper higher-order chromatin structure [48–50]. BRD4 is a member of the bromodomain and extraterminal domain (BET) family of bromodomain proteins. Members of the BET family are distinguished by the presence of two functional domains—tandem bromodomains and a so-called extraterminal domain, the latter of which may serve to mediate protein-protein interactions [49]. BRD4 contains a third functional domain termed the P-TEFb-interacting domain (PID) [51]. The PID serves to recruit and activate the Tat cofactor P-TEFb, a heterodimer composed of cyclin T1 and CDK9 that when complexed with the HEXIM1 inhibitor is part of an inactive ribonucleoprotein complex found in HeLa cells and other tumor cell lines [52,53]. While BRD4 is an important factor recruiting P-TEFb to the HIV promoter in the absence of Tat, Tat and the BRD4 PID compete for P-TEFb binding, making BRD4 a negative factor in Tat transactivation [51,54]. In addition, BRD4 negatively regulates HIV transcription by inducing an inhibitory phosphorylation event on CDK9 [55].

The cyclin T1 subunit of P-TEFb is acetylated at four defined residues by KAT3B/p300 [56]. Three of the four acetylated residues (K380, K386, K390) bind the second bromodomain of BRD4 defining a second acetylation-dependent P-TEFb interaction site in BRD4 besides the PID. Interestingly, while this acetylation-dependent interaction is required for basal HIV LTR activity and cellular gene expression, it is not necessary for Tat-mediated transactivation of HIV transcription, supporting the model that Tat- and BRD4-mediated activities at the HIV promoter are mutually exclusive [51,54]. Vollmuth *et al.* determined the crystal structures of the two bromodomains of BRD4 and showed that acetylated K390 weakly bound to the second bromodomain of BRD4 [57]. This binding is markedly enhanced when K380 and K386 are also acetylated [52], supporting an emerging model that bromodomains of BET proteins have a preference for binding to multiply acetylated proteins.

3.1.4. Tripartite Motif-Containing Protein 28 (TRIM28)

TRIM28 was originally identified as an interaction partner of members of the family of Krüppel-associated box (KRAB) domain-containing zinc finger transcription factors. It is also named KRAB-associated protein 1 (KAP1), KRAB-A-interacting protein 1 (KRIP1), and transcription intermediary factor (TIF) 1β. Its protein architecture includes an *N*-terminal tripartite motif (TRIM) that acts as a protein-protein and oligomerization interface, and contains a RBCC (Ring finger, two B-box zinc fingers, and a coiled coil) domain, a central heterochromatin protein 1 (HP1)-binding domain, a TIF1 signature sequence (TSS) domain, and a *C*-terminal plant homeodomain (PHD) and bromodomain. The TRIM28 bromodomain is a 100-amino acid stretch consisting of four α-helices that, similar to other bromodomain-containing proteins, has a conserved hydrophobic core and recognizes the backbone of histone tails [58]. Structural analysis of the tandem PHD and bromodomain (PB) of TRIM28 between amino acids 624 and 812 revealed that both domains function as a cooperative unit to facilitate lysine sumoylation, which is required for TRIM28 co-repressor activity in gene silencing [58]. In a yeast two-hybrid screen, TRIM28 was identified as an interaction partner of acetylated HIV-1 integrase [59]. TRIM28 *in vitro* and *in vivo* preferentially binds integrase when acetylated at K264, K266 and K273, rather than the unmodified protein, implicating that this interaction is mediated by the TRIM28 bromodomain. Integrase K264, K266 and K273 are targeted for acetylation by KAT3B/p300, which is a prerequisite for the interaction of TRIM28 with integrase and leads to subsequent recruitment of HDAC1. As a consequence, TRIM28 inhibits HIV-1 integration through integrase deacetylation by HDAC1 (Figure 2) [60].

Figure 2. Role of bromodomain proteins in HIV infection. Bromodomain proteins implicated in HIV transcription, HIV integration, and cell cycle progression are schematized. Briefly, acetylated integrase displays enhanced enzymatic activity, yet generates an interaction interface for the TRIM28 bromodomain that in turn recruits the HDAC1 deacetylase, negatively impacting HIV integration. With respect to viral transcription, Tat acetylated at K50/51 interacts with BAF180 and Brg-1 within the PBAF complex to support viral transcription. Acetylated Tat also interacts with p300/CBP-Associated Factor (PCAF) to induce local acetylation of histones and potentially other factors at the site of viral transcription. BRD4 is present at the HIV long terminal repeat (LTR), yet is hypothesized as an intracellular competitor of Tat, while the role of BRD2 in HIV transcription is unknown. Tat also interacts with TAF1 to repress select cellular promoters. BRD4 and SP140 are both cell cycle regulators that interact with Vif, yet the bromodomain-dependence and functional significance of these interactions remain unclear.

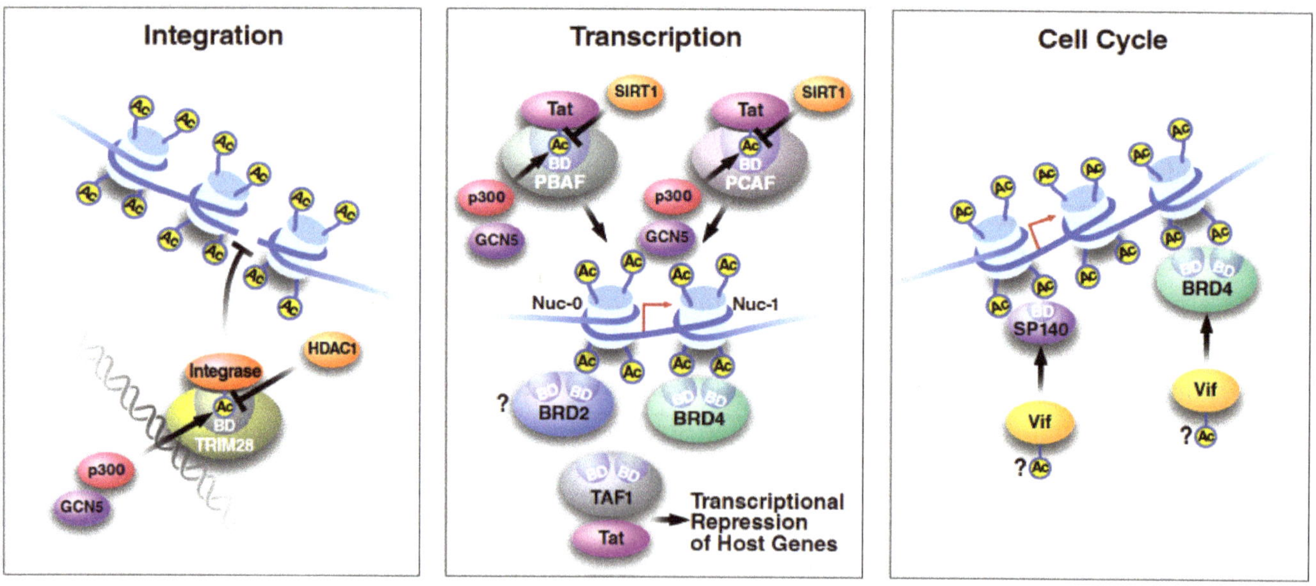

3.2. Other Interactions with Bromodomain-Containing Proteins

3.2.1. Transcription Initiation Factor TFIID, Subunit 1 (TAF1)

TAF1, also referred to as $TAF_{II}250$, is the largest component of transcription factor TFIID that is composed of TATA-binding protein (TBP) and a variety of TBP-associated factors. TAF1 contains *N*- and *C*-terminal serine/threonine kinase domains, but can also function as an acetyltransferase and an ubiquitin-activating/conjugating enzyme. It contains two tandem bromodomains, both located in the *C*-terminus of the protein. Structurally, the two bromodomains form two side-by-side, four-helix bundles, each with an acetyl lysine binding pocket at its center, recognized by diacetylated histone H4 peptides [61]. When Weissman *et al.* identified TAF1 as a Tat interaction partner, the interaction was mapped to amino acids 80 to 83 in Tat and a site in TAF1 that overlaps the acetyltransferase domain, inhibiting TAF1 acetyltransferase activity [62]. TAF1 was not required for Tat transactivation of the HIV LTR; instead, the interaction with TAF1 was linked to Tat-mediated transcriptional repression, *i.e.*, of the MHC class I promoter (Figure 2) [62]. These findings could be explained by a model in which the interaction with Tat inhibits TAF1 acetyltransferase activity, thereby recruiting an inactive Tat/TAF1 complex to actively transcribing gene promoters containing hyperacetylated histone H4.

3.2.2. Nuclear Body Protein SP140

SP140, also referred to as lymphoid-restricted homolog of Sp100 (LYSp100) is a component of a subset of nuclear bodies in lymphoid cells. It is involved in the pathogenesis of acute promyelocytic leukemia and has been shown to be an autoantigen in primary biliary cirrhosis [63–65]. Its protein architecture includes a *N*-terminal homogeneous staining region (HSR) domain, a central SAND domain which mediates DNA binding, a PHD-type zinc finger, and a *C*-terminal bromodomain. In a yeast two-hybrid screen, SP140 was identified as an interaction partner of the HIV Vif protein [66]. Vif enhances the infectivity of HIV virions released from so-called non-permissive cells by inducing the degradation of an antiviral restriction factor APOBEC3G [67]. SP140 was found specifically in non-permissive cells, and HIV-1 infection induced its dispersal from nuclear bodies into cytosolic colocalization with Vif [66]. SP140 interacts with the N-terminal and central regions of Vif (amino acids 1–112) in the yeast two-hybrid screen, and the SP140 prey cDNAs that were isolated encoded the *C*-terminal region between amino acids 527 and 836, which includes the SAND domain, the PHD-type zinc finger, and the bromodomain [66]. Further studies are needed to determine whether an acetyl-lysine-bromodomain interaction is involved in the interaction between Vif and SP140.

3.2.3. BRD2

BRD2, formerly named RING3 (really interesting new gene 3) or Fshrgl (female sterile homeotic related gene 1), is a nuclear serine/threonine kinase possessing chromatin binding and transcription activity. Along with BRD4, BRD2 is a member of the BET family, but lacks a *C*-terminal PID domain.

However, BRD2 was found to coimmunoprecipitate with CDK9/Cyclin T1 or Cyclin T2 [68]. BRD2 also functions as a Tat-independent suppressor of HIV transcription in latent cells [69]. In cell lines containing latent HIV, lentiviral shRNA-mediated depletion of BRD2 resulted in activation of the HIV LTR, and this effect was independent of Tat. The fact that BRD2 is known to bind co-repressor complexes including HDACs [70] supports a model whereby BRD2, by recruiting repressor complexes to the latent HIV LTR, directly suppresses HIV transcription. It remains to be seen whether BRD2, like BRD4, interacts with P-TEFb in an acetylation-dependent manner.

3.2.4. BRD4

In addition to its role in HIV transcription, BRD4 has been implicated in Vif-mediated cell-cycle progression. By mass spectrometry, Wang *et al.* identified BRD4 and CDK9 as Vif interactors required for Vif-mediated acceleration of cell-cycle transition from the G_1-to-S phase [71]. BRD4 also regulates the G_2-to-M transition and stimulates cell-cycle progression from G_1 to S through recruitment of P-TEFb to chromosomes and stimulation of G_1 gene expression during late mitosis [72,73]. It is unknown whether the Vif-BRD4 interaction involves the BRD4 bromodomains.

4. Bromodomain Inhibitors and HIV Infection

The characteristic architecture of the bromodomain-acetyl-lysine interface represents a potential target for the development of small-molecule inhibitors. In initial attempts to identify bromodomain inhibitors, NMR-based screens of commercial compound libraries were used to identify compounds that inhibit Tat transactivation at the Tat-PCAF interface [41]. Two lead compounds were discovered using this approach, both with relatively low IC_{50} values for the Tat-PCAF interaction *in vitro*. Recently, several high-affinity binding molecules for bromodomains of the BET family were described [74–78]. JQ1, a thienodiazepine derived from a BRD4 ligand developed by Mitsubishi Pharmaceuticals [79], was shown to bind the first bromodomain of BRD4 with high affinity and target the second bromodomain of BRD4, and those of BRD2, BRD3, and BRDT [75]. MS417, a BET inhibitor derived from JQ1, specifically targets the interaction between BRD4 and the acetylated p65/RelA subunit of the transcription factor NF-κB and has potent anti-inflammatory effects in a mouse model of HIV-associated kidney disease [78]. I-BET, a synthetic "histone mimic" identified using an ApoA1 reporter system, also functions as a potent anti-inflammatory agent that suppresses expression of pro-inflammatory genes in activated macrophages and confers protection against lipopolysaccharide-induced endotoxic shock and bacteria-induced sepsis [76]. These and other compounds are excellent tools to study BET protein function, but have also shown impressive preclinical promise for the treatment of the NUT midline carcinoma (JQ1, [75]), specific types of leukemia (JQ1 [80], I-BET151 [77]) inflammation (I-BET [76], MS417 [78]), and viral infections, including HIV.

Current antiretroviral therapy only suppresses viral replication, requiring life-long adherence to continuously limit viral loads, but does not eradicate virus from most infected people. Therefore, novel treatments that eliminate persistent viral reservoirs and thereby cure patients are needed. One approach is to reactivate proviral genomes in latently infected cells in order to "purge" viral reservoirs, either through the immune system or through the cytopathic effects associated with viral reactivation. HDAC inhibitors, including valproic acid and vorinostat (SAHA), show great promise as anti-latency therapeutics and have already begun to be tested in clinical trials [10,11,81,82]. Recently, a flood of publications demonstrated that BET bromodomain inhibitors reactivate HIV from latency in cell lines and primary T-cell models (summarized in Table 1). Notably, cells treated with drugs like JQ1 show little synergy with vorinostat, indicating that both drugs target similar pathways in HIV reactivation. However, it is unclear whether any of the current *ex vivo* models faithfully recapitulates the *in vivo* situation of latently infected cells; further studies are needed to evaluate the clinical potential of BET inhibitors in primary T cells.

Table 1. Selected reported bromodomain inhibitors tested in models of HIV latency.

Compound	Model of HIV latency	Effect	Reference
JQ1	Ach2	reactivation	[83]
JQ1	U1	reactivation	
JQ1	J-Lat 10.6	reactivation	
JQ1	Acutely infected primary $CD4^+$ cells	reactivation	
JQ1	JΔK	reactivation	[84]
JQ1	J-Lat A2	reactivation	[85]
JQ1	Jurkat 1G5	reactivation	
JQ1	HeLa NH1 and NH2	reactivation	
JQ1	HeLa-T4	reactivation	[86]
JQ1	Primary $CD4^+$ T cells	reactivation	
JQ1	Primary $CD4^+$ T cells	inhibition	
JQ1 + Prostratin or PMA	J-Lat 6.3	reactivation	
JQ1 + Prostratin or PMA	J-Lat 8.4	reactivation	
JQ1 + Prostratin or PMA	J-Lat 9.2	reactivation	
JQ1 + Prostratin or PMA	J-Lat 15.4	reactivation	
JQ1	J-Lat A2	reactivation	[87]
JQ1	J-Lat A72	reactivation	
JQ1	infected primary Bc12-transduced $CD4^+$ T cells	reactivation	
JQ1	infected primary nonpolarized T helper cells	no reactivation	
I-BET	infected primary Bc12-transduced $CD4^+$ T cells	reactivation	
I-BET	infected primary nonpolarized T helper cells	no reactivation	
I-Bet151	J-Lat A2	reactivation	
I-Bet151	J-Lat A72	reactivation	
I-Bet151	infected primary Bc12-transduced $CD4^+$ T cells	reactivation	
I-Bet151	infected primary nonpolarized T helper cells	no reactivation	
MS417	J-Lat A2	reactivation	
MS417	J-Lat A72	reactivation	
MS417	infected primary Bc12-transduced $CD4^+$ T cells	reactivation	
MS417	infected primary nonpolarized T helper cells	no reactivation	

5. Concluding Remarks

The acetyl-lysine-bromodomain interface, first therapeutically explored in HIV infection, represents an important regulatory axis that controls many aspects of HIV infection, including viral integration, Tat transactivation, HIV latency, cell-cycle progression of infected host cells, and virally induced inflammation. Furthermore, it is likely that new molecular functions for bromodomain-containing proteins in HIV infection await discovery. We expect that the use of existing and the development of novel bromodomain inhibitors will facilitate both the study and the treatment of HIV infection.

Acknowledgments

We thank John Carroll for assistance with graphics and Gary Howard for editorial assistance. We gratefully acknowledge support from the NIH (R01 AI083139 and CARE Collaboratory (U19AI096113) to M.O.). R.J.C. was supported in part by NIH Training Grant T32 GM007175.

References

1. Bannister, A.J.; Kouzarides, T. Regulation of chromatin by histone modifications. *Cell Res.* **2011**, *21*, 381–395.
2. Yang, X.J.; Seto, E. Lysine acetylation: Codified crosstalk with other posttranslational modifications. *Mol. Cell* **2008**, *31*, 449–461.
3. Choudhary, C.; Kumar, C.; Gnad, F.; Nielsen, M.L.; Rehman, M.; Walther, T.C.; Olsen, J.V.; Mann, M. Lysine acetylation targets protein complexes and co-regulates major cellular functions. *Science* **2009**, *325*, 834–840.
4. Sterner, D.E.; Berger, S.L. Acetylation of histones and transcription-related factors. *Microbiol. Mol. Biol. Rev.* **2000**, *64*, 435–459.
5. Dhalluin, C.; Carlson, J.E.; Zeng, L.; He, C.; Aggarwal, A.K.; Zhou, M.M. Structure and ligand of a histone acetyltransferase bromodomain. *Nature* **1999**, *399*, 491–496.
6. Filippakopoulos, P.; Knapp, S. The bromodomain interaction module. *FEBS Lett.* **2012**, *586*, 2692–2704.
7. Tamkun, J.W.; Deuring, R.; Scott, M.P.; Kissinger, M.; Pattatucci, A.M.; Kaufman, T.C.; Kennison, J.A. Brahma: A regulator of Drosophila homeotic genes structurally related to the yeast transcriptional activator SNF2/SWI2. *Cell* **1992**, *68*, 561–572.
8. Filippakopoulos, P.; Picaud, S.; Mangos, M.; Keates, T.; Lambert, J.P.; Barsyte-Lovejoy, D.; Felletar, I.; Volkmer, R.; Muller, S.; Pawson, T.; *et al.* Histone recognition and large-scale structural analysis of the human bromodomain family. *Cell* **2012**, *149*, 214–231.
9. Moriniere, J.; Rousseaux, S.; Steuerwald, U.; Soler-Lopez, M.; Curtet, S.; Vitte, A.L.; Govin, J.; Gaucher, J.; Sadoul, K.; Hart, D.J.; *et al.* Cooperative binding of two acetylation marks on a histone tail by a single bromodomain. *Nature* **2009**, *461*, 664–668.
10. Archin, N.M.; Liberty, A.L.; Kashuba, A.D.; Choudhary, S.K.; Kuruc, J.D.; Crooks, A.M.; Parker, D.C.; Anderson, E.M.; Kearney, M.F.; Strain, M.C.; *et al.* Administration of vorinostat disrupts HIV-1 latency in patients on antiretroviral therapy. *Nature* **2012**, *487*, 482–485.
11. Kent, S.J.; Reece, J.C.; Petravic, J.; Martyushev, A.; Kramski, M.; de Rose, R.; Cooper, D.A.; Kelleher, A.D.; Emery, S.; Cameron, P.U.; *et al.* The search for an HIV cure: Tackling latent infection. *Lancet Infect. Dis.* **2013**, doi:10.1016/S1473-3099(13)70043-4.
12. Contreras, X.; Schweneker, M.; Chen, C.S.; McCune, J.M.; Deeks, S.G.; Martin, J.; Peterlin, B.M. Suberoylanilide hydroxamic acid reactivates HIV from latently infected cells. *J. Biol. Chem.* **2009**, *284*, 6782–6789.

13. Edelstein, L.C.; Micheva-Viteva, S.; Phelan, B.D.; Dougherty, J.P. Short communication: Activation of latent HIV type 1 gene expression by suberoylanilide hydroxamic acid (SAHA), an HDAC inhibitor approved for use to treat cutaneous T cell lymphoma. *AIDS Res. Hum. Retroviruses* **2009**, *25*, 883–887.
14. Kelly, W.K.; Richon, V.M.; O'Connor, O.; Curley, T.; MacGregor-Curtelli, B.; Tong, W.; Klang, M.; Schwartz, L.; Richardson, S.; Rosa, E.; *et al.* Phase I clinical trial of histone deacetylase inhibitor: Suberoylanilide hydroxamic acid administered intravenously. *Clin. Cancer Res.* **2003**, *9*, 3578–3588.
15. Verdin, E.; Paras, P., Jr.; van Lint, C. Chromatin disruption in the promoter of human immunodeficiency virus type 1 during transcriptional activation. *EMBO J.* **1993**, *12*, 3249–3259.
16. Lusic, M.; Marcello, A.; Cereseto, A.; Giacca, M. Regulation of HIV-1 gene expression by histone acetylation and factor recruitment at the LTR promoter. *EMBO J.* **2003**, *22*, 6550–6561.
17. Sobhian, B.; Laguette, N.; Yatim, A.; Nakamura, M.; Levy, Y.; Kiernan, R.; Benkirane, M. HIV-1 Tat assembles a multifunctional transcription elongation complex and stably associates with the 7SK snRNP. *Mol. Cell* **2010**, *38*, 439–451.
18. He, N.; Liu, M.; Hsu, J.; Xue, Y.; Chou, S.; Burlingame, A.; Krogan, N.J.; Alber, T.; Zhou, Q. HIV-1 Tat and host AFF4 recruit two transcription elongation factors into a bifunctional complex for coordinated activation of HIV-1 transcription. *Mol. Cell* **2010**, *38*, 428–438.
19. Marzio, G.; Tyagi, M.; Gutierrez, M.I.; Giacca, M. HIV-1 tat transactivator recruits p300 and CREB-binding protein histone acetyltransferases to the viral promoter. *Proc. Natl. Acad. Sci. USA* **1998**, *95*, 13519–13524.
20. Coull, J.J.; Romerio, F.; Sun, J.M.; Volker, J.L.; Galvin, K.M.; Davie, J.R.; Shi, Y.; Hansen, U.; Margolis, D.M. The human factors YY1 and LSF repress the human immunodeficiency virus type 1 long terminal repeat via recruitment of histone deacetylase 1. *J. Virol.* **2000**, *74*, 6790–6799.
21. Williams, S.A.; Chen, L.F.; Kwon, H.; Ruiz-Jarabo, C.M.; Verdin, E.; Greene, W.C. NF-kappaB p50 promotes HIV latency through HDAC recruitment and repression of transcriptional initiation. *EMBO J.* **2006**, *25*, 139–149.
22. Imai, K.; Okamoto, T. Transcriptional repression of human immunodeficiency virus type 1 by AP-4. *J. Biol. Chem.* **2006**, *281*, 12495–12505.
23. Tyagi, M.; Karn, J. CBF-1 promotes transcriptional silencing during the establishment of HIV-1 latency. *EMBO J.* **2007**, *26*, 4985–4995.
24. Jiang, G.; Espeseth, A.; Hazuda, D.J.; Margolis, D.M. c-Myc and Sp1 contribute to proviral latency by recruiting histone deacetylase 1 to the human immunodeficiency virus type 1 promoter. *J. Virol.* **2007**, *81*, 10914–10923.
25. Van Lint, C.; Emiliani, S.; Ott, M.; Verdin, E. Transcriptional activation and chromatin remodeling of the HIV-1 promoter in response to histone acetylation. *EMBO J.* **1996**, *15*, 1112–1120.
26. Kiernan, R.E.; Vanhulle, C.; Schiltz, L.; Adam, E.; Xiao, H.; Maudoux, F.; Calomme, C.; Burny, A.; Nakatani, Y.; Jeang, K.T.; *et al.* HIV-1 tat transcriptional activity is regulated by acetylation. *EMBO J.* **1999**, *18*, 6106–6118.
27. Ott, M.; Schnolzer, M.; Garnica, J.; Fischle, W.; Emiliani, S.; Rackwitz, H.R.; Verdin, E. Acetylation of the HIV-1 Tat protein by p300 is important for its transcriptional activity. *Curr. Biol.* **1999**, *9*, 1489–1492.

28. Col, E.; Caron, C.; Seigneurin-Berny, D.; Gracia, J.; Favier, A.; Khochbin, S. The histone acetyltransferase, hGCN5, interacts with and acetylates the HIV transactivator, Tat. *J. Biol. Chem.* **2001**, *276*, 28179–28184.
29. Bres, V.; Kiernan, R.; Emiliani, S.; Benkirane, M. Tat acetyl-acceptor lysines are important for human immunodeficiency virus type-1 replication. *J. Biol. Chem.* **2002**, *277*, 22215–22221.
30. Kaehlcke, K.; Dorr, A.; Hetzer-Egger, C.; Kiermer, V.; Henklein, P.; Schnoelzer, M.; Loret, E.; Cole, P.A.; Verdin, E.; Ott, M. Acetylation of Tat defines a cyclinT1-independent step in HIV transactivation. *Mol. Cell* **2003**, *12*, 167–176.
31. Pagans, S.; Pedal, A.; North, B.J.; Kaehlcke, K.; Marshall, B.L.; Dorr, A.; Hetzer-Egger, C.; Henklein, P.; Frye, R.; McBurney, M.W.; *et al.* SIRT1 regulates HIV transcription via Tat deacetylation. *PLoS Biol.* **2005**, *3*, e41.
32. Huo, L.; Li, D.; Sun, X.; Shi, X.; Karna, P.; Yang, W.; Liu, M.; Qiao, W.; Aneja, R.; Zhou, J. Regulation of Tat acetylation and transactivation activity by the microtubule-associated deacetylase HDAC6. *J. Biol. Chem.* **2011**, *286*, 9280–9286.
33. Cereseto, A.; Manganaro, L.; Gutierrez, M.I.; Terreni, M.; Fittipaldi, A.; Lusic, M.; Marcello, A.; Giacca, M. Acetylation of HIV-1 integrase by p300 regulates viral integration. *EMBO J.* **2005**, *24*, 3070–3081.
34. Terreni, M.; Valentini, P.; Liverani, V.; Gutierrez, M.I.; Di Primio, C.; Di Fenza, A.; Tozzini, V.; Allouch, A.; Albanese, A.; Giacca, M.; *et al.* GCN5-dependent acetylation of HIV-1 integrase enhances viral integration. *Retrovirology* **2010**, *7*, 18.
35. Kino, T.; Gragerov, A.; Slobodskaya, O.; Tsopanomichalou, M.; Chrousos, G.P.; Pavlakis, G.N. Human immunodeficiency virus type 1 (HIV-1) accessory protein Vpr induces transcription of the HIV-1 and glucocorticoid-responsive promoters by binding directly to p300/CBP coactivators. *J. Virol.* **2002**, *76*, 9724–9734.
36. Nagy, Z.; Tora, L. Distinct GCN5/PCAF-containing complexes function as co-activators and are involved in transcription factor and global histone acetylation. *Oncogene* **2007**, *26*, 5341–5357.
37. Wang, C.Y.; Yang, S.F.; Wang, Z.; Tan, J.M.; Xing, S.M.; Chen, D.C.; Xu, S.M.; Yuan, W. PCAF acetylates Runx2 and promotes osteoblast differentiation. *J. Bone Miner. Metab.* **2013**, doi:10.1007/s00774-013-0428-y.
38. D'Orso, I.; Frankel, A.D. Tat acetylation modulates assembly of a viral-host RNA-protein transcription complex. *Proc. Natl. Acad. Sci. USA* **2009**, *106*, 3101–3106.
39. Dorr, A.; Kiermer, V.; Pedal, A.; Rackwitz, H.R.; Henklein, P.; Schubert, U.; Zhou, M.M.; Verdin, E.; Ott, M. Transcriptional synergy between Tat and PCAF is dependent on the binding of acetylated Tat to the PCAF bromodomain. *EMBO J.* **2002**, *21*, 2715–2723.
40. Mujtaba, S.; He, Y.; Zeng, L.; Farooq, A.; Carlson, J.E.; Ott, M.; Verdin, E.; Zhou, M.M. Structural basis of lysine-acetylated HIV-1 Tat recognition by PCAF bromodomain. *Mol. Cell* **2002**, *9*, 575–586.
41. Zeng, L.; Li, J.; Muller, M.; Yan, S.; Mujtaba, S.; Pan, C.; Wang, Z.; Zhou, M.M. Selective small molecules blocking HIV-1 Tat and coactivator PCAF association. *J. Am. Chem. Soc.* **2005**, *127*, 2376–2377.

42. Rafati, H.; Parra, M.; Hakre, S.; Moshkin, Y.; Verdin, E.; Mahmoudi, T. Repressive LTR nucleosome positioning by the BAF complex is required for HIV latency. *PLoS Biol.* **2011**, *9*, e1001206.
43. Mahmoudi, T. The BAF complex and HIV latency. *Transcription* **2012**, *3*, 171–176.
44. Van Duyne, R.; Guendel, I.; Narayanan, A.; Gregg, E.; Shafagati, N.; Tyagi, M.; Easley, R.; Klase, Z.; Nekhai, S.; Kehn-Hall, K.; *et al.* Varying modulation of HIV-1 LTR activity by Baf complexes. *J. Mol. Biol.* **2011**, *411*, 581–596.
45. Mahmoudi, T.; Parra, M.; Vries, R.G.; Kauder, S.E.; Verrijzer, C.P.; Ott, M.; Verdin, E. The SWI/SNF chromatin-remodeling complex is a cofactor for Tat transactivation of the HIV promoter. *J. Biol. Chem.* **2006**, *281*, 19960–19968.
46. Treand, C.; du Chene, I.; Bres, V.; Kiernan, R.; Benarous, R.; Benkirane, M.; Emiliani, S. Requirement for SWI/SNF chromatin-remodeling complex in Tat-mediated activation of the HIV-1 promoter. *EMBO J.* **2006**, *25*, 1690–1699.
47. Easley, R.; Carpio, L.; Dannenberg, L.; Choi, S.; Alani, D.; Van Duyne, R.; Guendel, I.; Klase, Z.; Agbottah, E.; Kehn-Hall, K.; *et al.* Transcription through the HIV-1 nucleosomes: Effects of the PBAF complex in Tat activated transcription. *Virology* **2010**, *405*, 322–333.
48. Dey, A.; Chitsaz, F.; Abbasi, A.; Misteli, T.; Ozato, K. The double bromodomain protein Brd4 binds to acetylated chromatin during interphase and mitosis. *Proc. Natl. Acad. Sci. USA* **2003**, *100*, 8758–8763.
49. Wu, S.Y.; Chiang, C.M. The double bromodomain-containing chromatin adaptor Brd4 and transcriptional regulation. *J. Biol. Chem.* **2007**, *282*, 13141–13145.
50. Hubner, M.R.; Eckersley-Maslin, M.A.; Spector, D.L. Chromatin organization and transcriptional regulation. *Curr. Opin. Genet. Dev.* **2012**, *23*, 89–95.
51. Bisgrove, D.A.; Mahmoudi, T.; Henklein, P.; Verdin, E. Conserved P-TEFb-interacting domain of BRD4 inhibits HIV transcription. *Proc. Natl. Acad. Sci. USA* **2007**, *104*, 13690–13695.
52. Schroder, S.; Cho, S.; Zeng, L.; Zhang, Q.; Kaehlcke, K.; Mak, L.; Lau, J.; Bisgrove, D.; Schnolzer, M.; Verdin, E.; *et al.* Two-pronged binding with bromodomain-containing protein 4 liberates positive transcription elongation factor b from inactive ribonucleoprotein complexes. *J. Biol. Chem.* **2012**, *287*, 1090–1099.
53. Yang, Z.; Zhu, Q.; Luo, K.; Zhou, Q. The 7SK small nuclear RNA inhibits the CDK9/cyclin T1 kinase to control transcription. *Nature* **2001**, *414*, 317–322.
54. Yang, Z.; Yik, J.H.; Chen, R.; He, N.; Jang, M.K.; Ozato, K.; Zhou, Q. Recruitment of P-TEFb for stimulation of transcriptional elongation by the bromodomain protein Brd4. *Mol. Cell* **2005**, *19*, 535–545.
55. Zhou, M.; Huang, K.; Jung, K.J.; Cho, W.K.; Klase, Z.; Kashanchi, F.; Pise-Masison, C.A.; Brady, J.N. Bromodomain protein Brd4 regulates human immunodeficiency virus transcription through phosphorylation of CDK9 at threonine 29. *J. Virol.* **2009**, *83*, 1036–1044.
56. Cho, S.; Schroeder, S.; Kaehlcke, K.; Kwon, H.S.; Pedal, A.; Herker, E.; Schnoelzer, M.; Ott, M. Acetylation of cyclin T1 regulates the equilibrium between active and inactive P-TEFb in cells. *EMBO J.* **2009**, *28*, 1407–1417.

57. Vollmuth, F.; Blankenfeldt, W.; Geyer, M. Structures of the dual bromodomains of the P-TEFb-activating protein Brd4 at atomic resolution. *J. Biol. Chem.* **2009**, *284*, 36547–36556.
58. Zeng, L.; Yap, K.L.; Ivanov, A.V.; Wang, X.; Mujtaba, S.; Plotnikova, O.; Rauscher, F.J., 3rd; Zhou, M.M. Structural insights into human KAP1 PHD finger-bromodomain and its role in gene silencing. *Nat. Struct. Mol. Biol.* **2008**, *15*, 626–633.
59. Allouch, A.; di Primio, C.; Alpi, E.; Lusic, M.; Arosio, D.; Giacca, M.; Cereseto, A. The TRIM family protein KAP1 inhibits HIV-1 integration. *Cell Host Microbe* **2011**, *9*, 484–495.
60. Allouch, A.; Cereseto, A. Identification of cellular factors binding to acetylated HIV-1 integrase. *Amino Acids* **2011**, *41*, 1137–1145.
61. Jacobson, R.H.; Ladurner, A.G.; King, D.S.; Tjian, R. Structure and function of a human TAFII250 double bromodomain module. *Science* **2000**, *288*, 1422–1425.
62. Weissman, J.D.; Brown, J.A.; Howcroft, T.K.; Hwang, J.; Chawla, A.; Roche, P.A.; Schiltz, L.; Nakatani, Y.; Singer, D.S. HIV-1 tat binds TAFII250 and represses TAFII250-dependent transcription of major histocompatibility class I genes. *Proc. Natl. Acad. Sci. USA* **1998**, *95*, 11601–11606.
63. Granito, A.; Yang, W.H.; Muratori, L.; Lim, M.J.; Nakajima, A.; Ferri, S.; Pappas, G.; Quarneti, C.; Bianchi, F.B.; Bloch, D.B.; Muratori, P. PML nuclear body component Sp140 is a novel autoantigen in primary biliary cirrhosis. *Am. J. Gastroenterol.* **2010**, *105*, 125–131.
64. Bloch, D.B.; de la Monte, S.M.; Guigaouri, P.; Filippov, A.; Bloch, K.D. Identification and characterization of a leukocyte-specific component of the nuclear body. *J. Biol. Chem.* **1996**, *271*, 29198–29204.
65. Dent, A.L.; Yewdell, J.; Puvion-Dutilleul, F.; Koken, M.H.; de The, H.; Staudt, L.M. LYSP100-associated nuclear domains (LANDs): Description of a new class of subnuclear structures and their relationship to PML nuclear bodies. *Blood* **1996**, *88*, 1423–1426.
66. Madani, N.; Millette, R.; Platt, E.J.; Marin, M.; Kozak, S.L.; Bloch, D.B.; Kabat, D. Implication of the lymphocyte-specific nuclear body protein Sp140 in an innate response to human immunodeficiency virus type 1. *J. Virol.* **2002**, *76*, 11133–11138.
67. Sheehy, A.M.; Gaddis, N.C.; Malim, M.H. The antiretroviral enzyme APOBEC3G is degraded by the proteasome in response to HIV-1 Vif. *Nat. Med.* **2003**, *9*, 1404–1407.
68. Malovannaya, A.; Lanz, R.B.; Jung, S.Y.; Bulynko, Y.; Le, N.T.; Chan, D.W.; Ding, C.; Shi, Y.; Yucer, N.; Krenciute, G.; *et al.* Analysis of the human endogenous coregulator complexome. *Cell* **2011**, *145*, 787–799.
69. Boehm, D.; Calvanese, V.; Dar, R.D.; Xing, S.; Schroeder, S.; Martins, L.; Aull, K.; Li, P.C.; Planelles, V.; Bradner, J.E.; *et al.* BET bromodomain-targeting compounds reactivate HIV from latency via a Tat-independent mechanism. *Cell Cycle* **2013**, *12*, 452–462.
70. Denis, G.V.; McComb, M.E.; Faller, D.V.; Sinha, A.; Romesser, P.B.; Costello, C.E. Identification of transcription complexes that contain the double bromodomain protein Brd2 and chromatin remodeling machines. *J. Proteome Res.* **2006**, *5*, 502–511.
71. Wang, J.; Reuschel, E.L.; Shackelford, J.M.; Jeang, L.; Shivers, D.K.; Diehl, J.A.; Yu, X.F.; Finkel, T.H. HIV-1 Vif promotes the G(1)- to S-phase cell-cycle transition. *Blood* **2011**, *117*, 1260–1269.

72. Yang, Z.; He, N.; Zhou, Q. Brd4 recruits P-TEFb to chromosomes at late mitosis to promote G1 gene expression and cell cycle progression. *Mol. Cell. Biol.* **2008**, *28*, 967–976.
73. Mochizuki, K.; Nishiyama, A.; Jang, M.K.; Dey, A.; Ghosh, A.; Tamura, T.; Natsume, H.; Yao, H.; Ozato, K. The bromodomain protein Brd4 stimulates G1 gene transcription and promotes progression to S phase. *J. Biol. Chem.* **2008**, *283*, 9040–9048.
74. Filippakopoulos, P.; Picaud, S.; Fedorov, O.; Keller, M.; Wrobel, M.; Morgenstern, O.; Bracher, F.; Knapp, S. Benzodiazepines and benzotriazepines as protein interaction inhibitors targeting bromodomains of the BET family. *Bioorg. Med. Chem.* **2012**, *20*, 1878–1886.
75. Filippakopoulos, P.; Qi, J.; Picaud, S.; Shen, Y.; Smith, W.B.; Fedorov, O.; Morse, E.M.; Keates, T.; Hickman, T.T.; Felletar, I.; *et al.* Selective inhibition of BET bromodomains. *Nature* **2010**, *468*, 1067–1073.
76. Nicodeme, E.; Jeffrey, K.L.; Schaefer, U.; Beinke, S.; Dewell, S.; Chung, C.W.; Chandwani, R.; Marazzi, I.; Wilson, P.; Coste, H.; *et al.* Suppression of inflammation by a synthetic histone mimic. *Nature* **2010**, *468*, 1119–1123.
77. Dawson, M.A.; Prinjha, R.K.; Dittmann, A.; Giotopoulos, G.; Bantscheff, M.; Chan, W.I.; Robson, S.C.; Chung, C.W.; Hopf, C.; Savitski, M.M.; *et al.* Inhibition of BET recruitment to chromatin as an effective treatment for MLL-fusion leukaemia. *Nature* **2011**, *478*, 529–533.
78. Zhang, G.; Liu, R.; Zhong, Y.; Plotnikov, A.N.; Zhang, W.; Zeng, L.; Rusinova, E.; Gerona-Nevarro, G.; Moshkina, N.; Joshua, J.; *et al.* Down-regulation of NF-kappaB transcriptional activity in HIV-associated kidney disease by BRD4 inhibition. *J. Biol. Chem.* **2012**, *287*, 28840–28851.
79. Miyoshi, S.; Ooike, S.; Iwata, K.; Hikawa, H.; Sugahara, K. International Patent PCT/JP2008/073864 (US2010/0286127 A1), 26 December 2008.
80. Zuber, J.; Shi, J.; Wang, E.; Rappaport, A.R.; Herrmann, H.; Sison, E.A.; Magoon, D.; Qi, J.; Blatt, K.; Wunderlich, M.; *et al.* RNAi screen identifies Brd4 as a therapeutic target in acute myeloid leukaemia. *Nature* **2011**, *478*, 524–528.
81. Routy, J.P.; Angel, J.B.; Spaans, J.N.; Trottier, B.; Rouleau, D.; Baril, J.G.; Harris, M.; Trottier, S.; Singer, J.; Chomont, N.; *et al.* Design and implementation of a randomized crossover study of valproic acid and antiretroviral therapy to reduce the HIV reservoir. *HIV Clin. Trials* **2012**, *13*, 301–307.
82. Routy, J.P.; Tremblay, C.L.; Angel, J.B.; Trottier, B.; Rouleau, D.; Baril, J.G.; Harris, M.; Trottier, S.; Singer, J.; Chomont, N.; *et al.* Valproic acid in association with highly active antiretroviral therapy for reducing systemic HIV-1 reservoirs: Results from a multicentre randomized clinical study. *HIV Med.* **2012**, *13*, 291–296.
83. Banerjee, C.; Archin, N.; Michaels, D.; Belkina, A.C.; Denis, G.V.; Bradner, J.; Sebastiani, P.; Margolis, D.M.; Montano, M. BET bromodomain inhibition as a novel strategy for reactivation of HIV-1. *J. Leukoc. Biol.* **2012**, *92*, 1147–1154.
84. Bartholomeeusen, K.; Xiang, Y.; Fujinaga, K.; Peterlin, B.M. Bromodomain and extra-terminal (BET) bromodomain inhibition activate transcription via transient release of positive transcription elongation factor b (P-TEFb) from 7SK small nuclear ribonucleoprotein. *J. Biol. Chem.* **2012**, *287*, 36609–36616.

85. Li, Z.; Guo, J.; Wu, Y.; Zhou, Q. The BET bromodomain inhibitor JQ1 activates HIV latency through antagonizing Brd4 inhibition of Tat-transactivation. *Nucleic Acids Res.* **2013**, *41*, 277–287.
86. Zhu, J.; Gaiha, G.D.; John, S.P.; Pertel, T.; Chin, C.R.; Gao, G.; Qu, H.; Walker, B.D.; Elledge, S.J.; Brass, A.L. Reactivation of Latent HIV-1 by Inhibition of BRD4. *Cell Rep.* **2012**, *2*, 807–816.
87. Boehm, D.; Calvanese, V.; Dar, R.D.; Xing, S.; Schroeder, S.; Martins, L.; Aull, K.; Li, P.C.; Planelles, V.; Bradner, J.E.; *et al*. BET bromodomain-targeting compounds reactivate HIV from latency via a Tat-independent mechanism. *Cell Cycle* **2013**, *12*, 452–462.

7

The Chromatin Landscape of Kaposi's Sarcoma-Associated Herpesvirus

Zsolt Toth *, Kevin Brulois and Jae U. Jung

Department of Molecular Microbiology and Immunology, Keck School of Medicine, University of Southern California, Harlyne J. Norris Cancer Research Tower, 1450 Biggy Street, Los Angeles, CA 90033, USA; E-Mails: brulois@usc.edu (K.B.); jaeujung@med.usc.edu (J.U.J.)

* Author to whom correspondence should be addressed: E-Mail: ztoth@usc.edu;

Abstract: Kaposi's sarcoma-associated herpesvirus is an oncogenic γ-herpesvirus that causes latent infection in humans. In cells, the viral genome adopts a highly organized chromatin structure, which is controlled by a wide variety of cellular and viral chromatin regulatory factors. In the past few years, interrogation of the chromatinized KSHV genome by whole genome-analyzing tools revealed that the complex chromatin landscape spanning the viral genome in infected cells has important regulatory roles during the viral life cycle. This review summarizes the most recent findings regarding the role of histone modifications, histone modifying enzymes, DNA methylation, microRNAs, non-coding RNAs and the nuclear organization of the KSHV epigenome in the regulation of latent and lytic viral gene expression programs as well as their connection to KSHV-associated pathogenesis.

Keywords: Kaposi's sarcoma-associated herpesvirus; KSHV; KS; viral chromatin; polycomb; EZH2; minichromosome; histone modifications; MLL/Set1; JMJD2A

---

1. Introduction

It is estimated that 15% of human cancers are caused by viral infections. Among the seven currently known human oncogenic viruses, two of them belong to the herpesvirus family: Kaposi's sarcoma-associated herpesvirus (KSHV or Human Herpesvirus 8, HHV-8) and Epstein-Barr virus (EBV or Human Herpesvirus 4, HHV-4). In 1994, KSHV was first discovered in Kaposi's sarcoma patients, who commonly present with cutaneous, neoplastic lesions of endothelial cell origin.

Subsequently, it was also linked to the development of two B cell lymphomas: primary effusion lymphoma (PEL) and Multicentric Castleman's disease [1,2]. Like other herpesviruses, KSHV establishes persistent infection in humans and alternates between two different life cycle phases: latency and lytic reactivation. In immunocompetent individuals KSHV establishes latency in $CD19^+$ B cells, where a highly restricted viral gene expression program is thought to be the primary means by which latently infected cells escape detection by the host immune system. On the other hand, immune suppression along with other environmental and physiological factors, including oxidative stress, inflammatory cytokines, hypoxia or infection by other pathogens, each can favorably contribute to the physiological conditions required for KSHV to transition from latency to viral reactivation and virus production [3–8].

The 160-175-kb KSHV genome is composed of a single, 140.5-kb long unique coding region (LUR), which is flanked by 20-35-kb long, GC-rich terminal repeats (TRs) [9]. The LUR encodes at least 86 protein-coding genes, 12 microRNAs and several non-coding and antisense RNAs. The majority of latent genes are located between ORF69 and K14 in the KSHV genome and their expression is driven by only a few promoters. On the other hand, lytic genes are spread across the entire KSHV genome and the expression of each is likely regulated by over 100 different promoters. Latent genes are constitutively expressed in KSHV-infected cells, regardless of whether the infection is in a latent or lytic phase. On the other hand, lytic gene expression is repressed during latency and is only activated upon lytic reactivation, during which the three classes of lytic genes, immediate early (IE), early (E) and late (L) are induced, respectively [10]. While a relatively clear picture of the life cycle-dependent gene expression patterns of KSHV has emerged, we still do not understand the mechanism(s) that allow latent genes to escape the transcriptional repression affecting the rest of the viral genes during latency and the regulatory processes that control the genome-wide repression and temporally-ordered transcription of lytic genes. The fact that lytic reactivation of KSHV can be induced by treating latently infected cells with chemicals that affect chromatin regulatory factors such as histone deacetylases (HDACs), DNA methyltransferases (DNMTs) and histone acetyltransferases (HATs) argues that chromatin and chromatin-associated factors must be involved in the control of viral gene expression [11–13]. Indeed, whereas the KSHV genome is linear and histone-free in the viral capsid, after infection, the viral DNA becomes a closed circular episome that associates with cellular histones and persists in the nucleus as a non-integrated minichromosome [14,15]. Micrococcal nuclease mapping studies and chromatin immunoprecipitations of various histones and chromatin regulatory proteins have demonstrated that KSHV gene expression is controlled by the dynamic modulation of nucleosomal structure, a finding reminiscent of the regulation of cellular genes on the host chromosome (see below).

The fundamental building block of chromatin is the nucleosome, which consists of 147 bp of DNA, which is wrapped around a histone octamer composed of two of each of the histones: H2A, H2B, H3 and H4 (Figure 1A). The N-terminal tail of histones protrudes from the nucleosomes and as such, is subject to various posttranslational modifications, including acetylation, methylation, phosphorylation and ubiquitination (Figure 1A). Depending on whether a gene is destined for activation or silencing, different histone modifying enzyme complexes are recruited to the gene promoter to generate specific posttranslational modifications on histones called histone marks, which function as key modulators of gene expression (Figure 1B) [16]. These histone marks can then be recognized by specific nuclear proteins that use histone mark recognizing modules [17]. These histone mark-readers can recruit additional transcription factors that either inhibit or activate transcription (Figure 1B). In addition to the histone marks, gene transcription can also be modulated by other structural features of chromatin, including the distribution of histone variants, the positioning of nucleosomes and the presence of cytosine 5-methylation of the CpG islands in the gene regulatory regions [18,19]. The nucleosome array of the DNA genome constitutes the primary structure of chromatin, which is further organized into a three-dimensional complex structure through expansive looping of the chromatinized DNA and large-scale compartmentalization in the nucleus [20]. This higher-order organization of the chromatin can influence genes within large chromosomal domains or co-regulate genes that are otherwise far from each other on the chromosome.

Figure 1. Chromatin components and their effect on gene expression. (**A**) The basic unit of chromatin is the nucleosome, which consists of 147 bp DNA wrapped around histones H2A, H2B, H3 and H4. The N terminus of histones is subject to different posttranslational modifications; (**B**) The levels and types of histone marks are dynamically regulated by antagonistic histone modifying enzymes (writers and erasers). Histone marks are recognized and interpreted by specific nuclear proteins (readers), resulting in the recruitment of either repressor or activator transcription regulatory complexes onto the target promoters. Some examples of repressive and activating chromatin modifications are listed in the boxed text.

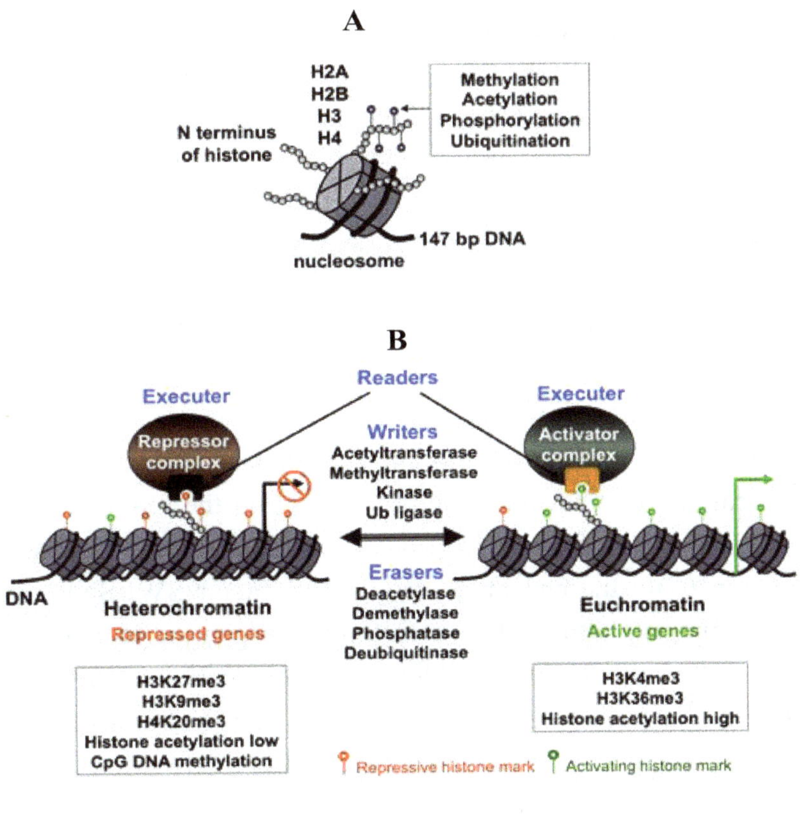

Chromatin immunoprecipitation combined with microarray technology (ChIP-on-chip), chromatin immunoprecipitation coupled with massively parallel DNA sequencing (ChIP-seq) and chromatin conformation capture assays have proved to be powerful techniques for the genome-wide mapping of histone marks, transcription factors and chromatin regulatory factors on the cellular genome and have provided a large amount data about the structural elements of the chromatin and their functional consequence for transcription. More and more studies have been emerging that also apply whole genome-analyzing tools for the interrogation of the epigenetic regulation of the KSHV genome, revealing an unexpectedly complex picture about the chromatin landscape of the viral genome in infected cells. In this review, we will mainly focus on the most recent studies that have investigated the regulation of chromatin on KSHV, including the relevant cellular and viral chromatin regulatory factors. Also, we will highlight some unanswered questions that require further investigation to better understand the fundamental chromatin-regulatory pathways involved in the control of the different stages of the KSHV lifecycle.

2. *De Novo* Infection and the Requirements for the Establishment of Latency

KSHV can infect a variety of cell types, including endothelial, fibroblast and epithelial cells, and establishes predominantly latent infections in cultured cells. However, without continuous drug selection, KSHV episomes get lost from most proliferating cells and only a subpopulation of cells can stably maintain the viral genome. Grundhoff and Ganem showed that the establishment of latency in these cells is not due to genetic mutations in the host or viral genome, but presumably epigenetic changes on the viral episome [21]. Such epigenetic alterations could involve the nucleosome structure, DNA methylation or histone modifications depositing onto the KSHV genome in the nucleus. Although we are getting a more and more detailed picture of the chromatin architecture of the latent KSHV genome, we still do not understand the processes by which naïve, histone-free KSHV genomes get chromatinized following *de novo* infection (Figure 2A).

Establishment of latency requires repression of lytic genes and continuous expression of latent genes after *de novo* infection. This picture became more complicated when it was shown that a limited number of lytic genes with immunomodulatory and antiapoptotic functions are temporarily expressed after infection, followed by a decline in their transcription as latent gene expression remains constant (Figure 2A) [22]. Interestingly, during this transient period of lytic gene expression, one of the lytic genes that is expressed is ORF50, which encodes an IE protein called Replication and Transcription Activator (RTA). RTA is a viral transcription factor that functions as the master switch between latency and the lytic gene expression programs and is both necessary and sufficient for the initiation of lytic replication as it can activate several lytic promoters and the replication of viral DNA (reviewed in [23]). In addition, RTA binds to several chromatin and transcription regulatory factors, including the histone acetyltransferase CBP, the chromatin remodeling factor SWI/SNF2 and the Mediator, all of which are involved in gene activation [24]. Interestingly, despite the induction of RTA during *de novo* infection, its expression does not lead to full-blown lytic replication in this setting, possibly due to the lack of sustained RTA expression. While the mechanisms responsible for the down-regulation of RTA are unknown, they likely involve the rapid inhibition of the RTA promoter as well as the lack of the activation of specific signaling pathways. In agreement with this, infection of telomerase-immortalized retinal pigment epithelial cells with a recombinant KSHV clone that expresses RTA from the constitutively active cellular phosphoglycerate kinase promoter results in constitutive lytic replication [25]. Thus, it appears that the RTA promoter is inherently prone to become transcriptionally inactive following *de novo* infection, a process that likely involves certain RTA promoter elements that orchestrate the recruitment of transcription repressor complexes and heterochromatin-associated epigenetic marks such as DNA methylation and repressive histone modifications. Indeed, several repressive chromatin-associated factors have been identified on the RTA promoter during latency (see details below) but the molecular events involved in their initial recruitment upon *de novo* infection are still not known.

Figure 2. Chromatinization of the KSHV episome and the role of the latent KSHV protein, LANA. (**A**) The KSHV genome is linear and histone-free in the viral capsid and becomes a closed circular episome following *de novo* infection. Subsequently, the viral DNA is organized into a nucleosome structure and it persists in the nucleus as a non-integrated minichromosome; (**B**) LANA is a constitutively expressed gene that is encoded within the major latency-associated locus of the KSHV genome. LANA binds to terminal repeat (TR) region of the viral genome and tethers the viral genome to the host chromosome by interacting with histones or other components of the cellular chromatin such as Brd4, MeCP2…*etc*. LANA also binds to several sites within the viral genome and it is involved in the recruitment of the H3K9me1/2 histone demethylase JMJD1A and repression of lytic genes. The posttranslational modifications of LANA play a critical role in the association of LANA with the KSHV genome and also regulate its activity in transcription regulation. During latency, LANA in maintained in an arginine methylated state resulting in its binding to the KSHV genome. Upon HDAC inhibitor (HDACi) treatment, LANA gets acetylated, which leads to its dissociation from the KSHV genome and the concomitant induction of lytic genes.

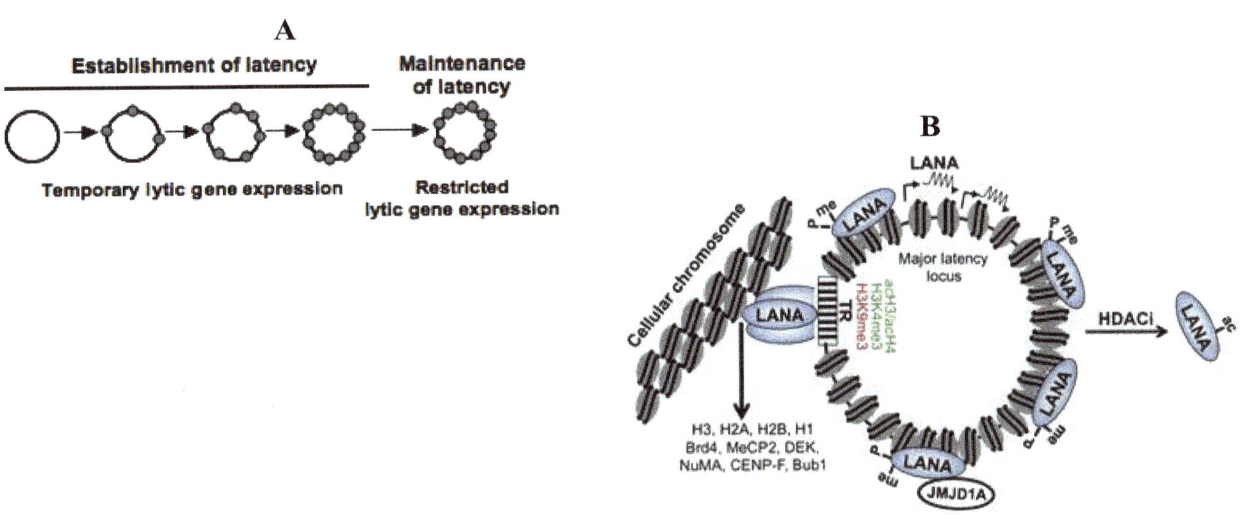

Since latent genes are rapidly induced after *de novo* infection and their expression persists during latency, it is plausible that latent proteins are involved in the repression of lytic genes. One of the latent proteins is the latency-associated nuclear antigen or LANA, which is a nuclear protein that binds to several sites on the KSHV genome, most notably the TR region (Figure 2B) [26–28]. It was shown that IE gene expression significantly increased in 293T cells following transfection of a LANA-deletion mutant of KSHV, suggesting that LANA plays a role in the downregulation of lytic genes during the establishment of latency [29]. Another group reported that HEK293 cells carrying a LANA-deletion KSHV mutant show increased expression of lytic genes, demonstrating that LANA can contribute to latency by repressing the expression of lytic genes [30]. The transcription repression activity of LANA can be attributed to its cellular binding partners, several of which are transcription repressors, including the heterochromatin protein HP1α, methyl-CpG-binding protein MeCP2, the H3K9me3 histone methyltransferase SUV39H1, histone deacetylase co-repressor mSin3 complex and DNA methyltransferases (DNMTs) [31–36]. LANA also interacts with and inhibits the enzymatic activity of the histone acetyltransferase CBP, resulting in repression of CBP target genes [37]. The functional consequences of the interaction of LANA with these chromatin regulatory proteins have been studied mainly in transcription reporter assays and not in the context of KSHV-infected cells. Therefore, it is currently unclear which of these protein-protein interactions has a role in the regulation of the viral chromatin and in repression of lytic KSHV genes.

Other important functions of LANA in the promotion of latency are the recruitment of cellular DNA replication factors onto TR and the tethering of the viral genome to the host chromosome during mitosis [14,38–40]. These LANA functions ensure that the replication of the KSHV genome occurs concurrently with that of the host genome and that viral episomes are disseminated to both daughter cells following mitosis. In accordance with this, a KSHV mutant lacking LANA was rapidly lost from cells after multiple cell divisions [41]. LANA interacts with histones H2A, H2B, H1 and cellular chromatin-associated factors such as Brd2, Brd4, MeCP2, DEK, nuclear mitotic apparatus protein (NuMA), centromeric protein F (CENP-F) and the kinetochore protein Bub1, all of which may be involved in the binding of LANA to the host chromosome [39,42–47]. Interestingly, LANA can associate with heterochromatin through binding to MeCP2 and this interaction might be involved in the downregulation of lytic genes during *de novo* infection, perhaps through tethering of the viral episome to a transcriptionally silenced host chromosomal regions [31,47]. Despite the ample number of cellular chromatin factors that bind to LANA, knowledge of the functional consequence of these interactions is limited, particularly in the setting of the LANA-mediated repression of lytic gene expression that occurs following *de novo* infection.

Posttranslational modifications of LANA also influence its function in the repression of lytic genes during latency by modulating its binding to the viral episome (Figure 2B). One group showed that arginine methylation in the histone-binding domain of LANA by the Protein arginine methyltransferase 1 (PRMT1) is associated with strong binding of LANA to the KSHV genome and repression of lytic genes [27]. Another group reported that treatment of KSHV-infected cells with histone deacetylase inhibitors causes the acetylation of LANA, which in turn results in the dissociation of LANA from the RTA promoter and the upregulation of RTA transcription [29]. Phosphorylation of LANA by Pim-1 and Pim-3 kinases can also counteract the transcription repressor activity of LANA on lytic genes [48]. Similarly, the phosphorylation of the histone-binding domain of LANA by different kinases can modulate association of LANA with the cellular chromatin [49]. These studies clearly show that the posttranslational modifications of the latent protein, LANA, play a critical role in the LANA-mediated inhibition of lytic genes during viral latency and presumably in the establishment of latency following *de novo* infection as well.

3. Regulation of the Chromatin Structure of KSHV during Latency and Lytic Reactivation

During latency the KSHV genome exists as a circular episome in the nucleus and has a nucleosome structure similar to the bulk cellular chromatin (Figure 2A) [12,15]. Since chromatin restricts the accessibility of transcription factors to promoters, modification of the chromatin architecture has a pivotal role in the control of gene expression. Histone modifying enzymes and ATP-dependent chromatin remodeling complexes each play a role in chromatin remodeling through the covalent modification of histones and the repositioning of nucleosomes, respectively. There is evidence that both classes of chromatin regulatory proteins are involved in the regulation of KSHV gene expression. However, only a few studies have investigated the effect of these chromatin regulatory factors on the entire KSHV genome. Most of what we know about the chromatin structure of KSHV is based on studies performed with PEL cells that carry KSHV in latency and can be readily reactivated upon stress stimuli. Here, we summarize the most recent results regarding the role of histone modifications, histone modifying enzymes, DNA methylation, miRNAs, non-coding RNAs and the nuclear organization of the KSHV epigenome in the regulation of latent and lyitc viral gene expression programs.

3.1. Activating and Repressive Histone Modifications on the KSHV Genome

Since lytic genes are repressed during latency it was presumed that they are associated with heterochromatin that is poised for rapid and ordered transition to a transcriptionally permissive state. The histone modifying enzyme complexes involved in the regulation of specific genes can be determined by the identification of their corresponding histone modifications associated with the genes. Two studies have used chromatin immunoprecipitation assays in conjunction with high-resolution KSHV-specific tiling microarrays (ChIP-on-chip) to shed light on the nature of the chromatin that is associated with the KSHV episomes in infected cells [50,51]. Specifically, these techniques were used to analyze chromatin from a KSHV-infected B cell lymphoma cell line called BCBL1 and a latently infected adherent cell line called SLKp, providing the first genome-wide views of the KSHV epigenetic landscape, including the occupancy of total histone H3 and several of its modified forms: the activating marks, H3K4me3 and acetylated H3K9/K14 (acH3) as well as the repressive H3K9me3 and H3K27me3 histone modifications. While H3 turned out to be uniformly distributed, the histone modifications show distinct patterns along the KSHV genome (Figure 3A). Specifically, in certain regions of the KSHV genome, the genomic localization of H3K4me3 overlaps with acH3 and the majority of H3K27me3 co-localizes with H3K9me3 on the viral episome. In contrast, other regions of the genome showed mutually exclusive enrichment of activating and repressive histone marks. Latent genes have H3K4me3/acH3-rich chromatin during latency and reactivation, a finding that is consistent with the presence of transcriptionally active RNA polymerase II (RNAPII) on the latent promoters and their constitutively active transcription (Figure 3A) [50,52]. Interestingly, the chromatin of IE and the majority of E genes also displays high level of H3K4me3 and acH3 during latency, despite the absence of IE and E gene expression. During latency, the promoter region of the IE genes, RTA and ORF48, shows a characteristic bivalent chromatin, defined by the concomitant presence of H3K4me3 and H3K27me3 [50,51]. Although bivalent chromatin is not permissive for gene expression, it is associated with genes that are in a poised state of transcription activation, as is the case for IE and E genes. In contrast to the IE/E gene-rich genomic regions of KSHV, the parts of the viral genome that encode many of the late genes are mainly associated with the repressive H3K9me3 and H3K27me3 and these chromatin marks are presumably responsible for the inhibition of late gene expression during latency and also during the early phase of reactivation. High expression of late genes only occurs upon viral DNA replication and is accompanied by the dissociation of heterochromatin from the KSHV genome [50]. These observations imply that the activation of late gene expression may be triggered by the de-chromatinization of the KSHV genome upon viral DNA replication. In addition, recent studies with MHV68 showed that deletion of certain viral genes can abrogate the induction of late genes, without affecting viral DNA replication, suggesting that viral proteins with transcription regulatory activity are also involved in the regulation of late genes [53–55].

Strikingly, while H3K9me3 is restricted to two loci that encode mainly late genes, H3K27me3 is widespread across the entire KSHV genome, with the exception of the latency locus (Figure 3A) [50,51]. In addition, lytic reactivation leads to the decline of H3K27me3 on lytic genes, while the level of H3K9me3 remains constant [50]. In keeping with this, the H3K27me3 histone methyltransferase of Polycomb repressive complex 2 (PRC2), called EZH2, binds to the KSHV genome and colocalizes with H3K27me3 during latency. Upon reactivation, EZH2 dissociation from the KSHV genome is initiated and correlates with the concomitant decline of H3K27me3, increase of H3K4me3/acH3, and induction of IE and E gene expression [50]. A number of additional experiments were used to examine how viral gene expression is affected by the presence of EZH2 and its corresponding histone mark, H3K27me3 on the KSHV episome. The inhibition of EZH2 expression with either shRNA knockdown or the chemical compound, DZNep triggered the induction of lytic genes in latently infected PEL cells [50]. Conversely, the transient expression of enzymatically active H3K27me3 demethylases, such as UTX or JMJD3, could induce lytic genes in latently infected cells, while the H3K9me3 demethylase JMJD2A failed to do so [50,51]. These data suggest that the PRC2 complex maintains a H3K27me3-enriched heterochromatin on lytic genes to repress their expression during latency (Figure 3B). Moreover, viral reactivation triggers the dissociation of PRC2 from the KSHV genome and the concomitant deposition of activating histone modifications and RNAPII on viral promoters, resulting in the induction of the IE and E genes [50–52].

Figure 3. The chromatin landscape of KSHV during latency. (**A**) Schematic of the KSHV genome and the genome-wide distribution of different histone marks along the viral genome. There are distinct chromatin domains on the viral episome, which are characterized by different histone modification patterns indicating the targeted recruitment of specific cellular chromatin modifying enzyme complexes to different sites of the viral genome. The cellular chromatin modifying factors associated with each histone mark are listed to the right. The position of the latency locus and examples of an IE gene (RTA), some early genes (viral interferon regulatory factors or vIRFs and the OriLytL-K7 locus) and L genes (ORF25 and ORF64) are indicated at the top; (**B**) The PRC2 complex co-localizes with H3K27me3-rich chromatin domains, while the binding of the H3K9me3 histone demethylase JMJD2A overlaps with the H3K4me3/acH3-enriched chromatin regions that have a low level of H3K9me3. PRC2 is involved in the inhibition of ORF50 (RTA) expression during latency.

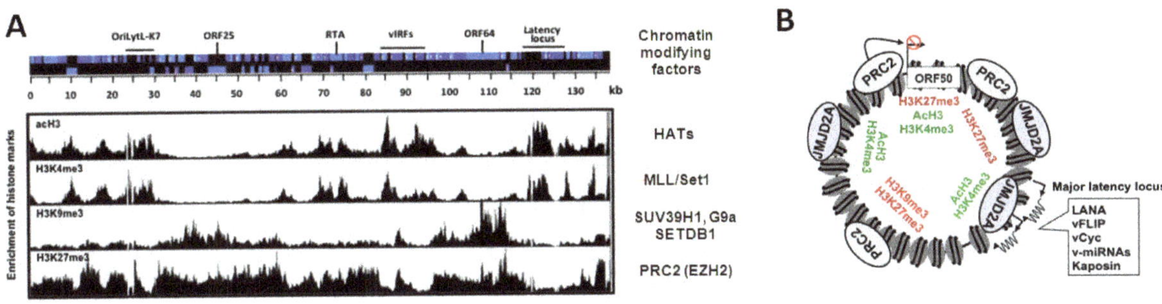

3.2. The Polycomb Connections

Polycomb group (PcG) proteins are cellular transcription repressors, which form two enzymatically distinct complexes called PRC2 and PRC1, both of which have been shown to inhibit transcription [56]. A number of different transcriptional silencing mechanisms contribute to PcG-mediated inhibition of transcription, including induction of chromatin condensation, inhibition of transcription initiation, blocking transcription elongation and recruitment of H3K4me3 histone demethylases to the target promoters [57–60]. PcG proteins are required for the inhibition of number of genes involved in development, cell proliferation and differentiation [56]. Importantly, there are several examples of human cancers in which increased expression of PcG proteins, specific point mutations or translocations of PcG gene loci have been observed [61]. Increased expression of specific PcG proteins have been shown to contribute transformation, indicating that PcG proteins can have oncogenic properties [62]. The PRC2 complex includes several subunits: EED, SUZ12, RbAp46/48, as well as EZH2, which catalyzes the di- and trimethylation of H3K27. In Drosophila, PRC2 has been shown to bind to target promoters through polycomb responsive DNA elements (PREs) [56]. In mammals, on the other hand, the recruitment of PRC2 to its target sites appears to be mediated mainly by various non-coding RNAs and distinct transcription factors [56]. The association of PRC2 with the chromatin is often extended beyond the target promoters in mammalian cells and overlaps with the distribution of

H3K27me3 along the target genes. This was explained by the finding that PRC2 could be recruited to H3K27me3 via EED, a PRC2 subunit that can recognize and bind to this histone mark [63,64]. Similarly, the localization of the PRC2 components, EZH2 and SUZ12, on the KSHV episome is not restricted to specific sites but spread across the entire genome [50]. While we have a clear picture of PRC2 occupancy during the latent and early lytic phases of the KSHV lifecycle, the events that enable the initial recruitment of PRC2 to the KSHV genome following *de novo* infection and its maintenance on the latent genome are still not understood.

It has been shown that most polycomb target genes are repressed by both PRC2 and PRC1 complexes. Recently, a comprehensive proteomic and genomic analysis revealed that there are six major PRC1 complexes comprising a distinct set of proteins [65]. However, all six of these PRC1 complexes harbor a common subunit called RING1A/B, which are E3 mono-ubiquitin ligases that generate H2AK119ub. In most cases the binding of PRC1 to target genes depends on the activity of PRC2 and the presence of its corresponding histone mark, H3K27me3, a histone modification that is recognized by PRC1 and used for its recruitment. Nevertheless, it should be noted that PRC1 can also be recruited to number of target sites that lack H3K27me3 [66]. Indeed, the subunit composition of the individual PRC1 complexes affects their genomic localizations, indicating that different recruitment mechanisms exist for each PRC1 complex [65]. Specific components of both PRC2 and PRC1 have been found to interact with lytic promoters of Herpes simplex virus type 1 (HSV-1) during latency, suggesting that not only PRC2, but also PRC1 might be involved in the control the heterochromatin of KSHV [67,68]. However, whether PRC1 also binds to the KSHV genome and plays a role in the repression of lytic genes has not yet been addressed.

Another interesting aspect of KSHV epigenetic regulation is the process by which PcG protein-mediated repression of lytic gene expression is reversed during reactivation. Importantly, the lysine 27 residue on histone H3 (H3K27) can either be acetylated (H3K27ac) or mono-, di-, or trimethylated. H3K27ac is associated with the activation of genes and is catalyzed by the histone acetyltransferases CBP/p300 in mammals [69]. The induction of lytic genes upon the overexpression of H3K27me3 demethylases UTX and JMJD3 in latently infected cells suggests that the modulation of posttranslational modifications of H3K27 must be critical for the regulation of lytic genes [50,51]. RTA, which binds to and activates number of lytic promoters during reactivation, has been shown to interact with CBP [24]. Furthermore, several RTA responsive promoters can be found in the viral genomic regions where H3K27me3 declines during reactivation, suggesting that RTA may recruit CBP to these sites, resulting in a transition from H3K27me3 to H3K27ac. In addition, the mixed-lineage leukemia (MLL) protein-containing MLL/Set1 complexes mediate H3K4me3 and, like RTA, increase at the same sites where H3K27me3 declines on the KSHV genome during lytic reactivation [50]. Moreover, MLL/Set1 complexes have been shown to interact with CBP as well as the H3K27me3 demethylase, UTX [70–72]. Therefore, it is possible that the H3K27me3 decline on IE and E genes during reactivation is the consequence of the recruitment of protein complexes to the viral promoters that can catalyze both demethylation and acetylation of H3K27 to induce lytic gene expression. In fact, a recent study showed that, a highly abundant KSHV non-coding RNA called polyadenylated nuclear

(PAN) RNA can interact with the RTA promoter and recruit the H3K27me3 demethylases, JMJD3 and UTX, as well as the H3K4me3 histone methyltransferase, MLL2 [73]. Since PAN RNA expression is dependent on IE genes, especially RTA, these data suggest that PAN RNA-mediated recruitment of chromatin factors to the RTA promoter may be part of a positive feedback regulatory mechanism that perpetuates RTA expression during later stages of reactivation. However, given that the expression of RTA is induced prior to that of PAN RNA (RTA is an IE gene and PAN RNA is an E gene), PAN RNA is not likely to be involved in the initial de-repression of PRC2-mediated inhibition of the RTA promoter during physiologically relevant reactivation conditions, *i.e.*, in the absence of exogenous PAN RNA expression. Thus, the means by which repressive histone marks are initially removed from the RTA promoter is still not understood.

The treatment of latently infected cells with histone deacetylase (HDAC) inhibitors can also trigger the induction of RTA and leads to the dissociation of EZH2 and the decline of H3K27me3 on the RTA promoter [74]. Several HDACs have been implicated in the repression of PcG target genes and may play a role in deacetylation of H3K27ac, allowing its trimethylation [75,76]. In fact, EED was found to interact with HDAC1, 2 and 3 in a yeast two-hybrid screen, suggesting a possible connection between PRC2 and HDACs [76]. Importantly, the HDAC inhibitor, trichostatin A (TSA), can induce the activation of PcG-silenced genes, including the expression of KSHV lytic genes [12,76]. Thus, HDACs can also be involved in the maintenance of PRC2-mediated lytic gene repression by promoting H3K27 deacetylation, thereby allowing PRC2 to catalyze the trimethylation of H3K27. Further experiments are required to see whether there are any specific HDACs that have a role in the regulation of PRC2-maintained KSHV latency.

3.3. Regulation of the Heterochromatin Mark H3K9me3 on the KSHV Genome

H3K9me3 occupies two specific regions of the KSHV genome, both of which encode primarily late genes (Figure 3A) [50,51,77]. Although H3K9me3 does not seem to be a major repressive histone mark for lytic genes, several studies found that H3K9me3 and its associated chromatin regulatory factors have important regulatory roles during the KSHV life cycle. Several histone methyltransferases (HMTs) can catalyze the methylation of H3K9, including G9a, SUV39H1 and SETDB1 [78]. SUV39H1 and the H3K9me3-binding protein HP1 have been shown to interact with LANA, resulting in their recruitment to the TR and some lytic promoters of KSHV, where they are involved in heterochromatinization during latency [33]. Since LANA ChIP-seq and ChIP-on-chip experiments revealed a number of LANA-binding sites on the KSHV genome, it would be important to know whether SUV39H1 can also be recruited to these LANA-binding sites and thereby facilitate H3K9me3 [26,27]. In addition, other H3K9me3 HMTs can also be recruited to the KSHV episome by cellular factors. Indeed, Hsing-Jien Kung's group has found that the cellular transcription repressor, KAP-1, is a novel regulator for KSHV latency, which is known to interact with SETDB1, a H3K9me3 HMT [79]. KAP-1 was found to be associated with a significant number of lytic promoters during latency, which becomes dissociated upon reactivation. Interestingly, KAP-1 is a substrate of the viral kinase encoded by ORF36 and the binding of KAP-1 to the KSHV genome is modulated by

ORF36-dependent phosphorylation [79]. The phosphorylation of KAP-1 causes the decline of its sumoylation, which decreases the ability of KAP-1 to bind to chromatin and repress genes. Importantly, the knockdown of KAP-1 by shRNA resulted in a 5-fold increase of RTA-mediated reactivation. Thus, KAP-1 could be one of the cellular transcription factors responsible for the recruitment of a H3K9me3 methyltransferase onto the KSHV genome, which is also involved in the inhibition of lytic genes during latency [79].

Two elegant studies have recently reported the genome-wide binding and functions of the H3K9 histone demethylases, JMJD2A and KDM3A/JMJD1A, on the latent KSHV genome, shedding light on the reasons behind the restricted localization pattern of H3K9me3 on the KSHV genome (Figures 2B and 3B) [77,80]. One of the studies showed that shRNA knockdown of JMJD2A resulted in attenuated lytic reactivation, while overexpression of an enzymatically active form of JMJD2A facilitated the induction of lytic genes [77]. Strikingly, the binding sites of JMJD2A on the viral episome inversely correlate with the presence of H3K9me3 and overlap with the H3K4me3/acH3-enriched genomic regions [77]. These results indicate that binding of JMJD2A to the IE and E genes during latency may be involved in preventing H3K9me3-marked heterochromatin formation on their promoters, thereby facilitating H3K9 acetylation and priming of the IE and E genes for robust induction upon reactivation. Based on the survey of several viral proteins, an IE/E protein called K-bZIP (K8) was found to interact with JMJD2A [77]. *In vitro* demethylase assays revealed that K-bZIP can inhibit the demethylase activity of JMJD2A. Moreover, it was shown that K-bZIP can recognize the H3K9me3 moiety and thereby interfere with the binding of JMJD2A with H3K9me3. Furthermore, K-bZIP could also block the demethylation of H3K9me3 caused by overexpressed JMJD2A in 293T cells. Despite of the robust expression of K-bZIP H3K9me3 level does not change significantly on the KSHV chromatin during reactivation. Thus, the effect of K-bZIP on H3K9me3 must be limited to a subset of K-bZIP target genes in infected cells. In fact, K-bZIP expression in KSHV-negative cells causes a global repression of host genes and increased H3K9me3-marked heterochromatin formation on cellular genes, including host immune-related genes [77,81].

Izumiya's group has recently reported that LANA forms a complex with KDM3A/JMJD1A, a cellular H3K9me1/2 histone demethylase, in KSHV infected cells [80]. The genome-wide occupancy of LANA and JMJD1A on the KSHV genome showed a high degree of overlap and was inversely correlated with the level of H3K9me2. Furthermore, depletion of LANA expression or overexpression of a JMJD1A-binding deficient LANA mutant in cells decreased the binding of JMJD1A to the viral episome, indicating that LANA recruits JMJD1A to the KSHV genome during latency. *In vitro* histone H3 peptide pull-down assays using purified LANA showed that LANA can interact with H3, H3K9me1 or H3K9me3 but not H3K9me2. Finally, the shRNA knockdown of JMJD1A resulted in decreased lytic reactivation, suggesting that JMJD1A is involved in the maintenance of H3K9 methylation-free chromatin on latent and a specific subset of lytic genes [80]. These studies altogether have shown that the regulation of H3K9me3 on the KSHV genome is indeed important for the proper induction of the lytic gene expression program [77,79,80].

3.4. H3K4me3 and the MLL/Set1 Family

Enrichment of H3K4me3 is typically present at the 5' end of transcriptionally induced genes. The first histone methyltransferase complex that can catalyze mono-, di- and trimethylation of H3K4 was identified in yeast and is called COMPASS (complex of proteins associated with Set1) [82,83]. The enzymatic subunit of COMPASS is Set1, which has at least 6 homologs in human, Set1A, Set1B, MLL1, MLL2, MLL3 and MLL4, all of which form different complexes and have distinct genomic localization [84]. In addition to their shared common subunits (Ash2, RbpBp5, Wdr5 and Dpy30), they differ in their enzymatic subunits and also have unique components. For instance, the tumor suppressor protein, Menin can only be found in complex with MLL1 or MLL2, while UTX, the Pax transactivation domain-interacting protein (PTIP), PTIP-associated protein 1 and nuclear receptor coactivator NCOA6 are exclusive components of the MLL3 and MLL4 complexes. In addition, Wdr82 is restricted to Set1A/Set1B complexes [84]. Whereas the Set1A/B complexes are the major H3K4 methylases responsible for the bulk H3K4me3 in mammalian cells, MLL1-4 play an important regulatory role for specific subsets of genes [85,86]. Mutations and random translocations of MLL genes are frequent occurrences in hematological malignancies like acute myeloid and lymphoid leukemia [87].

Regulation of H3K4me3 levels is important for controlling gene expression, particularly during lytic reactivation of KSHV, when lytic gene expression is rapidly induced. H3K4me3 is present on certain viral promoters during latency and is increased following reactivation (Figure 3) [50,51]. However, further studies are needed to identify the cellular factors that modulate H3K4me3 levels during the KSHV life cycle. It has been reported that while the binding of the core subunits of MLL/Set1 complexes, Ash2 and Wdr5, can increase on lytic promoters following reactivation, this was not observed on the latent LANA promoter [88]. Also, recruitment of Set1A could be detected on lytic promoters during reactivation but whether it is the sole H3K4me3 methylase responsible for the increase of H3K4me3 on lytic promoters has yet to be determined [88]. In addition, another group showed that MLL2 can interact with the RTA promoter through the viral non-coding PAN RNA, which raises the question whether distinct MLL/Set1 complexes can be targeted to different viral promoters [73]. Future studies using MLL/Set1 component-specific shRNAs as well as applying ChIP assays to test which of the unique subunits of MLL/Set1 complexes bind onto the KSHV episome will help to identify which of the MLL/Set1 complexes is responsible for the regulation of H3K4me3 on the KSHV genome during latency and following lytic reactivation.

There are a number of examples known of crosstalk between different histone modifications. For instance, H2B monoubiquitination at lysine 120 by the RAD6/BRE1 ubiquitin ligase complex is required for the methylation of H3K4 in human cells [89]. Furthermore, it was shown that the RNA polymerase II-associated factor (PAF) complex mediates the recruitment of RAD/BRE1 to the transcription machinery, where the monoubiquitination of H2B promotes Set1-mediated methylation of H3K4 in human cells [89]. Thus, it would be interesting to determine whether differential regulation of H2B ubiquitination is involved in the regulation of H3K4me3 levels on the KSHV episome.

3.5. Histone Acetylation and Deacetylation on the KSHV Genome

Acetylation and deacetylation of lysine residues of histone tails have antagonistic effect on gene transcription. While acetylation of histones by histone acetyltransferases (HATs) unravels chromatin and activates transcription, histone deacetylases (HDACs) induce chromatin condensation and gene silencing [90,91]. Shortly after the discovery of KSHV, it was found that lytic genes of KSHV can be induced from latency by treating latently infected cells with various HDAC inhibitors, highlighting the importance of histone acetylation in the regulation of lytic gene expression. Histone acetylation can occur at more than 20 different lysine residues positioned within histones. To date, 19 different HATs are known and each one is part of distinct transcription activator complexes. The majority of HATs can acetylate histones at multiple positions and likewise, the same lysine residue can be acetylated by various HATs. This redundancy makes it difficult to pinpoint the HAT(s) involved in a given histone acetylation on the KSHV chromatin (Figure 3A). Two ChIP-on-chip studies revealed that H3K9/K14ac are enriched on several lytic promoters during latency and are further increased upon lytic reactivation [50,51]. Using luciferase reporter assays, several cellular transcription factors that interact with HATs or HDACs (e.g., C/EBPα, AP1, Oct-1, STAT3 and RBP-Jκ) have been implicated in the regulation of specific lytic promoters such as RTA [23,92,93]. Nevertheless, comprehensive studies of histone acetylation on the KSHV epigenome during latency and reactivation are needed in order to provide more detailed insight into the role of histone acetylation and ultimately pave the way toward the identification of the HATs involved in viral gene regulation during the KSHV life cycle.

The interplay between HATs and HDACs in the regulation of RTA transcription was examined in detail. Lieberman's group analyzed the chromatin structure of the core promoter of RTA in the presence or absence of the HDAC inhibitors (HDACi) such as sodium butyrate (NaB) and trichostatin A (TSA) [12]. They found that the RTA promoter is highly inducible by these HDACs and a NaB responsive element was mapped to a short GC-box DNA sequence that binds Sp1 and Sp3. Micrococcal nuclease (MNase) mapping and restriction endonuclease accessibility assays revealed that there is a stably positioned nucleosome at the transcriptional initiation site of RTA during latency, which rapidly changes upon NaB treatment [12]. Furthermore, it was also observed that HDAC1, 5 and 7 bound to the RTA promoter, resulting in hypoacetylation of the viral chromatin during latency, while reactivation resulted in the hyperacetylation of histones H3 and H4 concomitantly with the recruitment of components of the SWI/SNF2 ATP-dependent chromatin-remodeling complex onto the RTA promoter (Figure 4). Ectopic expression of the CREB-binding HAT, CBP, resulted in 10-fold induction of the RTA promoter as determined by luciferase reporter assay, whereas expression of other HATs such as p300, PCAF, GCN5 and TIP60 had no such effect. The CBP-mediated promoter stimulation depends on the Sp1/3-binding site, suggesting that CBP can be recruited to the RTA promoter via interaction with Sp1/3 during reactivation, resulting in the acetylation of both H3 and H4 [12]. In agreement with this, others also showed that NaB treatment could induce an Sp1-binding site-dependent recruitment of CBP and p300 onto the RTA promoter. Moreover, the increased Sp1-binding on the viral promoter is transient during reactivation [94]. The role of CBP and SWI/SNF2 in the regulation of the RTA promoter was further detailed by Gwack and his co-workers [24]. They showed that the C-terminal activation domain of RTA forms a complex with the Mediator, SWI/SNF2 and CBP in cells. During reactivation RTA recruits these cellular factors onto the RTA promoter and other RTA-responsive lytic promoters resulting in their transcriptional activation [24]. These studies altogether show that reactivation of lytic genes requires the recruitment of HATs by cellular and viral transcription factors to the viral promoters, resulting in the remodeling of the chromatin structure of the virus (Figure 4).

Figure 4. Regulation of the RTA promoter during latency and reactivation. The H3K27me3 histone methyltransferase complex PRC2 as well as specific histone deacetylases (HDAC1, 5 and 7) are critical transcriptional repressors that are present on the RTA promoter during latency. The bivalent chromatin of the RTA promoter is indicated by the presence of both activating (H3K4me3 and acH3) and repressive (H3K27me3) histone marks. After reactivation RTA binds to its own promoter via CBF-1 (also called RBP-Jκ) and recruits several cellular transcription factors such as the Mediator, the ATP-dependent chromatin remodeling complex SWI/SNF2 and the histone acetyltransferase CBP. The induction of transcription is accompanied by the rapid recruitment of RNA polymerase II (RNAPII) and increased binding of Sp1 to the promoter. The KSHV non-coding PAN RNA can also interact with the RTA promoter and recruit the H3K4me3 histone methyltransferase MLL2 as well as the H3K27me3 histone demthylases UTX and JMJD3. The Sp1/3-binding sites play an important role in the HDAC inhibitor-mediated reactivation of the RTA promoter. While these sites contribute to the LANA-mediated repression of the RTA promoter during latency, they are also involved in recruitment of CBP, which can catalyze the hyperacetylation of histones on the viral promoter during reactivation.

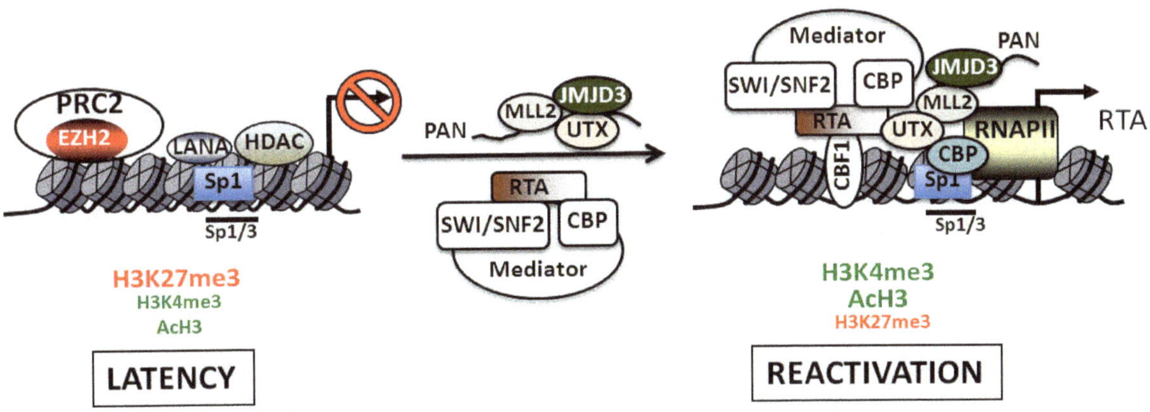

Histone acetylation and nucleosome positioning also play a critical role in the regulation of the chromatin structure of the origin of latent replication (Ori-P), which is embedded in the GC-rich TR region of the KSHV genome. Ori-P contains two LANA-binding sites, where LANA binds and recruits the cellular DNA replication proteins, ORC2 and MCM, to facilitate the replication of the viral genome concomitantly with the replication of the host genome during mitosis [38,40]. It was shown that Ori-P is enriched with hyperacetylated histones H3 and H4 and that this enrichment is due to the activity of LANA, which recruits HATs such as HBO1 or CBP, to the Ori-P (Figure 2B) [40]. In addition, the bromodomain-containing cellular protein, Brd2, which binds to acetylated histones and is a known LANA-binding protein, is also recruited to the Ori-P, and may also be involved in the maintenance of the hyperacetylation of histones in Ori-P. Nucleosome mapping assays revealed a highly ordered nucleosome array in Ori-P that becomes disorganized in a cell cycle-dependent manner [40]. The current model is that the maintenance of a hyperacetylated chromatin in Ori-P facilitates the assembly of the DNA replication complex.

3.6. DNA Methylation of the KSHV Genome

In mammalian cells, DNA methylation occurs mainly on cytidine residues in the context of CpG dinucleotides. Methylated CpGs are often found in clusters called CpG islands [95]. Hypermethylated CpG islands in the 5' regulatory regions of genes are associated with gene silencing. Methylation of DNA inhibits gene expression either by impeding the binding of transcription factors to the promoter or by the action of methyl-CpG-binding proteins (e.g., MeCP2), which bind to methylated CpG islands and recruit HDACs and other transcription repressors to the gene to turn off its expression [96]. The maintenance of DNA methylation during cell division is mediated by DNA methyltransferase 1 (DNMT1), which copies the DNA methylation pattern to the daughter strands during DNA replication, while DNMT3a and DNMT3b are *de novo* DNA methyltransferases [97].

It has been shown that the treatment of PEL cells with the DNA methyltransferase inhibitor 5-AzaC can induce lytic reactivation of KSHV, suggesting that DNA methylation of lytic promoters is involved in the suppression of lytic genes during latency [11]. Recently, the global DNA methylation pattern of KSHV was determined in different latently infected cell lines by using immunoprecipitation of methylated DNA (MeDIP) in conjunction with KSHV specific high-resolution tiling microarray [51]. These experiments showed that KSHV is subject to extensive DNA methylation during latency. Like the H3K27me3 pattern on the latent KSHV genome, DNA methylation was excluded from the transcriptionally active latency-associated locus, while most of the lytic genes were associated with DNA hypermethylation. Surprisingly, the RTA promoter was not methylated in most of the cell lines, suggesting that DNA methylation is unlikely to be involved in the inhibition of RTA expression during latency [51]. In addition, while the latency-specific histone modification patterns were rapidly deposited on the viral episome following *de novo* infection, DNA methylation patterns were established comparatively slower, indicating that DNA methylation does not play a role in establishment of latency. On the other hand, DNA methylation may reinforce the inhibition of lytic genes at late timepoints of infection [51].

3.7. Nuclear Organization of the KSHV Genome

It is known that the KSHV episome is tethered to the cellular chromosome by LANA, which interacts with histones and several components of the cellular chromatin. One question that remains is whether tethering of the KSHV genome is random or prone to localize on specific regions of the host chromosome. Infected cells harbor approximately 30–80 copies of the KSHV genome and ChIP-seq analysis has revealed at least 256 LANA-binding sites on the cellular genome, suggesting that not all LANA proteins may be involved in tethering the viral genome [26]. An interesting hypothesis is that the viral genome could be tethered to heterochromatin-enriched nuclear regions during latency and may relocate to a transcriptionally favorable nuclear compartment upon reactivation. Microscope analysis of the nuclear distribution of LANA in latently infected B cells showed that LANA preferentially associates with the border of heterochromatin, inviting speculation that close proximity to heterochromatin-rich regions of the host cell may be critical for the formation and maintenance of heterochromatin on the KSHV genome [98].

The structural organization of chromatin domains in the cellular genome plays an important role in the regulation cellular gene expression. Similarly, the chromatinized KSHV episome is also compartmentalized into different chromatin domains, which can interact with each other by a looping mechanism mediated by cellular factors that bind to the KSHV genome [99]. The maintenance of viral latency requires the separation of the latent genes from the lytic genes-encoding part of the KSHV genome so that the latent genes can be continuously expressed, while the lytic genes are repressed during latency. Lieberman's group found that CTCF and the cohesion complex, which are known chromatin boundary factors separating active and inactive chromatin domains, bound to several sites of the KSHV genome and they are involved in the transcription regulation of both latent and IE genes during latency [100,101]. One of the CTCF-binding sites (CBS) can be found in the intron of the latent gene, LANA. Deletion of CBS disrupted cohesin binding to the KSHV genome and caused viral episome instability and increased expression of lytic genes [100]. In addition, chromatin conformation capture (3C) assays provided evidence for the first time that the latent LANA promoter physically interacts with the lytic RTA promoter during latency, which is mediated by the CTCF/cohesin complex in the intron of LANA [99]. In agreement with this, CBS mutation, siRNA depletion of CTCF or the cohesin complex component RAD21 diminished the interaction between these latent and lytic promoters and deregulated the latent gene expression program. This viral chromosome looping was also disrupted during lytic reactivation suggesting that the CTCF/cohesin-mediated looping in the viral genome is dynamic and involved in the regulation of latent and lytic gene expression [99]. The CTCF/cohesin complex in the intron of LANA also plays a critical role in the regulation of transcription elongation and nucleosome organization in the latency locus [102,103].

Every KSHV infected cell carries multiple copies of KSHV genomes, which raises the question whether they all have the same nucleosome structure during latency, which change simultaneously during reactivation or they show diversity. To answer this question a recent study used single-molecule footprinting assays called MAPit (Methyltransferase Accessibility Protocol for individual templates), which allows the detection of multiple chromatin states at selected loci within a cell population [104]. The chromatin architecture of the promoter of the constitutively expressed latent gene, LANA, the promoter of the IE gene, RTA and the promoter of the early gene, K2 was investigated. Their analysis showed diverse chromatin at each of these promoters, which ranged from closed to open conformations. Interestingly, the induction of lytic gene expression program resulted in the remodeling of the viral chromatin only on a fraction of the viral episomes. These results indicate that KSHV genomes possess diverse chromatin conformations in infected cells during both latency and reactivation. Furthermore, local chromatin condensations caused by epigenetic drift can restrict the expression of any viral genes irrespectively of what gene expression classes (IE, E, L or latent) they belong to [104].

4. Reprogramming of the Host Transcriptome during KSHV Infection

In vitro experiments have shown that KSHV infection of endothelial cells results in transcriptional reprogramming such that infected lymphatic endothelial cells are driven toward a blood vessel endothelial cell phenotype and vice versa [105,106]. In addition, KSHV infection can also induce the transcriptional reprogramming of lymphatic endothelial cells to mesenchymal cells [107]. These observations imply that viral factors may be involved by either deregulating the expression of cell type-specific transcription factors or modulating their functions, which results in altered cellular gene expression profile. Both LANA and viral miRNAs, for example, have been implicated to play a role in changing the expression of specific cellular genes encoding master transcription factors [106,108]. These viral factors can use different ways to regulate cellular genes. For example, LANA recruits DNA methyltransferases to specific cellular promoters such as that of H-cadherin and TGF-β type II receptor, resulting in hypermethylation and transcriptional repression of these promoters [32,109]. Because LANA has been shown to interact with a wide variety of chromatin-associated regulatory proteins, it can affect large number of cellular genes. Recent ChIP-seq analysis revealed 256 LANA-binding sites on the cellular genome, several of which are linked to p53-, TNF- or IFN-γ regulated genes [26].

KSHV encodes 12 miRNA genes that produce 25 mature miRNAs. These are small non-coding gene regulatory RNAs that can bind to mRNAs resulting in translational block or their degradation to repress genes [110]. A recent study showed that the KSHV miRNA miR-K12-11 shares significant sequence homology with the cellular miRNA called miR-155, which is often overexpressed in human tumors [111]. Strikingly, when miR-K12-11 was expressed in bone marrow cells, it caused the downregulation of Jarid2, a component of the PRC2 complex [111]. Thus, this viral miRNA can potentially deregulate the expression of PRC2 target genes such as that are involved in cell cycle control, for example, which can contribute to the development of KSHV-associated malignancies. Another KSHV miRNA, miR-K12-4-5p targets the retinoblastoma-like protein 2 (Rbl2), which is a repressor of the *de novo* DNA methyltransefarses DNMT3a and DNMT3b genes [112]. Expression of miR-K12-4-5p reduces Rbl2 expression resulting in the increased expression of DNMTs that can globally affect cellular gene expression in infected cells. PAN RNA of KSHV that is abundantly expressed in the nucleus during reactivation has been reported to downregulate the expression of many immunomodulatory genes [113]. PAN RNA can bind to gene promoters and recruit different histone modifying enzymes, which can be involved in the PAN RNA-mediated cellular gene regulation observed in infected cells [73,113].

Viral proteins often targets cellular histone modifying enzymes to relocate them on the cellular genome, modulate their enzymatic activity or their expression, which can affect the expression of a large number of cellular genes, all of which serve the needs of the virus for efficient infection of the host. Several KSHV proteins such as LANA, K8 and vIRF1 can bind to the histone acetyltransferase CBP/p300 and inhibit CBP/p300-mediated cellular transcription [37,114,115]. In contrast, RTA can use CBP to robustly activate gene transcription but it is still unclear how widely RTA uses CBP in activation of cellular genes [24]. K8 also interacts with the H3K9me3 histone demethylase JMJD2A and blocks its activity, which could play a role in the observed K8-mediated global cellular gene repression [77]. LANA forms a complex with the H3K9me1/2 histone demethylase JMJD1A in infected cells, which raises the question whether LANA uses JMJD1A to activate any of its cellular target genes [80].

EZH2, the H3K27me3 histone methyltransferase of the PRC2 complex has been shown to be overexpressed in KSHV-infected cells in Kaposi's sarcoma (KS), suggesting that KSHV could be involved in EZH2 upregulation [116]. Indeed, KSHV infection of endothelial cells *in vitro* can induce the expression of EZH2, and this is mainly mediated by the KSHV latent proteins LANA and vFLIP via the upregulation of the NF-κB pathway [116]. Importantly, the increased expression of EZH2 turned out to be essential for KSHV-induced angiogenesis in KSHV-infected cells [116].

KSHV infection of B cells in human can lead to the development of the KSHV-associated primary effusion lymphoma (PEL), which is characterized by the disruption of the B-cell specific transcriptional program. Protein expression of several transcription factors that are essential for B-cell development is significantly altered in PEL cells compared to uninfected B-cells [117]. While PEL cells constitutively express IRF4, the protein level of other B-cell transcription factors such as Pax5, Oct-2, PU.1 and IRF-8 was completely abolished [117]. The viral factors involved in the reprogramming of the B-cell-specific transcription factor network have not yet been identified.

5. Outlook

ChIP-on-chip analysis of the KSHV episome revealed distinct chromatin domains on the viral genome, which are characterized by different histone modification and DNA methylation patterns indicative of targeted recruitment of specific cellular chromatin modifying enzyme complexes (Figure 3). The benefit of such compartmentalization of the KSHV genome might be the use of common transcription regulatory mechanisms for expression of genes that have related functions during the lifecycle of the virus. Strikingly, the IE and most of E genes are marked by activating histone marks while the majority of late genes, which are transcribed only following viral DNA replication, are associated with heterochromatin that remains unaltered during the early phase of reactivation [50,51]. These observations suggest that the type of chromatin structure associated with each viral gene can play a role in the regulation of their expression. Two recent papers have reported that H2AX, an isoform of the canonical histone H2A and the phosphorylation of histone H3 at serine 10 residue are also components of the viral chromatin landscape and regulate the persistence of viral episome in infected cells as well as the reactivation of the lytic gene expression program, respectively [118,119]. These studies also demonstrate that we only see the tip of the iceberg regarding to the components and the organization of the KSHV chromatin in infected cells.

Currently, at least 130 different posttranslational modification sites have been identified on histones and there are at least 150 histone-modifying enzymes known [120]. Because of the unique DNA sequence elements, the close proximity of genes and overlapping gene regulatory regions in the KSHV genome, KSHV may utilize unique mechanisms to regulate its genome. Also, the modulation of the function of cellular chromatin modifying enzymes by viral proteins allows the reprogramming of the cellular transcriptome in a way that becomes beneficial for persistent infection as well as the development of KSHV-associated malignancies. It has been demonstrated that drugs targeting of histone modifying enzymes is a viable strategy for controlling HSV-1 and Human cytomegalovirus (HCMV) infections [121–123]. Therefore, identifying the relevant cellular and viral factors involved in the chromatin control of KSHV infection may bring new opportunities for pharmacological control of KSHV infection and KSHV-associated diseases.

Acknowledgments

This work was partly supported by CA082057, CA31363, CA115284, DE019085, AI073099, Hastings Foundation, and Fletcher Jones Foundation (JUJ). We thank Jung's lab members for their support and discussions.

References

1. Cesarman, E.; Moore, P.S.; Rao, P.H.; Inghirami, G.; Knowles, D.M.; Chang, Y. *In vitro* establishment and characterization of two acquired immunodeficiency syndrome-related lymphoma cell lines (BC-1 and BC-2) containing Kaposi's sarcoma-associated herpesvirus-like (KSHV) DNA sequences. *Blood* **1995**, *86*, 2708–2714.

2. Chang, Y.; Cesarman, E.; Pessin, M.S.; Lee, F.; Culpepper, J.; Knowles, D.M.; Moore, P.S. Identification of herpesvirus-like DNA sequences in AIDS-associated Kaposi's sarcoma. *Science* **1994**, *266*, 1865–1869.

3. Lu, C.; Zeng, Y.; Huang, Z.; Huang, L.; Qian, C.; Tang, G.; Qin, D. Human herpesvirus 6 activates lytic cycle replication of Kaposi's sarcoma-associated herpesvirus. *Am. J. Pathol.* **2005**, *166*, 173–183.

4. Merat, R.; Amara, A.; Lebbe, C.; de The, H.; Morel, P.; Saib, A. HIV-1 infection of primary effusion lymphoma cell line triggers Kaposi's sarcoma-associated herpesvirus (KSHV) reactivation. *Int. J. Cancer* **2002**, *97*, 791–795.

5. Mercader, M.; Taddeo, B.; Panella, J.R.; Chandran, B.; Nickoloff, B.J.; Foreman, K.E. Induction of HHV-8 lytic cycle replication by inflammatory cytokines produced by HIV-1-infected T cells. *Am. J. Pathol.* **2000**, *156*, 1961–1971.
6. Vieira, J.; O'Hearn, P.; Kimball, L.; Chandran, B.; Corey, L. Activation of Kaposi's sarcoma-associated herpesvirus (human herpesvirus 8) lytic replication by human cytomegalovirus. *J. Virol.* **2001**, *75*, 1378–1386.
7. Ye, F.; Zhou, F.; Bedolla, R.G.; Jones, T.; Lei, X.; Kang, T.; Guadalupe, M.; Gao, S.J. Reactive oxygen species hydrogen peroxide mediates Kaposi's sarcoma-associated herpesvirus reactivation from latency. *PLoS Pathog.* **2011**, *7*, e1002054.
8. Davis, D.A.; Rinderknecht, A.S.; Zoeteweij, J.P.; Aoki, Y.; Read-Connole, E.L.; Tosato, G.; Blauvelt, A.; Yarchoan, R. Hypoxia induces lytic replication of Kaposi sarcoma-associated herpesvirus. *Blood* **2001**, *97*, 3244–3250.
9. Russo, J.J.; Bohenzky, R.A.; Chien, M.C.; Chen, J.; Yan, M.; Maddalena, D.; Parry, J.P.; Peruzzi, D.; Edelman, I.S.; Chang, Y.; *et al.* Nucleotide sequence of the Kaposi sarcoma-associated herpesvirus (HHV8). *Proc. Natl. Acad. Sci. USA* **1996**, *93*, 14862–14867.
10. Jenner, R.G.; Alba, M.M.; Boshoff, C.; Kellam, P. Kaposi's sarcoma-associated herpesvirus latent and lytic gene expression as revealed by DNA arrays. *J. Virol.* **2001**, *75*, 891–902.
11. Chen, J.; Ueda, K.; Sakakibara, S.; Okuno, T.; Parravicini, C.; Corbellino, M.; Yamanishi, K. Activation of latent Kaposi's sarcoma-associated herpesvirus by demethylation of the promoter of the lytic transactivator. *Proc. Natl. Acad. Sci. USA* **2001**, *98*, 4119–4124.
12. Lu, F.; Zhou, J.; Wiedmer, A.; Madden, K.; Yuan, Y.; Lieberman, P.M. Chromatin remodeling of the Kaposi's sarcoma-associated herpesvirus ORF50 promoter correlates with reactivation from latency. *J. Virol.* **2003**, *77*, 11425–11435.
13. Xie, J.; Ajibade, A.O.; Ye, F.; Kuhne, K.; Gao, S.J. Reactivation of Kaposi's sarcoma-associated herpesvirus from latency requires MEK/ERK, JNK and p38 multiple mitogen-activated protein kinase pathways. *Virology* **2008**, *371*, 139–154.
14. Ballestas, M.E.; Chatis, P.A.; Kaye, K.M. Efficient persistence of extrachromosomal KSHV DNA mediated by latency-associated nuclear antigen. *Science* **1999**, *284*, 641–644.
15. Renne, R.; Lagunoff, M.; Zhong, W.; Ganem, D. The size and conformation of Kaposi's sarcoma-associated herpesvirus (human herpesvirus 8) DNA in infected cells and virions. *J. Virol.* **1996**, *70*, 8151–8154.
16. Zentner, G.E.; Henikoff, S. Regulation of nucleosome dynamics by histone modifications. *Nat. Struct. Mol. Biol.* **2013**, *20*, 259–266.
17. Yun, M.; Wu, J.; Workman, J.L.; Li, B. Readers of histone modifications. *Cell Res.* **2011**, *21*, 564–578.
18. Cedar, H.; Bergman, Y. Programming of DNA methylation patterns. *Annu. Rev. Biochem.* **2012**, *81*, 97–117.
19. Loyola, A.; Almouzni, G. Marking histone H3 variants: How, when and why? *Trends Biochem. Sci.* **2007**, *32*, 425–433.

20. Holwerda, S.; de Laat, W. Chromatin loops, gene positioning, and gene expression. *Front. Genet.* **2012**, *3*, e217.
21. Grundhoff, A.; Ganem, D. Inefficient establishment of KSHV latency suggests an additional role for continued lytic replication in Kaposi sarcoma pathogenesis. *J. Clin. Investig.* **2004**, *113*, 124–136.
22. Krishnan, H.H.; Naranatt, P.P.; Smith, M.S.; Zeng, L.; Bloomer, C.; Chandran, B. Concurrent expression of latent and a limited number of lytic genes with immune modulation and antiapoptotic function by Kaposi's sarcoma-associated herpesvirus early during infection of primary endothelial and fibroblast cells and subsequent decline of lytic gene expression. *J. Virol.* **2004**, *78*, 3601–3620.
23. Guito, J.; Lukac, D.M. KSHV Rta promoter specification and viral reactivation. *Front. Microbiol.* **2012**, *3*, e30.
24. Gwack, Y.; Baek, H.J.; Nakamura, H.; Lee, S.H.; Meisterernst, M.; Roeder, R.G.; Jung, J.U. Principal role of TRAP/mediator and SWI/SNF complexes in Kaposi's sarcoma-associated herpesvirus RTA-mediated lytic reactivation. *Mol. Cell. Biol.* **2003**, *23*, 2055–2067.
25. Budt, M.; Hristozova, T.; Hille, G.; Berger, K.; Brune, W. Construction of a lytically replicating Kaposi's sarcoma-associated herpesvirus. *J. Virol.* **2011**, *85*, 10415–10420.
26. Lu, F.; Tsai, K.; Chen, H.S.; Wikramasinghe, P.; Davuluri, R.V.; Showe, L.; Domsic, J.; Marmorstein, R.; Lieberman, P.M. Identification of host-chromosome binding sites and candidate gene targets for Kaposi's sarcoma-associated herpesvirus LANA. *J. Virol.* **2012**, *86*, 5752–5762.
27. Campbell, M.; Chang, P.C.; Huerta, S.; Izumiya, C.; Davis, R.; Tepper, C.G.; Kim, K.Y.; Shevchenko, B.; Wang, D.H.; Jung, J.U.; *et al.* Protein arginine methyltransferase 1-directed methylation of Kaposi sarcoma-associated herpesvirus latency-associated nuclear antigen. *J. Biol. Chem.* **2012**, *287*, 5806–5818.
28. Barbera, A.J.; Chodaparambil, J.V.; Kelley-Clarke, B.; Luger, K.; Kaye, K.M. Kaposi's sarcoma-associated herpesvirus LANA hitches a ride on the chromosome. *Cell Cycle* **2006**, *5*, 1048–1052.
29. Lu, F.; Day, L.; Gao, S.J.; Lieberman, P.M. Acetylation of the latency-associated nuclear antigen regulates repression of Kaposi's sarcoma-associated herpesvirus lytic transcription. *J. Virol.* **2006**, *80*, 5273–5282.
30. Li, Q.; Zhou, F.; Ye, F.; Gao, S.J. Genetic disruption of KSHV major latent nuclear antigen LANA enhances viral lytic transcriptional program. *Virology* **2008**, *379*, 234–244.
31. Matsumura, S.; Persson, L.M.; Wong, L.; Wilson, A.C. The latency-associated nuclear antigen interacts with MeCP2 and nucleosomes through separate domains. *J. Virol.* **2010**, *84*, 2318–2330.
32. Shamay, M.; Krithivas, A.; Zhang, J.; Hayward, S.D. Recruitment of the *de novo* DNA methyltransferase Dnmt3a by Kaposi's sarcoma-associated herpesvirus LANA. *Proc. Natl. Acad. Sci. USA* **2006**, *103*, 14554–14559.

33. Sakakibara, S.; Ueda, K.; Nishimura, K.; Do, E.; Ohsaki, E.; Okuno, T.; Yamanishi, K. Accumulation of heterochromatin components on the terminal repeat sequence of Kaposi's sarcoma-associated herpesvirus mediated by the latency-associated nuclear antigen. *J. Virol.* **2004**, *78*, 7299–7310.

34. Viejo-Borbolla, A.; Kati, E.; Sheldon, J.A.; Nathan, K.; Mattsson, K.; Szekely, L.; Schulz, T.F. A Domain in the C-terminal region of latency-associated nuclear antigen 1 of Kaposi's sarcoma-associated Herpesvirus affects transcriptional activation and binding to nuclear heterochromatin. *J. Virol.* **2003**, *77*, 7093–7100.

35. Lim, C.; Lee, D.; Seo, T.; Choi, C.; Choe, J. Latency-associated nuclear antigen of Kaposi's sarcoma-associated herpesvirus functionally interacts with heterochromatin protein 1. *J. Biol. Chem.* **2003**, *278*, 7397–7405.

36. Krithivas, A.; Young, D.B.; Liao, G.; Greene, D.; Hayward, S.D. Human herpesvirus 8 LANA interacts with proteins of the mSin3 corepressor complex and negatively regulates Epstein-Barr virus gene expression in dually infected PEL cells. *J. Virol.* **2000**, *74*, 9637–9645.

37. Lim, C.; Gwack, Y.; Hwang, S.; Kim, S.; Choe, J. The transcriptional activity of cAMP response element-binding protein-binding protein is modulated by the latency associated nuclear antigen of Kaposi's sarcoma-associated herpesvirus. *J. Biol. Chem.* **2001**, *276*, 31016–31022.

38. Lim, C.; Sohn, H.; Lee, D.; Gwack, Y.; Choe, J. Functional dissection of latency-associated nuclear antigen 1 of Kaposi's sarcoma-associated herpesvirus involved in latent DNA replication and transcription of terminal repeats of the viral genome. *J. Virol.* **2002**, *76*, 10320–10331.

39. Cotter, M.A., 2nd; Robertson, E.S. The latency-associated nuclear antigen tethers the Kaposi's sarcoma-associated herpesvirus genome to host chromosomes in body cavity-based lymphoma cells. *Virology* **1999**, *264*, 254–264.

40. Stedman, W.; Deng, Z.; Lu, F.; Lieberman, P.M. ORC, MCM, and histone hyperacetylation at the Kaposi's sarcoma-associated herpesvirus latent replication origin. *J. Virol.* **2004**, *78*, 12566–12575.

41. Ye, F.C.; Zhou, F.C.; Yoo, S.M.; Xie, J.P.; Browning, P.J.; Gao, S.J. Disruption of Kaposi's sarcoma-associated herpesvirus latent nuclear antigen leads to abortive episome persistence. *J. Virol.* **2004**, *78*, 11121–11129.

42. Xiao, B.; Verma, S.C.; Cai, Q.; Kaul, R.; Lu, J.; Saha, A.; Robertson, E.S. Bub1 and CENP-F can contribute to Kaposi's sarcoma-associated herpesvirus genome persistence by targeting LANA to kinetochores. *J. Virol.* **2010**, *84*, 9718–9732.

43. Si, H.; Verma, S.C.; Lampson, M.A.; Cai, Q.; Robertson, E.S. Kaposi's sarcoma-associated herpesvirus-encoded LANA can interact with the nuclear mitotic apparatus protein to regulate genome maintenance and segregation. *J. Virol.* **2008**, *82*, 6734–6746.

44. Ottinger, M.; Christalla, T.; Nathan, K.; Brinkmann, M.M.; Viejo-Borbolla, A.; Schulz, T.F. Kaposi's sarcoma-associated herpesvirus LANA-1 interacts with the short variant of BRD4 and releases cells from a BRD4- and BRD2/RING3-induced G1 cell cycle arrest. *J. Virol.* **2006**, *80*, 10772–10786.

45. Barbera, A.J.; Chodaparambil, J.V.; Kelley-Clarke, B.; Joukov, V.; Walter, J.C.; Luger, K.; Kaye, K.M. The nucleosomal surface as a docking station for Kaposi's sarcoma herpesvirus LANA. *Science* **2006**, *311*, 856–861.
46. Viejo-Borbolla, A.; Ottinger, M.; Bruning, E.; Burger, A.; Konig, R.; Kati, E.; Sheldon, J.A.; Schulz, T.F. Brd2/RING3 interacts with a chromatin-binding domain in the Kaposi's Sarcoma-associated herpesvirus latency-associated nuclear antigen 1 (LANA-1) that is required for multiple functions of LANA-1. *J. Virol.* **2005**, *79*, 13618–13629.
47. Krithivas, A.; Fujimuro, M.; Weidner, M.; Young, D.B.; Hayward, S.D. Protein interactions targeting the latency-associated nuclear antigen of Kaposi's sarcoma-associated herpesvirus to cell chromosomes. *J. Virol.* **2002**, *76*, 11596–11604.
48. Cheng, F.; Weidner-Glunde, M.; Varjosalo, M.; Rainio, E.M.; Lehtonen, A.; Schulz, T.F.; Koskinen, P.J.; Taipale, J.; Ojala, P.M. KSHV reactivation from latency requires Pim-1 and Pim-3 kinases to inactivate the latency-associated nuclear antigen LANA. *PLoS Pathog.* **2009**, *5*, e1000324.
49. Woodard, C.; Shamay, M.; Liao, G.; Zhu, J.; Ng, A.N.; Li, R.; Newman, R.; Rho, H.S.; Hu, J.; Wan, J.; *et al.* Phosphorylation of the chromatin binding domain of KSHV LANA. *PLoS Pathog.* **2012**, *8*, e1002972.
50. Toth, Z.; Maglinte, D.T.; Lee, S.H.; Lee, H.R.; Wong, L.Y.; Brulois, K.F.; Lee, S.; Buckley, J.D.; Laird, P.W.; Marquez, V.E.; *et al.* Epigenetic analysis of KSHV latent and lytic genomes. *PLoS Pathog.* **2010**, *6*, e1001013.
51. Gunther, T.; Grundhoff, A. The epigenetic landscape of latent Kaposi sarcoma-associated herpesvirus genomes. *PLoS Pathog.* **2010**, *6*, e1000935.
52. Toth, Z.; Brulois, K.F.; Wong, L.Y.; Lee, H.R.; Chung, B.; Jung, J.U. Negative elongation factor-mediated suppression of RNA polymerase II elongation of Kaposi's sarcoma-associated herpesvirus lytic gene expression. *J. Virol.* **2012**, *86*, 9696–9707.
53. Wu, T.T.; Park, T.; Kim, H.; Tran, T.; Tong, L.; Martinez-Guzman, D.; Reyes, N.; Deng, H.; Sun, R. ORF30 and ORF34 are essential for expression of late genes in murine gammaherpesvirus 68. *J. Virol.* **2009**, *83*, 2265–2273.
54. Wong, E.; Wu, T.T.; Reyes, N.; Deng, H.; Sun, R. Murine gammaherpesvirus 68 open reading frame 24 is required for late gene expression after DNA replication. *J. Virol.* **2007**, *81*, 6761–6764.
55. Arumugaswami, V.; Wu, T.T.; Martinez-Guzman, D.; Jia, Q.; Deng, H.; Reyes, N.; Sun, R. ORF18 is a transfactor that is essential for late gene transcription of a gammaherpesvirus. *J. Virol.* **2006**, *80*, 9730–9740.
56. Simon, J.A.; Kingston, R.E. Mechanisms of polycomb gene silencing: Knowns and unknowns. *Nat. Rev. Mol. Cell Biol* **2009**, *10*, 697–708.
57. Stock, J.K.; Giadrossi, S.; Casanova, M.; Brookes, E.; Vidal, M.; Koseki, H.; Brockdorff, N.; Fisher, A.G.; Pombo, A. Ring1-mediated ubiquitination of H2A restrains poised RNA polymerase II at bivalent genes in mouse ES cells. *Nat. Cell Biol.* **2007**, *9*, 1428–1435.

58. Francis, N.J.; Kingston, R.E.; Woodcock, C.L. Chromatin compaction by a polycomb group protein complex. *Science* **2004**, *306*, 1574–1577.
59. Dellino, G.I.; Schwartz, Y.B.; Farkas, G.; McCabe, D.; Elgin, S.C.; Pirrotta, V. Polycomb silencing blocks transcription initiation. *Mol. Cell* **2004**, *13*, 887–893.
60. Pasini, D.; Hansen, K.H.; Christensen, J.; Agger, K.; Cloos, P.A.; Helin, K. Coordinated regulation of transcriptional repression by the RBP2 H3K4 demethylase and Polycomb-Repressive Complex 2. *Genes Dev.* **2008**, *22*, 1345–1355.
61. Mills, A.A. Throwing the cancer switch: Reciprocal roles of polycomb and trithorax proteins. *Nat. Rev. Cancer* **2010**, *10*, 669–682.
62. Raaphorst, F.M. Deregulated expression of Polycomb-group oncogenes in human malignant lymphomas and epithelial tumors. *Hum. Mol. Genet.* **2005**, *14*, R93–R100.
63. Margueron, R.; Justin, N.; Ohno, K.; Sharpe, M.L.; Son, J.; Drury, W.J., 3rd; Voigt, P.; Martin, S.R.; Taylor, W.R.; De Marco, V.; *et al.* Role of the polycomb protein EED in the propagation of repressive histone marks. *Nature* **2009**, *461*, 762–767.
64. Hansen, K.H.; Bracken, A.P.; Pasini, D.; Dietrich, N.; Gehani, S.S.; Monrad, A.; Rappsilber, J.; Lerdrup, M.; Helin, K. A model for transmission of the H3K27me3 epigenetic mark. *Nat. Cell Biol.* **2008**, *10*, 1291–1300.
65. Gao, Z.; Zhang, J.; Bonasio, R.; Strino, F.; Sawai, A.; Parisi, F.; Kluger, Y.; Reinberg, D. PCGF homologs, CBX proteins, and RYBP define functionally distinct PRC1 family complexes. *Mol. Cell.* **2012**, *45*, 344–356.
66. Tavares, L.; Dimitrova, E.; Oxley, D.; Webster, J.; Poot, R.; Demmers, J.; Bezstarosti, K.; Taylor, S.; Ura, H.; Koide, H.; *et al.* RYBP-PRC1 complexes mediate H2A ubiquitylation at polycomb target sites independently of PRC2 and H3K27me3. *Cell* **2012**, *148*, 664–678.
67. Kwiatkowski, D.L.; Thompson, H.W.; Bloom, D.C. The polycomb group protein Bmi1 binds to the herpes simplex virus 1 latent genome and maintains repressive histone marks during latency. *J. Virol.* **2009**, *83*, 8173–8181.
68. Cliffe, A.R.; Garber, D.A.; Knipe, D.M. Transcription of the herpes simplex virus latency-associated transcript promotes the formation of facultative heterochromatin on lytic promoters. *J. Virol.* **2009**, *83*, 8182–8190.
69. Pasini, D.; Malatesta, M.; Jung, H.R.; Walfridsson, J.; Willer, A.; Olsson, L.; Skotte, J.; Wutz, A.; Porse, B.; Jensen, O.N.; *et al.* Characterization of an antagonistic switch between histone H3 lysine 27 methylation and acetylation in the transcriptional regulation of Polycomb group target genes. *Nucleic Acids Res.* **2010**, *38*, 4958–4969.
70. Smith, E.R.; Lee, M.G.; Winter, B.; Droz, N.M.; Eissenberg, J.C.; Shiekhattar, R.; Shilatifard, A. Drosophila UTX is a histone H3 Lys27 demethylase that colocalizes with the elongating form of RNA polymerase II. *Mol. Cell Biol.* **2008**, *28*, 1041–1046.
71. Lee, M.G.; Villa, R.; Trojer, P.; Norman, J.; Yan, K.P.; Reinberg, D.; Di Croce, L.; Shiekhattar, R. Demethylation of H3K27 regulates polycomb recruitment and H2A ubiquitination. *Science* **2007**, *318*, 447–450.

72. Ernst, P.; Wang, J.; Huang, M.; Goodman, R.H.; Korsmeyer, S.J. MLL and CREB bind cooperatively to the nuclear coactivator CREB-binding protein. *Mol. Cell Biol.* **2001**, *21*, 2249–2258.

73. Rossetto, C.C.; Pari, G. KSHV PAN RNA associates with demethylases UTX and JMJD3 to activate lytic replication through a physical interaction with the virus genome. *PLoS Pathog.* **2012**, *8*, e1002680.

74. Toth, Z.; Jung, J. University of Southern California, Los Angeles, CA, USA. Unpublished work, 2013.

75. Reynolds, N.; Salmon-Divon, M.; Dvinge, H.; Hynes-Allen, A.; Balasooriya, G.; Leaford, D.; Behrens, A.; Bertone, P.; Hendrich, B. NuRD-mediated deacetylation of H3K27 facilitates recruitment of Polycomb Repressive Complex 2 to direct gene repression. *EMBO J.* **2012**, *31*, 593–605.

76. Van der Vlag, J.; Otte, A.P. Transcriptional repression mediated by the human polycomb-group protein EED involves histone deacetylation. *Nat. Genet.* **1999**, *23*, 474–478.

77. Chang, P.C.; Fitzgerald, L.D.; Hsia, D.A.; Izumiya, Y.; Wu, C.Y.; Hsieh, W.P.; Lin, S.F.; Campbell, M.; Lam, K.S.; Luciw, P.A.; *et al.* Histone demethylase JMJD2A regulates Kaposi's sarcoma-associated herpesvirus replication and is targeted by a viral transcriptional factor. *J. Virol.* **2011**, *85*, 3283–3293.

78. Fritsch, L.; Robin, P.; Mathieu, J.R.; Souidi, M.; Hinaux, H.; Rougeulle, C.; Harel-Bellan, A.; Ameyar-Zazoua, M.; Ait-Si-Ali, S. A subset of the histone H3 lysine 9 methyltransferases Suv39h1, G9a, GLP, and SETDB1 participate in a multimeric complex. *Mol. Cell* **2010**, *37*, 46–56.

79. Chang, P.C.; Fitzgerald, L.D.; Van Geelen, A.; Izumiya, Y.; Ellison, T.J.; Wang, D.H.; Ann, D.K.; Luciw, P.A.; Kung, H.J. Kruppel-associated box domain-associated protein-1 as a latency regulator for Kaposi's sarcoma-associated herpesvirus and its modulation by the viral protein kinase. *Cancer Res.* **2009**, *69*, 5681–5689.

80. Kim, K.Y.; Huerta, S.B.; Izumiya, C.; Wang, D.H.; Martinez, A.; Shevchenko, B.; Kung, H.J.; Campbell, M.; Izumiya, Y. Kaposi's Sarcoma-Associated Herpesvirus (KSHV) latency associated nuclear antigen regulates KSHV epigenome by association with histone demethylase, KDM3A. *J. Virol.* **2013**, doi:10.1128/JVI.00011-13.

81. Lefort, S.; Gravel, A.; Flamand, L. Repression of interferon-alpha stimulated genes expression by Kaposi's sarcoma-associated herpesvirus K-bZIP protein. *Virology* **2010**, *408*, 14–30.

82. Miller, T.; Krogan, N.J.; Dover, J.; Erdjument-Bromage, H.; Tempst, P.; Johnston, M.; Greenblatt, J.F.; Shilatifard, A. COMPASS: A complex of proteins associated with a trithorax-related SET domain protein. *Proc. Natl. Acad. Sci. USA* **2001**, *98*, 12902–12907.

83. Briggs, S.D.; Bryk, M.; Strahl, B.D.; Cheung, W.L.; Davie, J.K.; Dent, S.Y.; Winston, F.; Allis, C.D. Histone H3 lysine 4 methylation is mediated by Set1 and required for cell growth and rDNA silencing in Saccharomyces cerevisiae. *Genes Dev.* **2001**, *15*, 3286–3295.

84. Shilatifard, A. The COMPASS family of histone H3K4 methylases: Mechanisms of regulation in development and disease pathogenesis. *Annu. Rev. Biochem.* **2012**, *81*, 65–95.

85. Wang, P.; Lin, C.; Smith, E.R.; Guo, H.; Sanderson, B.W.; Wu, M.; Gogol, M.; Alexander, T.; Seidel, C.; Wiedemann, L.M.; *et al.* Global analysis of H3K4 methylation defines MLL family member targets and points to a role for MLL1-mediated H3K4 methylation in the regulation of transcriptional initiation by RNA polymerase II. *Mol. Cell Biol.* **2009**, *29*, 6074–6085.
86. Wu, M.; Wang, P.F.; Lee, J.S.; Martin-Brown, S.; Florens, L.; Washburn, M.; Shilatifard, A. Molecular regulation of H3K4 trimethylation by Wdr82, a component of human Set1/COMPASS. *Mol. Cell Biol.* **2008**, *28*, 7337–7344.
87. Krivtsov, A.V.; Armstrong, S.A. MLL translocations, histone modifications and leukaemia stem-cell development. *Nat. Rev. Canc.* **2007**, *7*, 823–833.
88. Jong, J.E.; Cha, S.; Jang, J.H.; Seo, T. Alteration of histone H3 lysine 4 trimethylation on putative lytic gene promoters by human Set1 complex during reactivation of Kaposi's Sarcoma-Associated Herpesvirus. *Intervirology* **2013**, *56*, 91–103.
89. Kim, J.; Guermah, M.; McGinty, R.K.; Lee, J.S.; Tang, Z.; Milne, T.A.; Shilatifard, A.; Muir, T.W.; Roeder, R.G. RAD6-Mediated transcription-coupled H2B ubiquitylation directly stimulates H3K4 methylation in human cells. *Cell* **2009**, *137*, 459–471.
90. Gallinari, P.; di Marco, S.; Jones, P.; Pallaoro, M.; Steinkuhler, C. HDACs, histone deacetylation and gene transcription: From molecular biology to cancer therapeutics. *Cell Res.* **2007**, *17*, 195–211.
91. Sterner, D.E.; Berger, S.L. Acetylation of histones and transcription-related factors. *Microbiol Mol. Biol. Rev.* **2000**, *64*, 435–459.
92. Wang, S.E.; Wu, F.Y.; Chen, H.; Shamay, M.; Zheng, Q.; Hayward, G.S. Early activation of the Kaposi's sarcoma-associated herpesvirus RTA, RAP, and MTA promoters by the tetradecanoyl phorbol acetate-induced AP1 pathway. *J. Virol.* **2004**, *78*, 4248–4267.
93. Wang, S.E.; Wu, F.Y.; Fujimuro, M.; Zong, J.; Hayward, S.D.; Hayward, G.S. Role of CCAAT/enhancer-binding protein alpha (C/EBPalpha) in activation of the Kaposi's sarcoma-associated herpesvirus (KSHV) lytic-cycle replication-associated protein (RAP) promoter in cooperation with the KSHV replication and transcription activator (RTA) and RAP. *J. Virol.* **2003**, *77*, 600–623.
94. Ye, J.; Shedd, D.; Miller, G. An Sp1 response element in the Kaposi's sarcoma-associated herpesvirus open reading frame 50 promoter mediates lytic cycle induction by butyrate. *J. Virol.* **2005**, *79*, 1397–1408.
95. Jones, P.A. Functions of DNA methylation: Islands, start sites, gene bodies and beyond. *Nat. Rev. Genet.* **2012**, *13*, 484–492.
96. Jin, B.; Li, Y.; Robertson, K.D. DNA methylation: Superior or subordinate in the epigenetic hierarchy? *Genes Canc.* **2011**, *2*, 607–617.
97. Denis, H.; Ndlovu, M.N.; Fuks, F. Regulation of mammalian DNA methyltransferases: A route to new mechanisms. *EMBO Rep.* **2011**, *12*, 647–656.
98. Szekely, L.; Kiss, C.; Mattsson, K.; Kashuba, E.; Pokrovskaja, K.; Juhasz, A.; Holmvall, P.; Klein, G. Human herpesvirus-8-encoded LNA-1 accumulates in heterochromatin-associated nuclear bodies. *J. Gen. Virol.* **1999**, *80*, 2889–2900.

99. Kang, H.; Wiedmer, A.; Yuan, Y.; Robertson, E.; Lieberman, P.M. Coordination of KSHV latent and lytic gene control by CTCF-cohesin mediated chromosome conformation. *PLoS Pathog.* **2011**, *7*, e1002140.

100. Stedman, W.; Kang, H.; Lin, S.; Kissil, J.L.; Bartolomei, M.S.; Lieberman, P.M. Cohesins localize with CTCF at the KSHV latency control region and at cellular c-myc and H19/Igf2 insulators. *EMBO J.* **2008**, *27*, 654–666.

101. Chen, H.S.; Wikramasinghe, P.; Showe, L.; Lieberman, P.M. Cohesins repress Kaposi's sarcoma-associated herpesvirus immediate early gene transcription during latency. *J. Virol.* **2012**, *86*, 9454–9464.

102. Kang, H.; Cho, H.; Sung, G.H.; Lieberman, P.M. CTCF regulates Kaposi's Sarcoma-Associated Herpesvirus latency transcription by nucleosome displacement and RNA polymerase programming. *J. Virol.* **2013**, *87*, 1789–1799.

103. Kang, H.; Lieberman, P.M. Mechanism of glycyrrhizic acid inhibition of Kaposi's sarcoma-associated herpesvirus: Disruption of CTCF-cohesin-mediated RNA polymerase II pausing and sister chromatid cohesion. *J. Virol.* **2011**, *85*, 11159–11169.

104. Darst, R.P.; Haecker, I.; Pardo, C.E.; Renne, R.; Kladde, M.P. Epigenetic diversity of Kaposi's sarcoma-associated herpesvirus. *Nucleic Acids Res.* **2013**, *41*, 2993–3009.

105. Wang, H.W.; Trotter, M.W.; Lagos, D.; Bourboulia, D.; Henderson, S.; Makinen, T.; Elliman, S.; Flanagan, A.M.; Alitalo, K.; Boshoff, C. Kaposi sarcoma herpesvirus-induced cellular reprogramming contributes to the lymphatic endothelial gene expression in Kaposi sarcoma. *Nat. Genet.* **2004**, *36*, 687–693.

106. Hong, Y.K.; Foreman, K.; Shin, J.W.; Hirakawa, S.; Curry, C.L.; Sage, D.R.; Libermann, T.; Dezube, B.J.; Fingeroth, J.D.; Detmar, M. Lymphatic reprogramming of blood vascular endothelium by Kaposi sarcoma-associated herpesvirus. *Nat. Genet.* **2004**, *36*, 683–685.

107. Cheng, F.; Pekkonen, P.; Laurinavicius, S.; Sugiyama, N.; Henderson, S.; Gunther, T.; Rantanen, V.; Kaivanto, E.; Aavikko, M.; Sarek, G.; *et al.* KSHV-initiated notch activation leads to membrane-type-1 matrix metalloproteinase-dependent lymphatic endothelial-to-mesenchymal transition. *Cell Host Microbe* **2011**, *10*, 577–590.

108. Hansen, A.; Henderson, S.; Lagos, D.; Nikitenko, L.; Coulter, E.; Roberts, S.; Gratrix, F.; Plaisance, K.; Renne, R.; Bower, M.; *et al.* KSHV-encoded miRNAs target MAF to induce endothelial cell reprogramming. *Genes Dev.* **2010**, *24*, 195–205.

109. Di Bartolo, D.L.; Cannon, M.; Liu, Y.F.; Renne, R.; Chadburn, A.; Boshoff, C.; Cesarman, E. KSHV LANA inhibits TGF-beta signaling through epigenetic silencing of the TGF-beta type II receptor. *Blood* **2008**, *111*, 4731–4740.

110. Qin, Z.; Jakymiw, A.; Findlay, V.; Parsons, C. KSHV-encoded MicroRNAs: Lessons for viral cancer pathogenesis and emerging concepts. *Int. J. Cell Biol.* **2012**, *2012*, 603961.

111. Dahlke, C.; Maul, K.; Christalla, T.; Walz, N.; Schult, P.; Stocking, C.; Grundhoff, A. A microRNA encoded by Kaposi sarcoma-associated herpesvirus promotes B-cell expansion *in vivo*. *PLoS One* **2012**, *7*, e49435.

112. Lu, F.; Stedman, W.; Yousef, M.; Renne, R.; Lieberman, P.M. Epigenetic regulation of Kaposi's sarcoma-associated herpesvirus latency by virus-encoded microRNAs that target Rta and the cellular Rbl2-DNMT pathway. *J. Virol.* **2010**, *84*, 2697–2706.
113. Rossetto, C.C.; Tarrant-Elorza, M.; Verma, S.; Purushothaman, P.; Pari, G.S. Regulation of viral and cellular gene expression by Kaposi's sarcoma associated herpesvirus (KSHV) PAN RNA. *J. Virol.* **2013**, 87, 5540–5553.
114. Hwang, S.; Gwack, Y.; Byun, H.; Lim, C.; Choe, J. The Kaposi's sarcoma-associated herpesvirus K8 protein interacts with CREB-binding protein (CBP) and represses CBP-mediated transcription. *J. Virol.* **2001**, *75*, 9509–9516.
115. Li, M.; Damania, B.; Alvarez, X.; Ogryzko, V.; Ozato, K.; Jung, J.U. Inhibition of p300 histone acetyltransferase by viral interferon regulatory factor. *Mol. Cell Biol.* **2000**, *20*, 8254–8263.
116. He, M.; Zhang, W.; Bakken, T.; Schutten, M.; Toth, Z.; Jung, J.U.; Gill, P.; Cannon, M.; Gao, S.J. Cancer angiogenesis induced by Kaposi sarcoma-associated herpesvirus is mediated by EZH2. *Canc. Res.* **2012**, *72*, 3582–3592.
117. Arguello, M.; Sgarbanti, M.; Hernandez, E.; Mamane, Y.; Sharma, S.; Servant, M.; Lin, R.; Hiscott, J. Disruption of the B-cell specific transcriptional program in HHV-8 associated primary effusion lymphoma cell lines. *Oncogene* **2003**, *22*, 964–973.
118. Jha, H.C.; Upadhyay, S.K.; Aj, M.P.; Lu, J.; Cai, Q.; Saha, A.; Robertson, E.S. H2AX phosphorylation is important for LANA mediated KSHV episome persistence. *J. Virol.* **2013**, 87, 5255–5269.
119. Dillon, P.J.; Gregory, S.M.; Tamburro, K.; Sanders, M.K.; Johnson, G.L.; Raab-Traub, N.; Dittmer, D.P.; Damania, B. Tousled-like kinases modulate reactivation of gammaherpesviruses from latency. *Cell Host Microbe* **2013**, *13*, 204–214.
120. Tan, M.; Luo, H.; Lee, S.; Jin, F.; Yang, J.S.; Montellier, E.; Buchou, T.; Cheng, Z.; Rousseaux, S.; Rajagopal, N.; *et al.* Identification of 67 histone marks and histone lysine crotonylation as a new type of histone modification. *Cell* **2011**, *146*, 1016–1028.
121. Liang, Y.; Vogel, J.L.; Arbuckle, J.H.; Rai, G.; Jadhav, A.; Simeonov, A.; Maloney, D.J.; Kristie, T.M. Targeting the JMJD2 histone demethylases to epigenetically control herpesvirus infection and reactivation from latency. *Sci. Transl. Med.* **2013**, *5*, 167ra165.
122. Liang, Y.; Quenelle, D.; Vogel, J.L.; Mascaro, C.; Ortega, A.; Kristie, T.M. A novel selective LSD1/KDM1A inhibitor epigenetically blocks herpes simplex virus lytic replication and reactivation from latency. *MBio* **2013**, *4*, e00558-12.
123. Liang, Y.; Vogel, J.L.; Narayanan, A.; Peng, H.; Kristie, T.M. Inhibition of the histone demethylase LSD1 blocks alpha-herpesvirus lytic replication and reactivation from latency. *Nat. Med.* **2009**, *15*, 1312–1317.

8

Regulation of Human Cytomegalovirus Transcription in Latency: Beyond the Major Immediate-Early Promoter

Matthew Reeves * and John Sinclair

Department of Medicine, University of Cambridge, Addenbrooke's Hospital, Hills Road, Cambridge, CB2 0QQ, UK; E-Mail: js152@cam.ac.uk

* Author to whom correspondence should be addressed; E-Mail: mbr23@cam.ac.uk;

Abstract: Lytic infection of differentiated cell types with human cytomegalovirus (HCMV) results in the temporal expression of between 170–200 open reading frames (ORFs). A number of studies have demonstrated the temporal regulation of these ORFs and that this is orchestrated by both viral and cellular mechanisms associated with the co-ordinated recruitment of transcription complexes and, more recently, higher order chromatin structure. Importantly, HCMV, like all herpes viruses, establishes a lifelong latent infection of the host—one major site of latency being the undifferentiated haematopoietic progenitor cells resident in the bone marrow. Crucially, the establishment of latency is concomitant with the recruitment of cellular enzymes that promote extensive methylation of histones bound to the major immediate early promoter. As such, the repressive chromatin structure formed at the major immediate early promoter (MIEP) elicits inhibition of IE gene expression and is a major factor involved in maintenance of HCMV latency. However, it is becoming increasingly clear that a distinct subset of viral genes is also expressed during latency. In this review, we will discuss the mechanisms that control the expression of these latency-associated transcripts and illustrate that regulation of these latency-associated promoters is also subject to chromatin mediated regulation and that the instructive observations previously reported regarding the negative regulation of the MIEP during latency are paralleled in the regulation of latent gene expression.

Keywords: cytomegalovirus; latency; gene expression; chromatin

---

1. Introduction

Human cytomegalovirus (HCMV) is an opportunistic pathogen that, like all herpes viruses, can establish a latent infection that persists for the lifetime of the host. In healthy individuals both primary infection and the reactivation of latent virus rarely causes any significant clinical symptoms due to a robust immune response in the host [1,2]. In contrast, infection or reactivation in immuno-suppressed transplant patients or immune-compromised late stage AIDS sufferers represents a major source of morbidity and mortality [3–5]. Furthermore, HCMV infection in utero remains the leading viral cause of infectious congenital disease [6]. As it is now clear that a major contribution to HCMV-mediated disease is due to the reactivation of latent virus, [2,4,7–9] a number of laboratories have studied intensively the mechanisms that activate and repress viral immediate early gene expression during lytic and latent infection, respectively.

2. Histones, Chromatin and Gene Expression

The 'histone code hypothesis' predicts that the signature of the post-translational modifications of histone proteins directly impacts on the transcriptional activity of the cell [10–12]. In the broadest terms, a promoter can be transcriptionally active or transcriptionally silent and this is influenced principally by the acetylation and methylation states of its associated histones [13–15]. As such, pan acetylation of histones H3 and H4 is directly linked with a promoter that is capable of transcription [14]. In contrast, trimethlyation at lysine residues 9 and 27 on histone H3 and the subsequent recruitment of heterochromatin protein 1 (HP1) or polycomb proteins, respectively, is indicative of a transcriptionally repressed promoter [16–19]. As with all biological systems caveats do exist. For instance, histone methylation is not exclusively indicative of repression—dimethylation at lysine residue 4 on histone H3 is a marker of a promoter that has been recently active [20]. Additionally, histone phosphorylation, which occurs at serine (10 & 28) and threonine (11 & 29) residues in the N terminal of histone H3, has been linked with both transcriptional activation and repression of promoter activity depending on the phase of the cell cycle [21].

The regulation of the major immediate early promoter (MIEP) during latency and reactivation has been the subject of a number of recent reviews and, thus, it will not be covered extensively, here. Suffice to say, the regulation of the MIEP during latency and reactivation exhibits many hallmarks associated with chromatin-mediated regulation of eukaryotic gene expression. The MIEP in latently infected CD34+ haematopoietic cells or circulating monocytes isolated from healthy seropositive donors is predominantly associated with HP1 [22]—a marker of a transcriptionally silenced promoter that is recruited to promoters via an interaction with histone H3 trimethylated on lysine 9 (H3K9) [19]. However, differentiation to a mature dendritic cell (DC) phenotype is concomitant with high levels of acetylation of the histones bound to the MIEP and a lack of HP1 binding [22]. Importantly, the differences in the pattern of the modifications of the histones bound to the MIEP in undifferentiated or differentiated myeloid cells correlates directly with the ability to detect of IE gene expression in these different cell types in healthy individuals [22–26].

It is now well accepted that differentiation-dependent changes in the post-translational modifications of histones around the MIEP regulate latency-associated repression and reactivation of MIEP activity. However, much less is known about viral gene expression associated with latent infection and whether this is also regulated by histone modifications. With the advent of more sensitive high throughput screening techniques, the identification of a small number of latency associated transcripts (which, in most cases, are also expressed during lytic infection) has been possible. These transcripts expressed during latent infection are from viral genes dispersed throughout the viral genome, suggesting that no one region is particularly 'latently active' but rather that latency-associated transcripts are regulated independently by specific promoters.

In this short review, we will present the current status of our knowledge regarding the regulation of expression of the latency associated transcripts of HCMV and its relationship to post-translational modifications of histones.

3. Human Cytomegalovirus Latent Gene Products

A key biological property of all herpes viruses is their ability to undergo latent infection during which time only a subset of viral genes are expressed. Latent herpes simplex virus (HSV) gene expression is predominantly restricted to one locus—the latency associated transcript (LAT) region [27]. Alternate splicing generates multiple non-coding RNAs with functions ranging from anti-apoptosis [28], anti-sense mediated inhibition of lytic gene expression [27,29] and the generation of miRNAs that influence gene expression during latency [30]. In contrast, a number of patterns of Epstein-Barr virus (EBV) latent gene expression have been reported based on the phenotype of the infected lymphocyte [31]. The initial infection and transformation of a resting B cell (latency III) is concomitant with the expression of a number of gene products including EBNA-1, -2, 3A-C, EBNA-LP, LMP-1, 2A and B, as well as the untranslated EBER transcripts. It is hypothesised, based on studies of cell lines and the analysis of tissue ex vivo that the level of EBV latent gene expression is down-regulated (latency II - EBNA-1, LMP-1, LMP-2A and the EBERs) with the LMP proteins thought to drive the differentiation into latently infected memory B cells [32–36]. Consistent with this, circulating immunoblastic lymphomas (latency III) are rarely detected *in vivo* likely due to the robust immune response directed against EBV in the host promoting their elimination. Indeed, the most common phenotype (latency 0) is genome carriage in the absence of latent gene expression [37]—although LMP-2A transcripts have been detected in these cells [38]. However, dividing memory B cells that display a latency I phenotype (EBNA-1) have also been detected *in vivo* [35].

In contrast to HSV and EBV, the analysis of latent HCMV gene expression is in its relative infancy. Latent transcripts arising from the major immediate early region had been identified in specific populations of granulocyte-macrophage progenitors by the Mocarski laboratory in the 1990s [39,40] and US28 transcripts were also reported in an experimentally infected THP1 leukaemia cell line [41], but the application of high throughput molecular approaches led to the identification of a number of novel latent transcripts. Microarray technology employed by the Shenk and Slobedman laboratories detected transcription from a number of different loci in experimentally latently infected myeloid progenitor cells [42,43]. Subsequent work confirmed that some of these products were also expressed during natural latency and included UL138 [44], UL111A [43] as well as the UL81-82 anti-sense transcript (UL81-82ast) [45,46]. Although it is worth noting that the latent transcriptomes reported by these studies are not entirely overlapping, likely due to different cell types and viral strains used in the analyses. Indeed, the possible effects of using different viral strains is no better illustrated than by recent work showing that the expression of UL144 during latency appears to be dependent on the strain of virus used [47] and is discussed in more detail later.

The selective expression of viral genes during latent infection is likely to depend on similar mechanisms known to modulate the MIEP during latent and lytic infection. Importantly, aberrant expression of viral gene products not required during latency would likely risk triggering a robust host immune response, from the high memory T cell population known to recognise lytic antigens in normal HCMV carriers, with no benefit to the virus. Consequently, tight control of viral gene expression during latency is likely to be of some import. Since, most of the viral genes expressed during lytic infection are regulated by the prodigious activity of the IE72 and IE86 proteins [48–52], a failure to express a number of genes during latency can likely be attributed to the lack of IE expression resulting from extensive silencing of the MIEP which is clearly observed in latently infected myeloid progenitor cells (reviewed in [53]). Clearly then, gene expression during latency must be subject to mechanisms of regulation which are independent of the functions of viral IE gene products. In this review, we will use the regulation of two gene products—UL81-82ast and UL144—to illustrate potential mechanisms for the control of latent gene expression by HCMV in myeloid progenitor cells.

4. The UL81-82 Antisense Transcript—LUNA

Of all the putative latent transcripts, the factors controlling expression of the UL81-82 antisense transcript (UL81-82ast) during latent and lytic infection are arguably the best understood [46,47,54]. UL81-82ast was identified by Bego *et al.* [45] whilst searching for the UL81 transcription detected in the previous study by Goodrum *et al.* [42]. Bego *et al.* identified RNAs spanning the UL81 region in naturally latent monocytes and showed that transcription of this RNA actually occurs from the opposite strand encoding UL81 (hence the designation UL81-82ast), giving rise to a putative 133aa serine rich protein called LUNA (Latency Unique Nuclear Antigen). Although there is no known function attributed to LUNA during natural latency, there is some recent evidence that expression of LUNA may impact on HCMV carriage and reactivation *in vitro* [55].

Superficially, at least, the regulation of LUNA promoter activity during lytic [54] and latent [46,47] infection appears to be mediated by very different mechanisms. However, closer scrutiny reveals that a number of the key proteins involved in latent or lytic LUNA transcriptional regulation actually exhibit overlapping functions—this provides an interesting model for the complex regulation of herpes virus gene promoters during different phases of infection.

4.1. Regulation of LUNA during Latent Infection

After confirmation that the expression of LUNA could be detected in experimentally and naturally latent CD34+ cells, a very simple question was asked—is the LUNA promoter associated with histone proteins during latency and, if so, what post-translational modifications do these histones have? Chromatin Immunoprecipitation analyses of the LUNA promoter alongside the MIEP showed that the promoter is indeed associated with histones [46]. Furthermore, the LUNA promoter, in contrast to the MIEP, was associated with acetylated histones [22,46]. Thus, in the latent phase of infection, the LUNA promoter is associated with histone post-translational modifications that support gene expression.

4.2. Regulation of LUNA during Lytic Infection

Although classified as a latent transcript, LUNA, like other latency associated transcripts, is also expressed during lytic infection [45]. Broadly speaking, the regulation of viral gene expression during lytic infection is subject to regulation by histone proteins [56–61] and, consistent with this including LUNA, the transfected LUNA promoter is responsive to the histone deacetylase inhibitor, Trichostatin A (TSA). Furthermore, increased expression of LUNA was detectable in virally infected cells incubated with TSA [54]. Further investigation identified that the expression of IE72 was critical for LUNA expression during lytic infection. Interestingly, IE72 has been hypothesised to drive early and late viral gene expression via the sequestration of inhibitory histone deacetylase activity [59]. However, unlike reported for other IE72-responsive genes LUNA gene expression in an IE72 null background was not rescued by TSA alone [54] suggesting that, although histone proteins may play a role, additional regulatory mechanisms besides IE72-mediated sequestration of histone deacetylases were needed for LUNA promoter activation [54]. Further work showed that activation of the LUNA promoter during lytic infection involved IE72 overcoming the repressive activity of the cellular repressor hDaxx and its binding partner, ATRX [54] (Figure 1A,B). Both hDaxx and ATRX have also been shown by a number of groups to exert a profound phenotype on the activity of the MIEP and these cellular proteins are targeted by incoming tegument protein, pp71 [60,62–65].

These observations are consistent with the view that chromatin architecture, whilst providing the framework for controlling gene expression, is not the only factor involved in LUNA promoter regulation. Indeed, it is interesting to note that parallels occur in other herpes viruses. EBV encoded BNRF1 disrupts the hDaxx:ATRX interaction to relieve early gene expression from the transcriptional silencing imposed by this complex also [66].

4.3. LUNA Is Regulated by the GATA Transcription Factors during Latency

The obvious question that arises from these observations is what drives differential LUNA promoter activity during latent infection? During latency LUNA expression must be independent of IE72 (by definition) whereas LUNA gene expression during lytic infection is IE72-dependent. Clues to the regulation of the LUNA promoter during latency came from a bioinformatics approach identifying a number of putative transcription sites in the LUNA promoter, including the GATA family of transcription factors [47]. GATA transcription factors are expressed in the haematopoietic cell lineage and have differential expression profiles dependent on the cell fate [67]. GATA-2 is a transcription factor expressed in early myeloid progenitors and declines in levels as myeloid cells differentiate and is sometimes referred to as the 'master regulator' of haematopoietic progenitor cells [68,69]. Certainly, GATA-2 is essential for haematopoiesis providing credence for such a grandiose moniker [69]. Furthermore, a lack of GATA-2 results in a severe defect in the generation of the granulocyte/ macrophage progenitor population [68]—a cell type which represents an important site of HCMV latency in the myeloid lineage [24,39,70]. Pertinently, GATA-2, along with other family members, has been shown to interact with chromatin modifying enzymes [71,72]. Amongst these interaction partners are histone acetyltransferases (pCAF and CBP/p300) which are important for histone and non-histone protein acetylation, including the GATA proteins themselves [71–73]. Similarly, GATA proteins also interact with histone deacetylases (HDACs) with GATA-2 interacting with HDACs-3 and -5, but not HDAC-1 [74] and thus, like a number of proteins, GATA-2 can promote the deacetylation as well as acetylation of target proteins including itself.

Interestingly, the LUNA promoter is GATA-2 responsive in transfection assays [46,47] and we have observed that GATA-2 over expression can rescue LUNA gene expression in ΔIE72 virus infected cells (M.R. and J.S., unpublished observations). Furthermore, a study that assessed the impact of HCMV latency on the expression of cellular miRNAs identified that mir92a was down-regulated in latently infected cells [75]. Interestingly, a target of mir92a is GATA-2 and, consistent with this, GATA-2 expression levels were elevated in latently infected cells [75]. Thus, at least in latency, it can be argued that HCMV promotes a micro-environment that supports the expression of LUNA by modulating the availability of the GATA-2 transcription factor. Taken together, these observations argue that during latency high levels of GATA-2 bind to the LUNA promoter and propagate a chromatin environment that is pro-transcriptional. However, during lytic infection, depletion of hDaxx:ATRX complex is required for LUNA gene expression to occur [54]. A pertinent question is why, then, does this complex not repress LUNA promoter activity in myeloid progenitors? One possible explanation is that there are differences in the relative balance of transcriptional activators and repressors which determine the activity of the LUNA promoter in different cell types. The viral MIEP provides a paradigm for this type of differential regulation in undifferentiated and differentiated myeloid cells (Figure 1). High levels of transcriptional repressors that bind the MIEP are present in early myeloid progenitors (Figure 1C) [22,76–80]. Furthermore, HCMV binding and entry into undifferentiated myeloid cells has been suggested to up-regulate transcription factors that would promote an environment repressive for the MIEP [81]—an event that does not occur upon infection of permissive fibroblasts [82]. In contrast, myeloid cell differentiation is concomitant with changes in both the absolute levels of repressors as well as the activation of transcriptional activators of the MIEP [22,83–85]. In the context of the LUNA promoter, the hDaxx:ATRX complex is likely to be stable in many cell types.

Figure 1. A model for the regulation of the major immediate early promoter (MIEP) and Latency Unique Nuclear Antigen (LUNA) promoter during lytic and latent infection. (**A**,**B**) Lower levels of GATA-2 expression in permissive differentiated cell types favour the recruitment of ATRX/Daxx to GATA-2 binding sites in the LUNA promoter to establish a repressive phenotype. As the lytic infection proceeds (**B**), IE72 is expressed which sequesters ATRX/Daxx complexes thus removing them as binding competitors at the LUNA promoter. This potentially increased GATA-2 binding which would promote LUNA gene expression in differentiated cells; (**C**) Latency is established following the infection of non-permissive haematopoietic CD34+ cells. High levels of transcriptional repressors bind to the MIEP and promote the formation of a repressive chromatin structure via the recruitment of histone modifying enzymes (histone methyltransferases (HMT) and histone deacetylases (HDAC). The relatively lower availability of transcriptional activators is possibly exacerbated by the exclusion of the major MIEP transactivator, pp71, from the nucleus in CD34+ cells. In contrast, high levels of GATA-2 are present in CD34+ cells and thus promote LUNA gene expression. In lytic infection, the scales are tipped towards transcriptional activation of the MIEP by relatively higher levels of activators versus repressors and the co-operative activity of pp71.

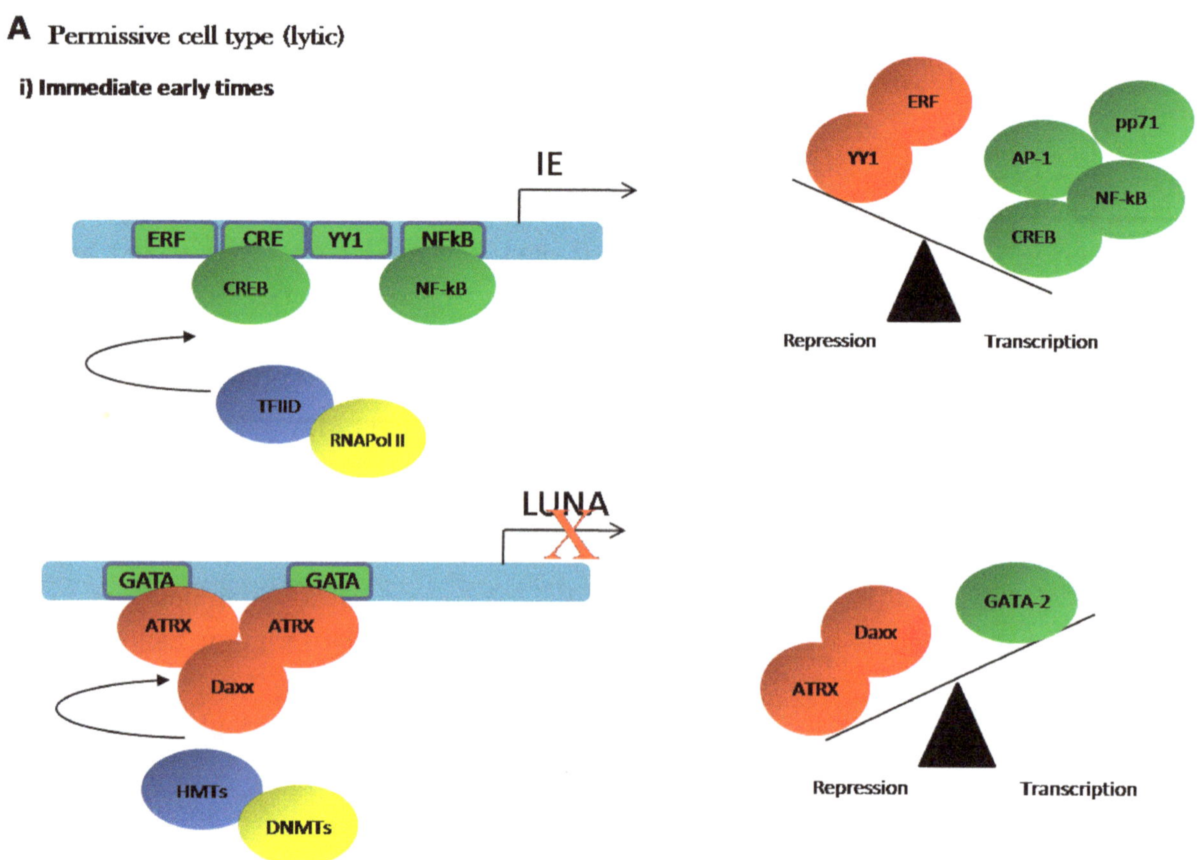

Figure 1. *Cont.*

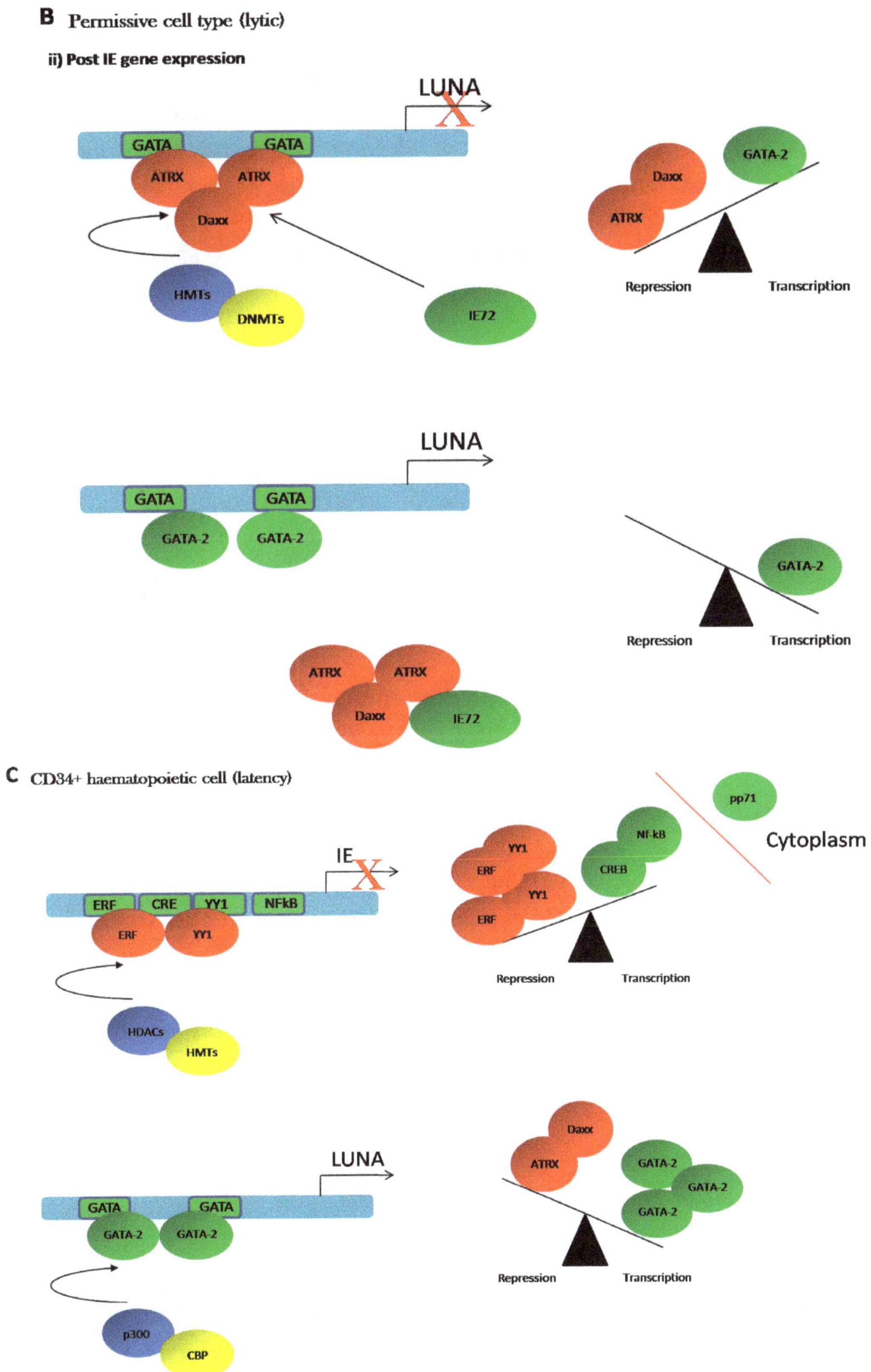

However, we hypothesise that in early myeloid cells high levels of GATA-2 (which would alone act as positive regulator of the LUNA promoter) out-compete the repressive hDaxx:ATRX complex (Figure 1C). In contrast, in more differentiated cells with functional levels of repressive hDaxx:ATRX, but lower levels of GATA-2, this GATA-2 mediated competition of hDaxx:ATRX repression would not occur (Figure 1B) and hDaxx:ATRX-mediated repression would need to be overcome by e.g., IE72 during lytic infection (Figure 1B). Consistent with this view, as stated above, over-expression of GATA-2 into ΔIE72 infected fibroblasts can drive LUNA gene expression. In essence, the low levels of GATA-2 in more differentiated cell types that HCMV lytically infects may result in the additional requirement of IE72 activity against hDaxx:ATRX to promote LUNA gene expression during lytic infection. Provocative evidence in support of the competition hypothesis is derived from a number of biological properties of ATRX. Firstly the N terminal region of ATRX encodes domains that bind to histones—particularly methylated histone H3 on lysine 9 [86] and, thus, associates with heterochromatic DNA where it establishes a functional interaction with the hDaxx protein [87] to promote transcriptional repression. Furthermore, in addition to encoding helicase and ATPase functions [88], the ATRX protein contains coiled-coiled regions that allow direct binding to DNA—with affinity for DNA regions encoding GATA protein binding sites [89] and thus could provide direct competition with GATA transcription factors for DNA promoter occupancy.

5. TNF Receptor Superfamily Member—UL144

The UL144 gene product was originally identified as an orthologue of the tumour necrosis factor receptor superfamily member, herpes virus entry mediator (HVEM) [90,91]. As such, UL144 like HVEM can interact with BTLA to inhibit the proliferation of activated T cells [92]. As well as this intercellular function, UL144 has been shown to modulate intracellular signalling to regulate further immune responses to infection by hijacking NF-kB signaling [93,94]. UL144 recruits cellular TRAF-6 to promote CCL22 expression [94]—a cytokine that has been shown to promote the migration of Th2 and T regulatory cells which could impact on immune-surveillance and clearance of infected cells by the Th1 T cell repertoire [95]. The activity of UL144 shares characteristics with the LMP2A gene product of EBV which is expressed in persistently infected B lymphocytes [32,35] and also results in increased CCL22 production [96]. Furthermore, although UL144 expression during latency was not identified in a previous study [42], the UL144-148 region of HCMV was shown to be important for more efficient establishment of latency in an *in vitro* system [44] and a subsequent re-investigation of UL144 expression during latent infection showed that UL144 was, indeed, expressed during HCMV latency [47].

5.1. UL144 Is Expressed during Latency in a Strain-Specific Manner

In lytic infection, the UL144 protein is expressed with early kinetics reaching steady state levels by 48 hours post infection [90]. Although suggestive that expression is dependent on IE gene expression during lytic infection, the first insights into the regulation of the UL144 promoter came from an analysis of different HCMV isolates during latent infection of myeloid progenitor cells and, interestingly, suggested some parallels to those observed with LUNA [47]. Analyses showed that UL144 expression did occur during latency but that this appeared to be isolate dependent [47]. Importantly, previous studies [42,43] that had failed to identify UL144 expression during latency were performed using strains of HCMV that were either UL144 deficient (AD169) or UL144 null for expression during latency expression (TB40/e and VR1814) - based on the these recent observations of Poole *et al.* [47]. In contrast, the HCMV sequence reference strain, Merlin [97], was UL144 positive for expression during latency. Thus the differences between these and previous data were easily reconciled and, furthermore, provided a level of cross validation for the respective studies.

5.2. UL144 Expression during Latency Is Dependent on GATA-2 Binding Sites

The observation by Poole *et al.* [47] that all the HCMV isolates analysed routinely expressed UL144 during lytic infection, even though this was not the case for latent infection, suggested that differential expression of UL144 during latency was a function of UL144 promoter activity specifically in myeloid progenitor cells. Sequence analysis of UL144 promoters showed that, although a high level of conservation was evident, a UL144 positive phenotype during latency correlated with the presence of putative GATA-2 binding sites in the UL144 promoter. Consistent with this, UL144 reporter constructs based on the Merlin Ul144 promoter were GATA-2 responsive whereas TB40/e-based UL144 reporter constructs were not. Additionally, the deletion of the putative GATA-2 sequences was sufficient to render the Merlin UL144 promoter inactive [47].

Direct evidence for a physical interaction between GATA-2 and UL144 promoter correlating with gene expression was also obtained by performing chromatin immunoprecipitation assays on infected myeloid cells. Crucially, GATA-2 immuno-precipitation with the UL144 promoter was only observed in cells infected with strains of HCMV that supported UL144 expression [47]. Furthermore, GATA-2 binding correlated with the detection of histone H3 di-methylated at lysine 4 bound to the UL144 promoter. In themselves, these data argue that the UL144 promoter is regulated by post-translational histone modifications around the UL144 promoter during latent infection likely modulated by GATA-2. Pertinently, the parallels with the LUNA promoter are overt [46]. Although LUNA expression during latency is independent of viral strain used, the LUNA promoter binds GATA-2 and is also responsive to GATA-2 in transfection assays [47].

6. Concluding Remarks

It is becoming increasingly clear that the regulation of cytomegalovirus gene expression during all phases of lytic infection involves post-translational modification of histone proteins (reviewed in [98]). Work from a number of laboratories has now demonstrated quite clearly that extensive chromatinisation of HCMV genomes occur [56–58,60,61,99,100] and that, during lytic infection, at least, the virus has to modify chromatin to control viral gene expression [59,101]. What is now also becoming clearer is that a complex interplay between cellular transcription factors and higher order chromatin structure with viral promoters is equally as important for the latency-associated regulation of viral gene expression [22,46,102].

Although the exact order of events controlling viral gene expression is still not fully understood, a model for the control of latent viral gene expression, based on a number of instructive observations, can be made. Firstly, the viral genome in the virion is naked—no histone proteins can be detected [56,58] consistent with a failure to detect histone proteins in purified virions by mass spectrometry [103]. This argues that the incoming viral genomes are subject to cellular responses that promote chromatinisation of the viral genome. Whether this is true for all foreign DNA is unclear but the association of plasmids and non-viral vector delivered DNA with histone proteins is documented *in vitro* [104] and *in vivo* [105]. The association of herpesvirus genomes with ND10 bodies—sites of extensive accumulation of histone modifying enzymes in the cell—is intrinsically repressive (reviewed in [106]). Indeed, the concerted attempt made by HCMV (and other herpes viruses) to disrupt these structures suggests they are anti-viral (reviewed in [107]). Consistent with a global repression of viral gene expression immediately post infection, studies of histone proteins at low MOIs show that a substantial number of incoming viral genomes are associated with methylated histone proteins [56] and that this response could be mediated by the action of a number of cellular proteins (*i.e.*, hDaxx, PML and Sp100) that accumulated at ND10 bodies. Consequently, the virus, through the action of pp71 [62,63,65,108] and subsequently IE72 [109–112] targets these ND10 structures to quickly overcome repression and initiate a lytic infection, especially at high MOIs.

During latent infection, however, it is likely that the same initial events occur—the genome is chromatinised immediately upon infection and that the same intrinsic immune defences are activated. However, the failure of pp71 to translocate to the nucleus and inactivate these defences upon infection of myeloid progenitors (Figure 1A) has been argued to be one possible mechanism to aid the establishment of latency [113]—although whether this is mediated solely by an interaction with hDaxx is still not clear [114]. Regardless of the exact mechanism, there is no doubt that the failure of a major viral transactivator of the MIEP (pp71) to enter the nucleus would have a significant impact upon activation of IE gene expression. Nevertheless, there are also longstanding observations that the MIEP—even after transfection—is transcriptionally less active in myeloid progenitors [77,115]. The prevailing hypothesis is that this latent phenotype is driven by the presence of high levels of transcriptional repressors in myeloid progenitors, such as YY1 and ERF, promoting long term silencing during latency via interactions with histone deacetylase and histone methyltransferase enzymes (Figure 1C). However, maybe a more refined model would suggest that levels of promoter occupancy and the recruitment of co-factors is critical to the establishment of latency rather than the absolute levels of ubiquitous transcription factors. Nevertheless, it is likely that the known interactions of YY1 and ERF with histone deacetylases and methyltransferases contribute significantly to the repressive ‘chromatin phenotype’ observed in naturally latent CD34+ haematopoietic cells around the viral MIEP [22].

It is also likely that these same mechanisms which promote silencing of the MIEP in latency are also important for driving viral latent gene expression. GATA-2 is, like YY1 and ERF, highly expressed in myeloid progenitor cells [68] and, while YY1 and ERF are binding to the MIEP mediating repression [76,79], GATA-2 binding to the LUNA and UL144 promoters drives their activity [47,54]. Interestingly, an in silico analysis of the promoters of other latently expressed genes identified putative GATA binding sites which may be important for the expression of the vIL10 and UL138 gene products. It is highly likely that histones are also recruited to latent promoters immediately post infection and, akin to the binding of ERF and YY1 to the MIEP resulting in the recruitment of histone deacetylases and histone methyltransferases, it is highly plausible that the binding of GATA-2 to the UL144 and LUNA promoters in latently infected monocytes [47] results in the recruitment of, for example histone acetyltransferases, generating the histone signature we observe in latently infected cells [46]. This 'open' chromatin conformation would support transcription and is consistent with viral latent gene transcription observed during HCMV latency [45–47]. Clearly, it remains to be seen whether GATA transcription factors are solely responsible for all the latent HCMV transcription that has been reported. Indeed, the regulation of UL138 gene expression during latency has been shown to be dependent on LUNA gene expression [55] in a long term monocyte culture model of latency [116] by, as of yet, an unidentified mechanism. However, the expression of viral genes containing binding sites for transcription factors highly expressed in the myeloid progenitor cells is highly plausible and provides further evidence for the key role cellular mechanisms of gene regulation play in the control of gene expression during persistent virus infection.

Acknowledgments

We are indebted to the contribution from members of the laboratory past and present and apologise to colleagues in the field we have not been able to cite for space reasons. Our own work is generously supported by grants from the UK Medical Research Council (M.B.R.; G:0900466 & J.H.S.; G:0701279) and the NIHR UK Biomedical Research Centre.

References

1. Pass, R.F.; Stagno, S.; Britt, W.J.; Alford, C.A. Specific cell-mediated immunity and the natural history of congenital infection with cytomegalovirus. *J. Infect. Dis.* **1983**, *148*, 953–961.

2. Zanghellini, F.; Boppana, S.B.; Emery, V.C.; Griffiths, P.D.; Pass, R.F. Asymptomatic primary cytomegalovirus infection: Virologic and immunologic features. *J. Infect. Dis.* **1999**, *180*, 702–707.

3. Griffiths, P.D. Cytomegalovirus in intensive care. *Rev. Med. Virol.* **2010**, *20*, 1–3.

4. Limaye, A.P.; Kirby, K.A.; Rubenfeld, G.D.; Leisenring, W.M.; Bulger, E.M.; Neff, M.J.; Gibran, N.S.; Huang, M.L.; Santo Hayes, T.K.; Corey, L.; *et al.* Cytomegalovirus reactivation in critically ill immunocompetent patients. *JAMA* **2008**, *300*, 413–422.

5. Crough, T.; Khanna, R. Immunobiology of human cytomegalovirus: From bench to bedside. *Clin. Microbiol. Rev.* **2009**, *22*, 76–98, Table of Contents.
6. Revello, M.G.; Gerna, G. Pathogenesis and prenatal diagnosis of human cytomegalovirus infection. *J. Clin. Virol.* **2004**, *29*, 71–83.
7. Kutza, A.S.; Muhl, E.; Hackstein, H.; Kirchner, H.; Bein, G. High incidence of active cytomegalovirus infection among septic patients. *Clin. Infect. Dis.* **1998**, *26*, 1076–1082.
8. Heininger, A.; Jahn, G.; Engel, C.; Notheisen, T.; Unertl, K.; Hamprecht, K. Human cytomegalovirus infections in nonimmunosuppressed critically ill patients. *Crit. Care Med.* **2001**, *29*, 541–547.
9. Chilet, M.; Aguilar, G.; Benet, I.; Belda, J.; Tormo, N.; Carbonell, J.A.; Clari, M.A.; Costa, E.; Navarro, D. Virological and immunological features of active cytomegalovirus infection in nonimmunosuppressed patients in a surgical and trauma intensive care unit. *J. Med. Virol.* **2010**, *82*, 1384–1391.
10. Strahl, B.D.; Allis, C.D. The language of covalent histone modifications. *Nature* **2000**, *403*, 41–45.
11. Doenecke, D.; Gallwitz, D. Acetylation of histones in nucleosomes. *Mol. Cell. Biochem.* **1982**, *44*, 113–128.
12. Lopez-Rodas, G.; Brosch, G.; Georgieva, E.I.; Sendra, R.; Franco, L.; Loidl, P. Histone deacetylase. A key enzyme for the binding of regulatory proteins to chromatin. *FEBS Lett.* **1993**, *317*, 175–180.
13. Lusser, A. Acetylated, methylated, remodeled: Chromatin states for gene regulation. *Curr. Opin. Plant Biol.* **2002**, *5*, 437–443.
14. Mizzen, C.A.; Allis, C.D. Linking histone acetylation to transcriptional regulation. *Cell. Mol. Life Sci.* **1998**, *54*, 6–20.
15. Zhang, Y.; Reinberg, D. Transcription regulation by histone methylation: Interplay between different covalent modifications of the core histone tails. *Genes Dev.* **2001**, *15*, 2343–2360.
16. Razin, A. CpG methylation, chromatin structure and gene silencing—A three-way connection. *EMBO J.* **1998**, *17*, 4905–4908.
17. Cao, R.; Wang, L.; Wang, H.; Xia, L.; Erdjument-Bromage, H.; Tempst, P.; Jones, R.S.; Zhang, Y. Role of histone H3 lysine 27 methylation in Polycomb-group silencing. *Science* **2002**, *298*, 1039–1043.
18. Peters, A.H.; Mermoud, J.E.; O'Carroll, D.; Pagani, M.; Schweizer, D.; Brockdorff, N.; Jenuwein, T. Histone H3 lysine 9 methylation is an epigenetic imprint of facultative heterochromatin. *Nat. Genet.* **2002**, *30*, 77–80.
19. Bannister, A.J.; Zegerman, P.; Partridge, J.F.; Miska, E.A.; Thomas, J.O.; Allshire, R.C.; Kouzarides, T. Selective recognition of methylated lysine 9 on histone H3 by the HP1 chromo domain. *Nature* **2001**, *410*, 120–124.

20. Wang, H.; Huang, Z.Q.; Xia, L.; Feng, Q.; Erdjument-Bromage, H.; Strahl, B.D.; Briggs, S.D.; Allis, C.D.; Wong, J.; Tempst, P.; *et al.* Methylation of histone H4 at arginine 3 facilitating transcriptional activation by nuclear hormone receptor. *Science* **2001**, *293*, 853–857.
21. Sawicka, A.; Seiser, C. Histone H3 phosphorylation—A versatile chromatin modification for different occasions. *Biochimie* **2012**, *94*, 2193–2201.
22. Reeves, M.B.; MacAry, P.A.; Lehner, P.J.; Sissons, J.G.; Sinclair, J.H. Latency, chromatin remodeling, and reactivation of human cytomegalovirus in the dendritic cells of healthy carriers. *Proc. Natl. Acad. Sci. USA* **2005**, *102*, 4140–4145.
23. Mendelson, M.; Monard, S.; Sissons, P.; Sinclair, J. Detection of endogenous human cytomegalovirus in CD34+ bone marrow progenitors. *J. Gen. Virol.* **1996**, *77*, 3099–3102.
24. Hahn, G.; Jores, R.; Mocarski, E.S. Cytomegalovirus remains latent in a common precursor of dendritic and myeloid cells. *Proc. Natl. Acad. Sci. USA* **1998**, *95*, 3937–3942.
25. Taylor-Wiedeman, J.; Sissons, P.; Sinclair, J. Induction of endogenous human cytomegalovirus gene expression after differentiation of monocytes from healthy carriers. *J. Virol.* **1994**, *68*, 1597–1604.
26. Soderberg-Naucler, C.; Fish, K.N.; Nelson, J.A. Reactivation of latent human cytomegalovirus by allogeneic stimulation of blood cells from healthy donors. *Cell* **1997**, *91*, 119–126.
27. Stevens, J.G.; Wagner, E.K.; Devi-Rao, G.B.; Cook, M.L.; Feldman, L.T. RNA complementary to a herpesvirus alpha gene mRNA is prominent in latently infected neurons. *Science* **1987**, *235*, 1056–1059.
28. Perng, G.C.; Jones, C.; Ciacci-Zanella, J.; Stone, M.; Henderson, G.; Yukht, A.; Slanina, S.M.; Hofman, F.M.; Ghiasi, H.; Nesburn, A.B.; *et al.* Virus-induced neuronal apoptosis blocked by the herpes simplex virus latency-associated transcript. *Science* **2000**, *287*, 1500–1503.
29. Mador, N.; Goldenberg, D.; Cohen, O.; Panet, A.; Steiner, I. Herpes simplex virus type 1 latency-associated transcripts suppress viral replication and reduce immediate-early gene mRNA levels in a neuronal cell line. *J. Virol.* **1998**, *72*, 5067–5075.
30. Umbach, J.L.; Kramer, M.F.; Jurak, I.; Karnowski, H.W.; Coen, D.M.; Cullen, B.R. MicroRNAs expressed by herpes simplex virus 1 during latent infection regulate viral mRNAs. *Nature* **2008**, *454*, 780–783.
31. Thorley-Lawson, D.A. Epstein-Barr virus: Exploiting the immune system. *Nat. Rev. Immunol.* **2001**, *1*, 75–82.
32. Tierney, R.J.; Steven, N.; Young, L.S.; Rickinson, A.B. Epstein-Barr virus latency in blood mononuclear cells: Analysis of viral gene transcription during primary infection and in the carrier state. *J. Virol.* **1994**, *68*, 7374–7385.
33. Babcock, G.J.; Decker, L.L.; Freeman, R.B.; Thorley-Lawson, D.A. Epstein-barr virus-infected resting memory B cells, not proliferating lymphoblasts, accumulate in the peripheral blood of immunosuppressed patients. *J. Exp. Med.* **1999**, *190*, 567–576.
34. Miyashita, E.M.; Yang, B.; Lam, K.M.; Crawford, D.H.; Thorley-Lawson, D.A. A novel form of Epstein-Barr virus latency in normal B cells *in vivo*. *Cell* **1995**, *80*, 593–601.

35. Hochberg, D.; Middeldorp, J.M.; Catalina, M.; Sullivan, J.L.; Luzuriaga, K.; Thorley-Lawson, D.A. Demonstration of the Burkitt's lymphoma Epstein-Barr virus phenotype in dividing latently infected memory cells *in vivo*. *Proc. Natl. Acad. Sci. USA* **2004**, *101*, 239–244.

36. Babcock, G.J.; Thorley-Lawson, D.A. Tonsillar memory B cells, latently infected with Epstein-Barr virus, express the restricted pattern of latent genes previously found only in Epstein-Barr virus-associated tumors. *Proc. Natl. Acad. Sci. USA* **2000**, *97*, 12250–12255.

37. Babcock, G.J.; Hochberg, D.; Thorley-Lawson, A.D. The expression pattern of Epstein-Barr virus latent genes *in vivo* is dependent upon the differentiation stage of the infected B cell. *Immunity* **2000**, *13*, 497–506.

38. Kuppers, R. B cells under influence: Transformation of B cells by Epstein-Barr virus. *Nat. Rev. Immunol.* **2003**, *3*, 801–812.

39. Kondo, K.; Kaneshima, H.; Mocarski, E.S. Human cytomegalovirus latent infection of granulocyte-macrophage progenitors. *Proc. Natl. Acad. Sci. USA* **1994**, *91*, 11879–11883.

40. Kondo, K.; Xu, J.; Mocarski, E.S. Human cytomegalovirus latent gene expression in granulocyte-macrophage progenitors in culture and in seropositive individuals. *Proc. Natl. Acad. Sci. USA* **1996**, *93*, 11137–11142.

41. Beisser, P.S.; Laurent, L.; Virelizier, J.L.; Michelson, S. Human cytomegalovirus chemokine receptor gene US28 is transcribed in latently infected THP-1 monocytes. *J. Virol.* **2001**, *75*, 5949–5957.

42. Goodrum, F.D.; Jordan, C.T.; High, K.; Shenk, T. Human cytomegalovirus gene expression during infection of primary hematopoietic progenitor cells: A model for latency. *Proc. Natl. Acad. Sci. USA* **2002**, *99*, 16255–16260.

43. Jenkins, C.; Abendroth, A.; Slobedman, B. A novel viral transcript with homology to human interleukin-10 is expressed during latent human cytomegalovirus infection. *J. Virol.* **2004**, *78*, 1440–1447.

44. Goodrum, F.; Reeves, M.; Sinclair, J.; High, K.; Shenk, T. Human cytomegalovirus sequences expressed in latently infected individuals promote a latent infection *in vitro*. *Blood* **2007**, *110*, 937–945.

45. Bego, M.; Maciejewski, J.; Khaiboullina, S.; Pari, G.; St Jeor, S. Characterization of an antisense transcript spanning the UL81-82 locus of human cytomegalovirus. *J. Virol.* **2005**, *79*, 11022–11034.

46. Reeves, M.B.; Sinclair, J.H. Analysis of latent viral gene expression in natural and experimental latency models of human cytomegalovirus and its correlation with histone modifications at a latent promoter. *J. Gen. Virol.* **2010**, *91*, 599–604.

47. Poole, E.; Walther, A.; Raven, K.; Benedict, C.A.; Mason, G.M.; Sinclair, J. The myeloid transcription factor GATA-2 regulates the viral UL144 gene during human cytomegalovirus latency in an isolate-specific manner. *J. Virol.* **2013**, doi: 10.1128/JVI.03497-12.

48. Hermiston, T.W.; Malone, C.L.; Witte, P.R.; Stinski, M.F. Identification and characterization of the human cytomegalovirus immediate-early region 2 gene that stimulates gene expression from an inducible promoter. *J. Virol.* **1987**, *61*, 3214–3221.

49. Malone, C.L.; Vesole, D.H.; Stinski, M.F. Transactivation of a human cytomegalovirus early promoter by gene products from the immediate-early gene IE2 and augmentation by IE1: Mutational analysis of the viral proteins. *J. Virol.* **1990**, *64*, 1498–1506.

50. Staprans, S.I.; Rabert, D.K.; Spector, D.H. Identification of sequence requirements and trans-acting functions necessary for regulated expression of a human cytomegalovirus early gene. *J. Virol.* **1988**, *62*, 3463–3473.

51. Greaves, R.F.; Mocarski, E.S. Defective growth correlates with reduced accumulation of a viral DNA replication protein after low-multiplicity infection by a human cytomegalovirus ie1 mutant. *J. Virol.* **1998**, *72*, 366–379.

52. Spector, D.H. Activation and regulation of human cytomegalovirus early genes. *Intervirology* **1996**, *39*, 361–377.

53. Reeves, M.; Sinclair, J. Aspects of human cytomegalovirus latency and reactivation. *Curr. Top. Microbiol. Immunol.* **2008**, *325*, 297–313.

54. Reeves, M.; Woodhall, D.; Compton, T.; Sinclair, J. Human cytomegalovirus IE72 protein interacts with the transcriptional repressor hDaxx to regulate LUNA gene expression during lytic infection. *J. Virol.* **2010**, *84*, 7185–7194.

55. Keyes, L.R.; Hargett, D.; Soland, M.; Bego, M.G.; Rossetto, C.C.; Almeida-Porada, G.; St Jeor, S. HCMV protein LUNA is required for viral reactivation from latently infected primary CD14(+) cells. *PLoS One* **2013**, *7*, e52827.

56. Groves, I.J.; Reeves, M.B.; Sinclair, J.H. Lytic infection of permissive cells with human cytomegalovirus is regulated by an intrinsic 'pre-immediate-early' repression of viral gene expression mediated by histone post-translational modification. *J. Gen. Virol.* **2009**, *90*, 2364–2374.

57. Cuevas-Bennett, C.; Shenk, T. Dynamic histone H3 acetylation and methylation at human cytomegalovirus promoters during replication in fibroblasts. *J. Virol.* **2008**, *82*, 9525–9536.

58. Nitzsche, A.; Paulus, C.; Nevels, M. Temporal dynamics of cytomegalovirus chromatin assembly in productively infected human cells. *J. Virol.* **2008**, *82*, 11167–11180.

59. Nevels, M.; Paulus, C.; Shenk, T. Human cytomegalovirus immediate-early 1 protein facilitates viral replication by antagonizing histone deacetylation. *Proc. Natl. Acad. Sci. USA* **2004**, *101*, 17234–17239.

60. Woodhall, D.L.; Groves, I.J.; Reeves, M.B.; Wilkinson, G.; Sinclair, J.H. Human Daxx-mediated repression of human cytomegalovirus gene expression correlates with a repressive chromatin structure around the major immediate early promoter. *J. Biol. Chem.* **2006**, *281*, 37652–37660.

61. Ioudinkova, E.; Arcangeletti, M.C.; Rynditch, A.; de Conto, F.; Motta, F.; Covan, S.; Pinardi, F.; Razin, S.V.; Chezzi, C. Control of human cytomegalovirus gene expression by differential histone modifications during lytic and latent infection of a monocytic cell line. *Gene* **2006**, *384*, 120–128.

62. Saffert, R.T.; Kalejta, R.F. Inactivating a cellular intrinsic immune defense mediated by Daxx is the mechanism through which the human cytomegalovirus pp71 protein stimulates viral immediate-early gene expression. *J. Virol.* **2006**, *80*, 3863–3871.

63. Lukashchuk, V.; McFarlane, S.; Everett, R.D.; Preston, C.M. Human cytomegalovirus protein pp71 displaces the chromatin-associated factor ATRX from nuclear domain 10 at early stages of infection. *J. Virol.* **2008**, *82*, 12543–12554.

64. Hofmann, H.; Sindre, H.; Stamminger, T. Functional interaction between the pp71 protein of human cytomegalovirus and the PML-interacting protein human Daxx. *J. Virol.* **2002**, *76*, 5769–5783.

65. Cantrell, S.R.; Bresnahan, W.A. Interaction between the human cytomegalovirus UL82 gene product (pp71) and hDaxx regulates immediate-early gene expression and viral replication. *J. Virol.* **2005**, *79*, 7792–7802.

66. Tsai, K.; Thikmyanova, N.; Wojcechowskyj, J.A.; Delecluse, H.J.; Lieberman, P.M. EBV tegument protein BNRF1 disrupts DAXX-ATRX to activate viral early gene transcription. *PLoS Pathog.* **2011**, *7*, e1002376.

67. Bresnick, E.H.; Katsumura, K.R.; Lee, H.Y.; Johnson, K.D.; Perkins, A.S. Master regulatory GATA transcription factors: Mechanistic principles and emerging links to hematologic malignancies. *Nucleic Acids Res.* **2012**, *40*, 5819–5831.

68. Tsai, F.Y.; Keller, G.; Kuo, F.C.; Weiss, M.; Chen, J.; Rosenblatt, M.; Alt, F.W.; Orkin, S.H. An early haematopoietic defect in mice lacking the transcription factor GATA-2. *Nature* **1994**, *371*, 221–226.

69. Ling, K.W.; Ottersbach, K.; van Hamburg, J.P.; Oziemlak, A.; Tsai, F.Y.; Orkin, S.H.; Ploemacher, R.; Hendriks, R.W.; Dzierzak, E. GATA-2 plays two functionally distinct roles during the ontogeny of hematopoietic stem cells. *J. Exp. Med.* **2004**, *200*, 871–882.

70. Slobedman, B.; Mocarski, E.S.; Arvin, A.M.; Mellins, E.D.; Abendroth, A. Latent cytomegalovirus down-regulates major histocompatibility complex class II expression on myeloid progenitors. *Blood* **2002**, *100*, 2867–2873.

71. Boyes, J.; Byfield, P.; Nakatani, Y.; Ogryzko, V. Regulation of activity of the transcription factor GATA-1 by acetylation. *Nature* **1998**, *396*, 594–598.

72. Hayakawa, F.; Towatari, M.; Ozawa, Y.; Tomita, A.; Privalsky, M.L.; Saito, H. Functional regulation of GATA-2 by acetylation. *J. Leukoc. Biol.* **2004**, *75*, 529–540.

73. Hung, H.L.; Lau, J.; Kim, A.Y.; Weiss, M.J.; Blobel, G.A. CREB-Binding protein acetylates hematopoietic transcription factor GATA-1 at functionally important sites. *Mol. Cell. Biol.* **1999**, *19*, 3496–3505.

74. Ozawa, Y.; Towatari, M.; Tsuzuki, S.; Hayakawa, F.; Maeda, T.; Miyata, Y.; Tanimoto, M.; Saito, H. Histone deacetylase 3 associates with and represses the transcription factor GATA-2. *Blood* **2001**, *98*, 2116–2123.

75. Poole, E.; McGregor Dallas, S.R.; Colston, J.; Joseph, R.S.; Sinclair, J. Virally induced changes in cellular microRNAs maintain latency of human cytomegalovirus in CD34(+) progenitors. *J. Gen. Virol.* **2011**, *92*, 1539–1549.

76. Wright, E.; Bain, M.; Teague, L.; Murphy, J.; Sinclair, J. Ets-2 repressor factor recruits histone deacetylase to silence human cytomegalovirus immediate-early gene expression in non-permissive cells. *J. Gen. Virol.* **2005**, *86*, 535–544.

77. Sinclair, J.H.; Baillie, J.; Bryant, L.A.; Taylor-Wiedeman, J.A.; Sissons, J.G. Repression of human cytomegalovirus major immediate early gene expression in a monocytic cell line. *J. Gen. Virol.* **1992**, *73*, 433–435.

78. Shelbourn, S.L.; Kothari, S.K.; Sissons, J.G.; Sinclair, J.H. Repression of human cytomegalovirus gene expression associated with a novel immediate early regulatory region binding factor. *Nucleic Acids Res.* **1989**, *17*, 9165–9171.

79. Liu, R.; Baillie, J.; Sissons, J.G.; Sinclair, J.H. The transcription factor YY1 binds to negative regulatory elements in the human cytomegalovirus major immediate early enhancer/promoter and mediates repression in non-permissive cells. *Nucleic Acids Res.* **1994**, *22*, 2453–2459.

80. Zweidler-Mckay, P.A.; Grimes, H.L.; Flubacher, M.M.; Tsichlis, P.N. Gfi-1 encodes a nuclear zinc finger protein that binds DNA and functions as a transcriptional repressor. *Mol. Cell. Biol.* **1996**, *16*, 4024–4034.

81. Slobedman, B.; Stern, J.L.; Cunningham, A.L.; Abendroth, A.; Abate, D.A.; Mocarski, E.S. Impact of human cytomegalovirus latent infection on myeloid progenitor cell gene expression. *J. Virol.* **2004**, *78*, 4054–4062.

82. Browne, E.P.; Wing, B.; Coleman, D.; Shenk, T. Altered cellular mRNA levels in human cytomegalovirus-infected fibroblasts: Viral block to the accumulation of antiviral mRNAs. *J. Virol.* **2001**, *75*, 12319–12330.

83. Keller, M.J.; Wu, A.W.; Andrews, J.I.; McGonagill, P.W.; Tibesar, E.E.; Meier, J.L. Reversal of human cytomegalovirus major immediate-early enhancer/promoter silencing in quiescently infected cells via the cyclic AMP signaling pathway. *J. Virol.* **2007**, *81*, 6669–6681.

84. Yuan, J.; Liu, X.; Wu, A.W.; McGonagill, P.W.; Keller, M.J.; Galle, C.S.; Meier, J.L. Breaking human cytomegalovirus major immediate-early gene silence by vasoactive intestinal peptide stimulation of the protein kinase A-CREB-TORC2 signaling cascade in human pluripotent embryonal NTera2 cells. *J. Virol.* **2009**, *83*, 6391–6403.

85. Prosch, S.; Wuttke, R.; Kruger, D.H.; Volk, H.D. NF-kappaB—A potential therapeutic target for inhibition of human cytomegalovirus (re)activation? *Biol. Chem.* **2002**, *383*, 1601–1609.

86. Dhayalan, A.; Tamas, R.; Bock, I.; Tattermusch, A.; Dimitrova, E.; Kudithipudi, S.; Ragozin, S.; Jeltsch, A. The ATRX-ADD domain binds to H3 tail peptides and reads the combined methylation state of K4 and K9. *Hum. Mol. Genet.* **2011**, *20*, 2195–2203.

87. Tang, J.; Wu, S.; Liu, H.; Stratt, R.; Barak, O.G.; Shiekhattar, R.; Picketts, D.J.; Yang, X. A novel transcription regulatory complex containing death domain-associated protein and the ATR-X syndrome protein. *J. Biol. Chem.* **2004**, *279*, 20369–20377.

88. De La Fuente, R.; Baumann, C.; Viveiros, M.M. Role of ATRX in chromatin structure and function: Implications for chromosome instability and human disease. *Reproduction* **2011**, *142*, 221–234.

89. Argentaro, A.; Yang, J.C.; Chapman, L.; Kowalczyk, M.S.; Gibbons, R.J.; Higgs, D.R.; Neuhaus, D.; Rhodes, D. Structural consequences of disease-causing mutations in the ATRX-DNMT3-DNMT3L (ADD) domain of the chromatin-associated protein ATRX. *Proc. Natl. Acad. Sci. USA* **2007**, *104*, 11939–11944.

90. Benedict, C.A.; Butrovich, K.D.; Lurain, N.S.; Corbeil, J.; Rooney, I.; Schneider, P.; Tschopp, J.; Ware, C.F. Cutting edge: A novel viral TNF receptor superfamily member in virulent strains of human cytomegalovirus. *J. Immunol.* **1999**, *162*, 6967–6970.

91. Montgomery, R.I.; Warner, M.S.; Lum, B.J.; Spear, P.G. Herpes simplex virus-1 entry into cells mediated by a novel member of the TNF/NGF receptor family. *Cell* **1996**, *87*, 427–436.

92. Cheung, T.C.; Humphreys, I.R.; Potter, K.G.; Norris, P.S.; Shumway, H.M.; Tran, B.R.; Patterson, G.; Jean-Jacques, R.; Yoon, M.; Spear, P.G.; *et al.* Evolutionarily divergent herpesviruses modulate T cell activation by targeting the herpesvirus entry mediator cosignaling pathway. *Proc. Natl. Acad. Sci. USA* **2005**, *102*, 13218–13223.

93. Poole, E.; Groves, I.; MacDonald, A.; Pang, Y.; Alcami, A.; Sinclair, J. Identification of TRIM23 as a cofactor involved in the regulation of NF-kappaB by human cytomegalovirus. *J. Virol.* **2009**, *83*, 3581–3590.

94. Poole, E.; King, C.A.; Sinclair, J.H.; Alcami, A. The UL144 gene product of human cytomegalovirus activates NFkappaB via a TRAF6-dependent mechanism. *EMBO J.* **2006**, *25*, 4390–4399.

95. Charlton, B.; Lafferty, K.J. The Th1/Th2 balance in autoimmunity. *Curr. Opin. Immunol.* **1995**, *7*, 793–798.

96. Nakayama, T.; Hieshima, K.; Nagakubo, D.; Sato, E.; Nakayama, M.; Kawa, K.; Yoshie, O. Selective induction of Th2-attracting chemokines CCL17 and CCL22 in human B cells by latent membrane protein 1 of Epstein-Barr virus. *J. Virol.* **2004**, *78*, 1665–1674.

97. Stanton, R.J.; Baluchova, K.; Dargan, D.J.; Cunningham, C.; Sheehy, O.; Seirafian, S.; McSharry, B.P.; Neale, M.L.; Davies, J.A.; Tomasec, P.; *et al.* Reconstruction of the complete human cytomegalovirus genome in a BAC reveals RL13 to be a potent inhibitor of replication. *J. Clin. Investig.* **2010**, *120*, 3191–3208.

98. Reeves, M.B. Chromatin-mediated regulation of cytomegalovirus gene expression. *Virus Res.* **2011**, *157*, 134–143.

99. Murphy, J.C.; Fischle, W.; Verdin, E.; Sinclair, J.H. Control of cytomegalovirus lytic gene expression by histone acetylation. *EMBO J.* **2002**, *21*, 1112–1120.

100. Sinclair, J. Chromatin structure regulates human cytomegalovirus gene expression during latency, reactivation and lytic infection. *Biochim. Biophys. Acta* **2009**, *1799*, 286–295.

101. Reeves, M.; Murphy, J.; Greaves, R.; Fairley, J.; Brehm, A.; Sinclair, J. Autorepression of the human cytomegalovirus major immediate-early promoter/enhancer at late times of infection is mediated by the recruitment of chromatin remodeling enzymes by IE86. *J. Virol.* **2006**, *80*, 9998–10009.

102. Reeves, M.B.; Lehner, P.J.; Sissons, J.G.; Sinclair, J.H. An *in vitro* model for the regulation of human cytomegalovirus latency and reactivation in dendritic cells by chromatin remodelling. *J. Gen. Virol.* **2005**, *86*, 2949–2954.

103. Varnum, S.M.; Streblow, D.N.; Monroe, M.E.; Smith, P.; Auberry, K.J.; Pasa-Tolic, L.; Wang, D.; Camp, D.G., 2nd; Rodland, K.; Wiley, S.; *et al.* Identification of proteins in human cytomegalovirus (HCMV) particles: The HCMV proteome. *J. Virol.* **2004**, *78*, 10960–10966.

104. Reeves, R.; Gorman, C.M.; Howard, B. Minichromosome assembly of non-integrated plasmid DNA transfected into mammalian cells. *Nucleic Acids Res.* **1985**, *13*, 3599–3615.

105. Riu, E.; Chen, Z.Y.; Xu, H.; He, C.Y.; Kay, M.A. Histone modifications are associated with the persistence or silencing of vector-mediated transgene expression *in vivo*. *Mol. Ther.* **2007**, *15*, 1348–1355.

106. Maul, G.G. Initiation of cytomegalovirus infection at ND10. *Curr. Top. Microbiol. Immunol.* **2008**, *325*, 117–132.

107. Tavalai, N.; Stamminger, T. Intrinsic cellular defense mechanisms targeting human cytomegalovirus. *Virus Res.* **2011**, *157*, 128–133.

108. Ishov, A.M.; Vladimirova, O.V.; Maul, G.G. Daxx-mediated accumulation of human cytomegalovirus tegument protein pp71 at ND10 facilitates initiation of viral infection at these nuclear domains. *J. Virol.* **2002**, *76*, 7705–7712.

109. Wilkinson, G.W.; Kelly, C.; Sinclair, J.H.; Rickards, C. Disruption of PML-associated nuclear bodies mediated by the human cytomegalovirus major immediate early gene product. *J. Gen. Virol.* **1998**, *79*, 1233–1245.

110. Tavalai, N.; Papior, P.; Rechter, S.; Leis, M.; Stamminger, T. Evidence for a role of the cellular ND10 protein PML in mediating intrinsic immunity against human cytomegalovirus infections. *J. Virol.* **2006**, *80*, 8006–8018.

111. Ahn, J.H.; Brignole, E.J., 3rd; Hayward, G.S. Disruption of PML subnuclear domains by the acidic IE1 protein of human cytomegalovirus is mediated through interaction with PML and may modulate a RING finger-dependent cryptic transactivator function of PML. *Mol. Cell. Biol.* **1998**, *18*, 4899–4913.

112. Ahn, J.H.; Hayward, G.S. The major immediate-early proteins IE1 and IE2 of human cytomegalovirus colocalize with and disrupt PML-associated nuclear bodies at very early times in infected permissive cells. *J. Virol.* **1997**, *71*, 4599–4613.

113. Saffert, R.T.; Kalejta, R.F. Human cytomegalovirus gene expression is silenced by Daxx-mediated intrinsic immune defense in model latent infections established *in vitro*. *J. Virol.* **2007**, *81*, 9109–9120.

114. Groves, I.J.; Sinclair, J.H. Knockdown of hDaxx in normally non-permissive undifferentiated cells does not permit human cytomegalovirus immediate-early gene expression. *J. Gen. Virol.* **2007**, *88*, 2935–2940.

115. Saffert, R.T.; Penkert, R.R.; Kalejta, R.F. Cellular and viral control over the initial events of human cytomegalovirus experimental latency in CD34+ cells. *J. Virol.* **2010**, *84*, 5594–5604.

116. Hargett, D.; Shenk, T.E. Experimental human cytomegalovirus latency in CD14+ monocytes. *Proc. Natl. Acad. Sci. USA* **2010**, *107*, 20039–20044.

9

Deregulation of Epigenetic Mechanisms by the Hepatitis B Virus X Protein in Hepatocarcinogenesis

Ourania M. Andrisani

Department of Basic Medical Science and Center for Cancer Research,
Purdue University West Lafayette, IN 47907, USA; E-Mail: andrisao@purdue.edu;

Abstract: This review focuses on the significance of deregulation of epigenetic mechanisms by the hepatitis B virus (HBV) X protein in hepatocarcinogenesis and HBV replication. Epigenetic mechanisms, DNA methylation, and specific histone modifications, e.g., trimethylation of H3 on lysine-27 or lysine-4, maintain 'cellular memory' by silencing expression of lineage-inducing factors in stem cells and conversely, of pluripotency factors in differentiated cells. The X protein has been reported to induce expression of DNA methyltransferases (DNMTs), likely promoting epigenetic changes during hepatocarcinogenesis. Furthermore, in cellular and animal models of X-mediated oncogenic transformation, protein levels of chromatin modifying proteins Suz12 and Znf198 are down-regulated. Suz12 is essential for the Polycomb Repressive Complex 2 (PRC2) mediating the repressive trimethylation of H3 on lysine-27 (H3K27me3). Znf198, stabilizes the LSD1-CoREST-HDAC complex that removes, via lysine demethylase1 (LSD1), the activating trimethylation of H3 on lysine-4 (H3K4me3). Down-regulation of Suz12 also occurs in liver tumors of woodchucks chronically infected by woodchuck hepatitis virus, an animal model recapitulating HBV-mediated hepatocarcinogenesis in humans. Significantly, subgroups of HBV-induced liver cancer re-express hepatoblast and fetal markers, and imprinted genes, suggesting hepatocyte reprogramming during oncogenic transformation. Lastly, down-regulation of Suz12 and Znf198 enhances HBV replication. Collectively, these observations suggest deregulation of epigenetic mechanisms by HBV X protein influences both the viral cycle and the host cell.

Keywords: Hepatitis B virus (HBV); HBV X protein; Hepatocellular Carcinoma (HCC); HBV replication; epigenetic regulation; DNA methylation; DNA methyl transferases (DNMTs); Polycomb Repressive complex 2 (PRC2); Suz12; suppressor of zeste 12 homolog (Drosophila); Znf198; zinc finger; MYM-type 2; LSD1-Co-REST-HDAC1

1. Introduction

Chronic hepatitis B virus (HBV) infection is a major etiologic factor in pathogenesis of hepatocellular carcinoma (HCC) [1,2]. Despite an HBV vaccine, the World Health Organization estimates 400 million people globally are chronically infected with HBV, and HCC has become the fifth most common cancer world-wide [3,4]. Liver tumors are highly heterogeneous, differing in genetic alterations, treatment, and prognosis [5]. Global transcriptome analyses of human liver tumors have identified distinct subgroups of HCCs associated with specific genetic changes and clinical prognosis [6]. In this review, of special interest is the HCC subgroup G1, identified and characterized by the transcriptome studies of Boyault *et al.* [7]. The G1 subgroup is associated with low titer HBV infection, high rate of chromosomal instability, poor prognosis, and high expression levels of AFP (alpha-fetoprotein), imprinted genes (IGFII, H19, PEG3 and PEG10), and transcription factor SOX9, a key regulator of pancreatobiliary ductal system development. Given that classification of tumors by histologic markers does not identify the cellular origin of the tumor, *i.e.*, differentiated *vs.* progenitor cell, in this review I explore mechanisms that could mediate the upregulated expression of the hepatoblast/fetal markers and imprinted genes observed in the G1 subgroup of HBV-mediated HCCs.

2. The HBV Life Cycle

Hepatitis B virus (HBV) is a small enveloped virus belonging to the hepadnavirus family [8]. It infects human hepatocytes causing acute and chronic liver infection and disease. Epidemiologic studies have established that chronic HBV infection, occurring in less than 5% of HBV infected patients, is associated with high risk of developing hepatocellular carcinoma by the fourth or fifth decade of life [1].

The HBV genome is partially double stranded and comprised of 3.2 Kb. It encodes the pre-S/S (surface antigen), the pre-C/C (core protein), the P (viral polymerase) and X open reading frames. The X protein is essential for viral transcription and replication [9,10]. Following infection of hepatocytes by the hepatitis B virus, the viral nucleocapsids are transported to the nuclear membrane where they become disassembled, releasing the viral genome into the nuclear compartment [11]. At this stage, the viral genome takes the form of relaxed, circular (RC), partially double-stranded DNA. The RC DNA is subsequently converted into covalently closed, circular DNA (cccDNA) which serves as template for transcription of the pregenomic RNA (pgRNA) and the RNA species that encode the viral proteins [12]. In turn, the pgRNA serves as the template for synthesis of the viral genome by virus-encoded reverse transcriptase [13]. This step occurs in viral capsids in the cytoplasm [14]. Importantly, the cccDNA in the nucleus of infected cells forms chromatin-like structure by association with nucleosomes [15]. Moreover, it has been clearly demonstrated that the histone modifications associated with the viral mini-chromosome determine its transcriptional activation or repression. Specifically, chromatin immunoprecipitation assays of the cccDNA/mini-chromosome have demonstrated that lysine acetylation of H3 and H4 correlates with viral replication which depends on transcription of the pgRNA, and the level of viremia in HBV-infected patients [16–18]. These results imply that changes in the activity of chromatin modifying complexes (*i.e.*, those that mediate epigenetic histone modifications in infected hepatocytes), influence the rate of transcription from the viral mini-chromosome, and in turn the rate of HBV replication.

3. HBV and Hepatocellular Carcinoma (HCC)

Chronic infection by HBV is associated with increased risk of liver cancer development (1). Factors contributing to pathogenesis of HBV-mediated HCC include chronic liver inflammation due to continued hepatocyte death and regeneration [19]. In addition, the functions of viral proteins X [20,21], S [22] and core [23] are likely contributors to HBV-mediated hepatocarcinogenesis. In this review I focus on the role of the X protein in HBV-mediated hepatocarcinogenesis.

HBV DNA integrates into the host genome at early steps of clonal tumor expansion, the majority of tumors displaying continued expression of pX [24]. Genomic aberrations frequently occur in HBV-mediated HCC [25], but the mechanism(s) that initiate and propagate these genomic changes are not yet understood. pX is a multifunctional protein essential for the viral life cycle. Involvement of the X protein in HCC pathogenesis is supported by data from animal models revealing pX acts as a weak oncogene or a co-factor in hepatocarcinogenesis [20,21]. pX activates cellular mitogenic pathways and induces transcription of select viral and cellular genes [26,27], thereby influencing cellular proliferation mechanisms. [The reader also is referred to recent comprehensive reviews of X protein functions and HBV-mediated hepatocarcinogenesis [28,29].

Pertinent to the weakly oncogenic potential of the X protein, it was shown in a cellular model of immortalized hepatocytes that inducible expression of pX promotes DNA re-replication-induced DNA damage, propagation of damaged DNA to daughter cells, and generation of partial polyploidy (>4 N DNA) [30,31]. In this cellular model, it was determined pX prematurely activates the mitotic polo-like-kinase1 (Plk1) in the G2 phase [32]. Plk1 is a cell cycle regulated gene [33], required for checkpoint recovery after completion of DNA repair [34], allowing mitotic entry and cell cycle progression [35]. Significantly, Plk1 is over-expressed in many human cancers, including liver cancer [36], and this up-regulation correlates with poor cancer prognosis. Elevated expression of Plk1 and of a cluster of proliferation genes was also observed by microarray analyses of human HCCs, including liver tumors from chronic HBV patients [37]. Importantly, in an *in vitro* cellular model of pX-mediated hepatocyte transformation, inhibition of Plk1 suppressed transformation [31], underscoring the importance of this enzyme in HBV-induced HCC. Recent studies have linked the increased expression of Plk1 during HCC progression to down-regulation of miR-100, a microRNA that targets Plk1 [38]. Whether miR-100 becomes down-regulated in HBV-mediated HCCs remains to be determined.

Proteomic studies have shown Plk1 phosphorylates substrates involved in a wide variety of processes [39]. A classic substrate of Plk1 is the protein claspin that participates in checkpoint activation by ATR [33]; in turn, upon completion of DNA repair, the G2/M DNA damage checkpoint is terminated by proteosomal degradation of claspin [34]. This step is initiated by phosphorylation of claspin by Plk1 at phosphodegron sites, signaling ubiquitination of the substrate and proteosomal destruction [34]. The mechanism by which Plk1 induction promotes pX-mediated oncogenic transformation remains to be determined.

4. Chromatin Modifying Proteins Suz12 and Znf198 in the X Protein Signaling Network

A genome-wide siRNA library screen performed in pX-expressing cells led to identification of nuclear proteins Suz12 and Znf198, both components of chromatin modifying complexes, as downstream players in the pX signaling network [40]. Specifically, siRNA-mediated knockdown of these proteins rescued X-expressing cells from DNA damage induced apoptosis, suggesting a role of these proteins in X-mediated hepatocyte transformation. Loss-of-function of Znf198 and Suz12 has been described in other human cancers [41,42]. More importantly, the ZNF198 gene located on chromosome 13q12.11 is frequently affected (~30% of cases) by loss of heterozygosity in early onset HCC, correlating with high tumor grade and HBV-related tumors [43,44]. Both Suz12 [45] and Znf198 [46] associate with promyelocytic leukemia (PML) nuclear bodies (NBs) [47]; Suz12 and Znf198 knockdown cell lines exhibit reduced numbers of PML NBs [40].

PML NBs are dynamic nuclear structures that change in composition during the cell cycle [47]; are sites of epigenetic regulation [48,49], p53 function [50], DNA repair [51]; and play a role in the innate immune response [52] and viral replication [53]. Indeed, Suz12 and Znf198 knockdown cell lines, similar to PML knockdown cell lines, exhibit reduced numbers of PML NBs, loss of p53-mediated apoptosis, and loss of DNA repair [40]. Moreover, knockdown of PML, Suz12, and Znf198 proteins by siRNA transfection enhances HBV replication [40], in a cellular model of HepAD38 cells engineered to support HBV replication in a tetracycline- inducible manner. Viruses employ various mechanisms to disrupt PML function, favoring enhanced viral replication [54] For example, an early event in Herpes Simplex Virus1 (HSV1) replication, mediated by the ICP0 protein, is dislodging of HDAC1/2 from the LSD1-CoREST-HDAC complex [55,56]. In HBV replication, PML NBs become altered in both number and morphology [57]. Furthermore, HBV replication depends on modifications of H3 and H4 associated with cccDNA, the template of pgRNA transcription [16–18]. As described above, pgRNA transcription determines the rate of HBV replication [8], and HDAC1 associated with cccDNA correlates with decline in HBV replication [18].

Interestingly, Znf198 stabilizes the LSD1-CoREST-HDAC1 chromatin modifying complex [58] that removes histone modifications associated with transcriptional activation (Figure 1). Specifically, lysine demethylase1 (LSD1) removes the activating trimethylation of histone 3 on lysine-4 (H3K4me3), and histone deacetylase 1(HDAC1) removes the activating acetylation of histones. Thus, loss of Znf198, destabilizing the LSD1-CoREST-HDAC1 chromatin modifying complex, will maintain the transcriptionally activating histone modifications of the host chromatin as well as the viral mini-chromosome, providing yet another example of how viruses hijack cellular mechanisms to the advantage of their life cycle.

Figure 1. Diagram shows Znf198 interacting and stabilizing the LSD1-Co-REST-HDAC1 complex [58]. LSD1 removes the transcriptionally activating trimethylation of H3 on K4. HDAC1 removes the transcriptionally activating acetylation of histones.

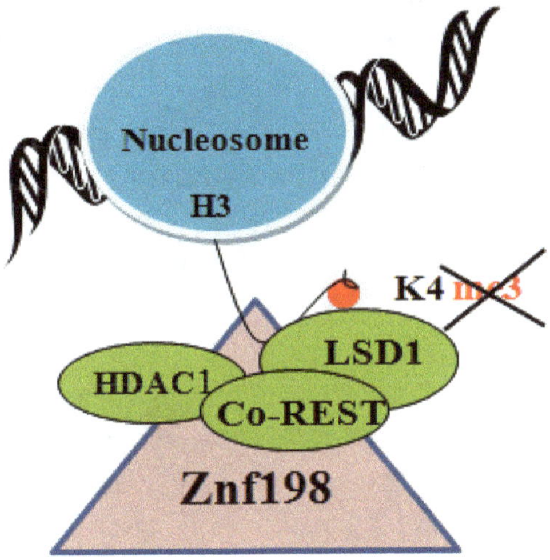

5. Suz12 Containing PRC2 Complex

Suz12 is an essential component for activity of the polycomb repressive complex PRC2, comprised of histone methylstransferase EZH2 and EED [59]. The PRC2 complex (Figure 2) mediates the trimethylation of histone 3 on lysine27 (H3K27me3), a mark of transcriptionally silent chromatin [60,61]. The PRC2 chromatin modifying complex regulates expression of many developmental and signaling genes in embryonic stem cells (ESCs). Accordingly, the PRC2 complex was proposed to have a role in the maintenance of stem cell pluripotency [62–65]. However, additional studies have refined our understanding of the role of the PRC2 complex in ESCs. Specifically, PRC2-deficient ESCs failed to maintain expression of lineage-specific genes, exhibiting impaired differentiation, lack of repression of ESC markers, and lack of activation of differentiation-specific genes [66]. These observations were interpreted to mean the PRC2 complex regulates cell fate transitions during lineage commitment [66–68].

In human embryonic fibroblasts, more than 1,000 genes are transcriptionally silenced by the PRC2 complex [62]. In untransformed hepatocytes, Suz12 chromatin immunoprecipitation assays identified a subset of genes that are repressed by the PRC2 complex, including: BAMBI, CCND2, DLK1, EpCAM, and IGFII [69]. Interestingly, Suz12 occupancy at the promoters of these genes was significantly reduced in X-transformed cells, and up-regulated expression of these genes was detected in liver tumors from animal models of X-mediated and HBV-mediated hepatocarcinogenesis [69,70]. Significantly, these genes are up-regulated in the G1 subgroup of HBV-mediated HCCs [7] and also are expressed in hepatic cancer initiating/stem cells [71]. Intriguingly, these genes are also markers of normal hepatoblasts [70], raising a question of the mechanism allowing re-expression of hepatoblast markers during oncogenic transformation of differentiated hepatocytes. One might predict up-regulation of genes supporting re-establishment of the hepatoblast phenotype, resulting in lineage mis-specification and reversal of the differentiated phenotype.

Figure 2. Diagram shows the essential components of the PRC2 complex, namely SUZ12, EED and EZH2. EZH2 is the histone methyltransferase enzyme that trimethylates H3 on K27. This modification silences transcription.

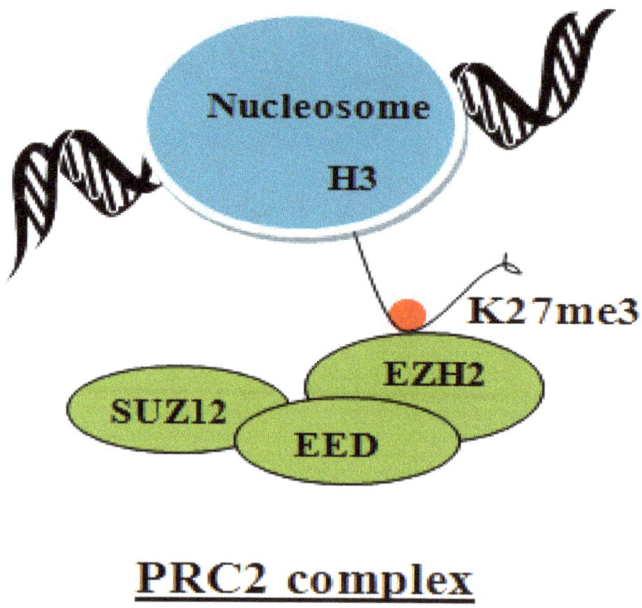

In this dynamic process of lineage change as in hepatocyte de-differentiation, it is not understood how the PRC2 complex selects genes for repression. Although several possibilities exist including interaction of the PRC2 complex with specific transcription factors, the PRC2 complex binding to specific long, noncoding RNAs [72] as well as to short RNAs transcribed from the 5' end of genes repressed by the PRC2 complex [73], suggests a likely mechanisms for target gene selection. For example, in embryonic stem cells, the PRC2 complex regulates expression of the imprinted DLK1 gene via interaction with the long noncoding RNA Gtl2 serving as cofactor [74]. Interestingly, the DLK1 gene is expressed in hepatic progenitors and hepatoblasts [70], as well as in the G1 subgroup of HBV-mediated HCCs [7]. Moreover, poor prognosis, HBV-mediated liver tumors, referred to as the C3 subgroup in the study by Toffanin *et al* [74] also re-express EpCAM and AFP, and exhibit elevated expression of a cluster of microRNAs encoded by the imprinted DLK1-DIO3 region. Taken together, both of these studies [7,74] have identified the re-expression of hepatoblast/fetal genes in the G1/C3 subgroups of HBV-mediated HCCs, significantly, genes repressed by the PRC2 complex in differentiated hepatocytes. Furthermore, these studies suggest the down-regulation of the PRC2 complex or of its activity in the G1/C3 subgroups of HBV-mediated HCCs, raising the question of how the PRC2 complex is regulated.

6. Regulation of the PRC2 Complex

Studies by independent groups have identified several mechanisms by which the PRC2 complex is regulated. (1) Suz12 protein can be down-regulated via the action of microRNAs. Specifically miR-200 targets the 3'UTR of Suz12 [75]; (2) Ezh2, the component of the PRC2 complex containing the histone methyltransferase enzymatic activity, is inactivated by Akt-mediated phosphorylation [76]. Importantly, poor prognosis HBV-mediated HCCs, such as those of the G1 subgroup, exhibit enhanced activation of Akt [7]; (3) Loss of the protein JARID, enabling association of the PRC2 complex with target genes [77]; (4) Induction of the H3K27 demethylase (JMJD3 or KD6M) could also result in removal of the transcriptionally repressive H3K27me3 modification, likely resulting in re-expression of the targeted genes. Interestingly, recent studies have shown induction of JMJD3 in Epstein Barr virus infected cells and associated Hodgkin's lymphoma [78]; (5) Lastly, an inverse relationship was noted between protein levels of Plk1 and Suz12/Znf198 in X-induced tumorigenesis [69], suggesting Suz12 and Znf198 are down-regulated via Plk1-mediated phosphorylation, promoting their proteasomal degradation. Suz12 is phosphorylated *in vivo* at a Plk1 consensus site [79] and both Suz12 and Znf198 are *in vitro* substrates of Plk1 (unpublished data). Since Plk1 is up-regulated in HBV-mediated HCCs, and the X protein activates Plk1, these chromatin modifying proteins undergo transient down-regulation during G2 and M phases of the cell cycle. The down-regulation of Suz12 and Znf198 suggests that the respective chromatin modifying complexes are concurrently inactivated. Importantly, the LSD1-CoREST-HDAC1 complex and the PRC2 complex are tethered together via the lincRNA HOTAIR, indicating that their activities are coupled, likely acting on the same gene [80]. In ESCs, genes that contain both H3K27me3 and H3K4me3 modifications are described as "poised or bivalent" genes, awaiting activation [81]. Down-regulation of these chromatin modifying complexes induces re-activation of specific genes in the respective knockdown cell lines, during progression to X-induced transformation and in animal models of X- and HBV-mediated liver cancer development [69].

The consequence of chronic HBV infection and continued expression of X, mediating down-regulation of these proteins through each cell cycle of an HBV infected hepatocyte, for many cell generations, is not yet understood. The gene expression program of differentiated cells is maintained after cell division by propagating the identical "chromatin landscape" of the parental cell to the daughter cell via heritable histone modifications known as epigenetic marks [82]. Recent studies in *Drosophila* have shown that propagation of the heritable chromatin landscape through cell division involves chromatin-modifying proteins including the Enhancer-of-Zeste, found to associate with newly synthesized DNA [83]. It was proposed that these histone modifying enzymes re-establish the heritable histone modifications on newly assembled unmethylated histones, serving as the epigenetic mark. Whether the PRC2 complex also serves as the epigenetic mark in mammalian cells is unknown. If that turns out to be the case, the down-regulation of Suz12 and Znf198 by pX in HBV infected hepatocytes not only alters the gene expression pattern of the hepatocyte, but its down-regulation has the potential to propagate to the subsequent cell generations an altered chromatin landscape.

7. Distinct Histone Modifications and DNA Methylation Landscapes in Pluripotent *vs.* Differentiated Cells

In addition to histone modifications described above, DNA methylation is another heritable modification that is linked to gene activity and maintenance of cellular memory. For example, DNA methylation at the promoter of the pluripotency factor Oct4 in a differentiated cell maintains the Oct4 gene repressed, ensuring maintenance of the differentiated state [84]. Large scale analyses examined the link between DNA methylation and histone modifications, showing that the methylation state of H3K4 is a good predictor of promoter DNA methylation. Specifically, methylation of H3K4 disrupts promoter DNA methylation by inhibiting contact between DNA methyl transferases (DNMTs) and histones [85,86]. Global comparison of the chromatin landscape between hESCs and differentiated cells [87] using Chip-Seq approaches showed the following: (1) Differentiated cells display extensive regions with repressive histone modifications (H3K27me3 and H3K9me3) in comparison to pluripotent cells; (2) In differentiated cells there is an association of H3K27me3 with promoter hypomethylation, also suggesting a connection between histone modifications and DNA methylation. Indeed, liver differentiation *in vivo* is characterized by specific demethylation in regions enriched in H3K27me3 [88]; (3) Transcribed exons in gene regions associated with H3K36me3 exhibit DNA hypermethylation [87]. Together, these results emphasize a strong connection between histone modifications and DNA methylation in determining cellular memory. Consequently, alterations in both histone modifying enzymes as well as in DNA methyltransferases (DNMTs) have the potential to alter the heritable epigenetic landscape of the cell, thereby altering its cellular memory and identity.

8. DNA Methylation and the X Protein

Several studies have reported increased levels of DNMT1, DNMT3A, and DNMT3B and aberrant DNA methylation in HBV infected cells and HBV-mediated liver tumors [89–91]. DNMT3A and DNMT3B are *de novo* DNA methyltransferases, and DNMT1 maintains the DNA methylation pattern of the daughter strand during DNA replication, and is referred to as the maintenance methyltransferase [92]. DNMTs catalyze the addition of a methyl group to the cytosine ring of the 5'-CpG dinucleotide.

The HBV X protein was reported to induce transcription of DNMT1, DNMT3A, and DNMT3B genes [89] and to directly interact and activate the *de novo* methyltransferase DNMT3A [90]. Specific gene promoters were shown to be methylated in HBV infected cells including the IL-4, metallothionein-1F, IGFBP3, SUFU, and TIRAP [90,93]. Moreover, these DNMTs also methylate the viral DNA, resulting in a reduction in viral replication [93–95]. The significance of these DNA modifications in the pathogenesis of HCC is not understood. Recent technological advances for identification of global CpG methylation patterns have been reported [96] and will undoubtedly be applied to determine the DNA methylome of HBV-mediated HCCs. It will be interesting to explore the link between pX-mediated down-regulation of the PRC2 complex and induction of DNMTs in the cellular reprogramming of HBV infected hepatocytes.

9. Conclusion

Since HBV infection occurs in differentiated hepatocytes, requiring the transcriptional activity of hepatocyte-specific transcription factors [97], it is intriguing that subgroups of HBV-induced HCCs express hepatoblast and fetal markers.

The evidence presented in this review discussed the down-regulation of Suz12/PRC2 and Znf198/LSD1-CoREST-HDAC1 chromatin modifying complexes in X-mediated tumorigenesis [69] and the induction of the DNMTs in HBV-induced HCCs [89–91]. A third epigenetic mechanism that is likely involved in this cellular reprogramming is deregulation of microRNAs, a topic not included in this review. In the cellular context of the HBV-infected hepatocyte, it is likely that the combination of the enhanced DNMTs expression, down-regulation of the two chromatin modifying complexes and deregulated expression of microRNAs induce epigenetic reprogramming of the differentiated hepatocyte into a de-differentiated state resembling a hepatoblast/hepatic progenitor cell. This leads to re-expression of hepatoblast, fetal and imprinted genes observed in the G1 subgroup of HCCs [7] along with acquisition of enhanced proliferative potential resembling self-renewing stem cells. Based on this scenario, I propose that this combination of X-induced epigenetic processes gives rise to hepatic cancer initiating stem cells. Recent studies have established a specific molecular sequence of events mediating cellular reprogramming of somatic cells into the induced pluripotency (iPS) cells [98]. Whether epigenetic reprogramming of chronically HBV-infected hepatocytes to HCC is a random or mechanism-specific process remains to be determined.

Acknowledgments

Supported by National Institutes of Health (NIH) Grant DK044533 to O.M.A. The author thanks R.L. Hullinger for critical review of this manuscript.

References

1. Beasley, R.P.; Hwang, L.Y.; Lin, C.C.; Chien, C.S. Hepatocellular carcinoma and hepatitis B virus. A prospective study of 22,707 men in Taiwan. *Lancet* **1981**, *2*, 1129–1133.
2. Bruix, J.; Boix, L.; Sala, M.; Llovet, J.M. Focus on hepatocellular carcinoma. *Cancer Cell.* **2004**, *5*, 215–219.
3. El-Serag, H.B.; Rudolph, K.L. Hepatocellular carcinoma: Epidemiology and molecular carcinogenesis. *Gastroenterology* **2007**, *132*, 2557–2576.
4. Parkin, D.M. International variation. *Oncogene* **2004**, *23*, 6329–6340.

5. Thomas, M.B.; Jaffe, D.; Choti, M.M.; Belghiti, J.; Curley, S.; Fong, Y.; Gores, G.; Kerlan, R.; Merle, P.; O'Neil, B.; *et al.* Hepatocellular carcinoma: Consensus recommendations of the National Cancer Institute Clinical Trials Planning Meeting. *J. Clin. Onocol.* **2010**, *28*, 3994–4005.

6. Hoshida, Y.; Nijman, S.M.; Kobayashi, M.; Chan, J.A.; Brunet, J.P.; Chiang, D.Y.; Villanueva, A.; Newell, P.; Ikeda, K.; Hashimoto, M.; *et al.* Integrative transcriptome analysis reveals common molecular subclasses of human hepatocellular carcinoma. *Cancer Res.* **2009**, *69*, 7385–7392.

7. Boyault, S.; Rickman, D.S.; de Reyniès, A.; Balabaud, C.; Rebouissou, S.; Jeannot, E.; Hérault, A.; Saric, J.; Belghiti, J.; Franco, D.; *et al.* Transcriptome classification of HCC is related to gene alterations and to new therapeutic targets. *Hepatology* **2007**, *45*, 42–52.

8. Seeger, C.; Mason, W.S. Hepatitis B virus biology. *Microbiol. Mol. Biol. Rev.* **2000**, *64*, 51–68.

9. Zoulim, F.; Saputelli, J.; Seeger, C. Woodchuck hepatitis virus X protein is required for viral infection *in vivo*. *J. Virol.* **1994**, *68*, 2026–2030.

10. Lucifora, J.; Arzberger, S.; Durantel, D.; Belloni, L.; Strubin, M.; Levrero, M.; Zoulim, F.; Hantz, O.; Protzer, U. Hepatitis B virus X protein is essential to initiate and maintain virus replication after infection. *J. Hepatol.* **2011**, *55*, 996–1003.

11. Rabe, B.; Vlachou, A.; Panté, N.; Helenius, A.; Kann, M. Nuclear import of hepatitis B virus capsids and release of the viral genome. *Proc. Natl. Acad. Sci. USA* **2003**, *100*, 9849–9854.

12. Weiser, B.; Ganem, D.; Seeger, C.; Varmus, H.E. Closed circular viral DNA and asymmetrical heterogeneous forms in livers of animals infected with ground squirrel hepatitis virus. *J. Virol.* **1983**, *48*, 1–9.

13. Summers, J.; Mason, W.S. Replication of the genome of a hepatitis B-like virus by reverse transcription of an RNA intermediate. *Cell* **1982**, *29*, 403–415.

14. Beck, J.; Nassal, M. Hepatitis B virus replication. *World J. Gastroenterol.* **2007**, *13*, 48–64.

15. Bock, C.T.; Schranz, P.; Schröder, C.H.; Zentgraf, H. Hepatitis B virus genome is organized into nucleosomes in the nucleus of the infected cell. *Virus Genes* **1994**, *8*, 215–229.

16. Pollicino, T.; Belloni, L.; Raffa, G.; Pediconi, N.; Squadrito, G.; Raimondo, G.; Levrero, M. Hepatitis B virus replication is regulated by the acetylation status of hepatitis B virus cccDNA-bound H3 and H4 histones. *Gastroenterology* **2006**, *130*, 827–837.

17. Levrero, M.; Pollicino, T.; Petersen, J.; Belloni, L.; Raimondo, G.; Dandri, M. Control of cccDNA function in hepatitis B virus infection. *J. Hepatol.* **2009**, *51*, 581–592.

18. Belloni, L.; Pollicino,T.; de Nicola, F., Guerrieri, F.; Raffa, G.; Fanciulli, M.; Raimondo, G.; Levrero, M. Nuclear HBx binds the HBV minichromosome and modifies the epigenetic regulation of cccDNA function. *Proc. Natl. Acad. Sci. USA* **2009**, *106*, 19975–19979.

19. Hagen, T.M.; Huang, S.; Curnutte, J.; Fowler, P.; Martinez, V.; Wehr, C.M.; Ames, B.N.; Chisari, F.V. Extensive oxidative DNA damage in hepatocytes of transgenic mice with chronic active hepatitis destined to develop hepatocellular carcinoma. *Proc. Natl. Acad. Sci. USA* **1994**, *91*, 12808–12812.

20. Terradillos, O.; Billet, O.; Renard, C.A.; Levy, R.; Molina, T.; Briand, P.; Buendia, M.A. The hepatitis B virus X gene potentiates c-myc-induced liver oncogenesis in transgenic mice. *Oncogene* **1997**, *14*, 395–404.
21. Madden, C.R.; Finegold, M.J.; Slagle, B.L. Hepatitis B virus X protein acts as a tumor promoter in development of diethylnitrosamine-induced preneoplastic lesions. *J. Virol.* **2001**, *75*, 3851–3858.
22. Yin, J.; Xie, J.; Zhang, H.; Shen, Q.; Han, L.; Lu, W.; Han, Y.; Li, C.; Ni, W.; Wang, H.; *et al.* Significant association of different preS mutations with hepatitis B-related cirrhosis or hepatocellular carcinoma. *J. Gastroenterol.* **2010**, *45*, 1063–1071.
23. Du, J.; Liang, X.; Liu, Y.; Qu, Z.; Gao, L.; Han, L.; Liu, S.; Cui, M.; Shi, Y.; Zhang, Z.; *et al.* Hepatitis B virus core protein inhibits TRAIL-induced apoptosis of hepatocytes by blocking DR5 expression. *Cell Death Differ.* **2009**, *16*, 219–229.
24. Su, Q.; Schröder, C.H.; Hofmann, W.J.; Otto, G.; Pichlmayr, R.; Bannasch, P. Expression of Hepatitis B virus X protein in HBV-infected human livers and hepatocellular carcinomas. *Hepatology* **1998**, *27*, 1109–1120.
25. Buendia, M.A. Genetics of hepatocellular carcinoma. *Semin. Cancer Biol.* **2000**, *10*, 185–200.
26. Andrisani, O.M.; Barnabas, S. The transcriptional function of the hepatitis B virus X protein and its role in hepatocarcinogenesis. *Int. J. Oncol.* **1999**, *15*, 373–379.
27. Bouchard, M.J.; Schneider, R.J. The enigmatic X gene of hepatitis B virus. *J. Virol.* **2004**, *78*, 12725–12734.
28. Ng, S.A.; Lee, C. Hepatitis B virus X gene and hepatocarcinogenesis. *J. Gastroenterol.* **2011**, *46*, 974–990.
29. Rawat, S.; Clippinger, A.J.; Bouchard, M.J. Modulation of apoptotic signaling by the hepatisis B virus X protein. *Viruses* **2012**, *4*, 2945–2972
30. Rakotomalala, L.; Studach, L.; Wang, W.H.; Gregori, G.; Hullinger, R.L.; Andrisani, O. Hepatitis B virus X protein increases the Cdt-1-to-geminin ratio inducing DNA re-replication and polyploidy. *J. Biol. Chem.* **2008**, *283*, 28729–28740.
31. Studach, L.L.; Rakotomalala, L.; Wang, W.H.; Hullinger, R.L.; Cairo, S.; Buendia, M.A.; Andrisani, O.M. Polo-like kinase 1 inhibition suppresses hepatitis B virus X protein-induced transformation in an *in vitro* model of liver cancer progression. *Hepatology* **2009**, *50*, 414–423.
32. Studach, L.; Wang, W.H.; Weber, G.; Tang, J.; Hullinger, R.L.; Malbrue, R.; Liu, X.; Andrisani, O. Polo-like kinase 1 activated by the hepatitis B virus X protein attenuates both the DNA damage checkpoint and DNA repair resulting in partial polyploidy. *J. Biol. Chem.* **2010**, *285*, 30282–30293.
33. Golsteyn, R.M.; Schultz, S.J.; Bartek, J.; Ziemiecki, A.; Ried, T.; Nigg, E.A. Cell cycle analysis and chromosomal localization of human Plk1, a putative homologue of the mitotic kinases *Drosophila polo* and *Saccharomyces cerevisiae* Cdc5. *J. Cell. Sci.* **1994**, *107*, 1509–1517.
34. Mamely, I.; van Vugt, M.A.; Smits, V.A.; Semple, J.I.; Lemmens, B.; Perrakis, A.; Medema, R.H.; Freire, R. Polo-like kinase-1 controls proteasome-dependent degradation of Claspin during checkpoint recovery. *Curr. Biol.* **2006**, *16*, 1950–1955.

35. Kumagai, A.; Dunphy, W.G. Purification and molecular cloning of Plx1, a Cdc25-regulatory kinase from *Xenopus* egg extracts. *Science* **1996**, *273*, 1377–80.
36. Pelegrino, R.; Calvisi, D.F.; Ladu, S.; Ehemann, V.; Staniscia, T.; Evert, M.; Dombrowski, F.; Schirmacher, P.; Longerich, T. Oncogenic and tumor suppressive roles of Polo-like kinases in human hepatocellular carcinoma. *Hepatology* **2010**, *51*, 857–868.
37. Petrelli, A.; Perra, A.; Schernhuber, K.; Cargnelutti, M.; Salvi, A.; Migliore, C.; Ghiso, E.; Benetti, A.; Barlati, S.; Ledda-Columbano, G.M.; *et al.* Sequential analysis of multistage hepatocarcinogenesis reveals that miR-100 and PLK1 dysregulation is an early event maintained along tumor progression. *Oncogene* **2012**, *31*, 4517–4526.
38. Chen, X.; Cheung, S.T.; So, S.; Fan, S.T.; Barry, C.; Higgins, J.; Lai, K.M.; Ji, J.; Dudoit, S.; Ng, I.O.; *et al.* Gene expression patterns in human liver cancers. *Mol. Biol. Cell* **2002**, *13*, 1929–1939.
39. Bruinsma, W.; Raaijmakers, J.A.; Medema, R.H. Switching Polo-like kinase-1 on and off in time and space. *Trends Biochem. Sci.* **2012**, *37*, 534–542.
40. Wang, W.H.; Studach, L.L.; Andrisani, O.M. Proteins ZNF198 and SUZ12 are down-regulated in hepatitis B virus (HBV) X protein-mediated hepatocyte transformation and in HBV replication. *Hepatology* **2011**, *53*, 1137–1147.
41. Xiao, S.; Nalabolu, S.; Aster, J.C.; Ma, J.; Abruzzo, L.; Jaffe, E.S.; Stone, R.; Weissman, S.M.; Hudson, T.J.; Fletcher, J.A. FGFR1 is fused with novel zinc-finger gene, ZNF198, in the t(8;13) leukaemia/lymphoma syndrome. *Nat. Genet.* **1998**, *18*, 84–87.
42. Li, H.; Ma, X.; Wang, J.; Koontz, J.; Nucci, M.; Sklar, J. Effects of rearrangement and allelic exclusion of JJAZ1/SUZ12 on cell proliferation and survival. *Proc. Natl. Acad. Sci. USA* **2007**, *104*, 20001–20006.
43. Moinzadeh, P.; Breuhahn, K.; Stützer, H.; Schirmacher, P. Chromosome alterations in human hepatocellular carcinomas correlate with aetiology and histological grade-results of an explorative CGH meta-analysis. *Br. J. Cancer* **2005**, *92*, 935–941.
44. Chen, C.F.; Yeh, S.H.; Chen, D.S.; Chen, P.J.; Jou, Y.S. Molecular genetic evidence supporting a novel human hepatocellular carcinoma tumor suppressor locus at 13q12.11. *Genes Chromosom. Cancer* **2005**, *44*, 320–328.
45. Villa, R.; Pasini, D.; Gutierrez, A.; Morey, L.; Occhionorelli, M.; Viré, E.; Nomdedeu, J.F.; Jenuwein, T.; Pelicci, P.J.; Minucci, S.; *et al.* Role of the polycomb repressive complex 2 in acute promyelocytic leukemia. *Cancer Cell* **2007**, *11*, 513–525.
46. Kunapuli, P.; Kasyapa, C.S.; Chin, S.F.; Caldas, C.; Cowell, J.K. ZNF198, a zinc finger protein rearranged in myeloproliferative disease, localizes to the PML nuclear bodies and interacts with SUMO-1 and PML. *Exp. Cell Res.* **2006**, *312*, 3739–3751.
47. Bernardi, R.; Pandolfi, P.P. Structure, dynamics and functions of promyelocytic leukaemia nuclear bodies. *Nat. Rev. Mol. Cell Biol.* **2007**, *8*, 1006–1016.
48. Torok, D.; Ching, R.W.; Bazett-Jones, D.P. PML nuclear bodies as sites of epigenetic regulation. *Front. Biosci.* **2009**, *14*, 1325–1336.

49. Cho, S.; Park, J.S.; Kang, Y.K. Dual functions of histone-lysine N-methyltransferase Setdb1 protein at promyelocytic leukemia-nuclear body (PML-NB): Maintaining PML-NB structure and regulating the expression of its associated genes. *J. Biol. Chem.* **2011**, *286*, 41115–41124.

50. Bernardi, R.; Papa, A.; Pandolfi, P.P. Regulation of apoptosis by PML and the PML-NBs. *Oncogene* **2008**, *27*, 6299–6312.

51. Dellaire, G.; Ching, R.W.; Ahmed, K.; Jalali, F.; Tse, K.C.; Bristow, R.G.; Bazett-Jones, D.P. Promyelocytic leukemia nuclear bodies behave as DNA damage sensors whose response to DNA double-strand breaks is regulated by NBS1 and the kinases ATM, Chk2, and ATR. *J. Cell. Biol.* **2006**, *175*, 55–66.

52. Everett, R.D.; Chelbi-Alix, M.K. PML and PML nuclear bodies: Implications in antiviral defence. *Biochimie* **2007**, *89*, 819–830.

53. Frappier, L. Viral disruption of promyelocytic leukemia (PML) nuclear bodies by hijacking host PML regulators. *Virulence* **2001**, *2*, 58–62.

54. Reineke, E.L.; Kao, H.Y. Targeting promyelocytic leukemia protein: A means to regulating PML nuclear bodies. *Int. J. Biol. Sci.* **2009**, *5*, 366–376.

55. Gu, H.; Roizman, B. The two functions of herpes simplex virus 1 ICP0, inhibition of silencing by the CoREST/REST/HDAC complex and degradation of PML are executed in tandem. *J. Virol.* **2009**, *83*, 181–187.

56. Gu, H.; Roizman, B. Engagement of the lysine-specific demethylase/HDAC1/CoREST/REST complex by herpes simplex virus 1. *J. Virol.* **2009**, *83*, 4376–4385.

57. Chung, Y.L.; Tsai, T.Y. Promyelocytic leukemia nuclear bodies link the DNA damage repair pathway to hepatitis B virus replication: Implications for hepatitis B virus exacerbation during chemotherapy and radiotherapy. *Mol. Cancer Res.* **2009**, *7*, 1672–1685.

58. Gocke, C.B.; Yu, H. ZNF198 stabilizes the LSD-1-CoREST-HDAC1 complex on chromatin through its MYM-type zinc fingers. *PLoS One* **2008**, *3*, e3255.

59. Cao, R.; Zhang, Y. SUZ12 is required for both the histone methyltransferase activity and the silencing function of the EED-EZH2 complex. *Mol. Cell* **2004**, *15*, 57–67.

60. Squazzo, S.L.; O'Geen, H.; Komashko, V.M.; Krig, S.R.; Jin, V.X.; Jang, S.W.; Margueron, R.; Reinberg, D.; Green, R.; Farnham, P.J. Suz12 binds to silenced regions of the genome in a cell-type-specific manner. *Genome Res.* **2006**, *16*, 890–900.

61. Simon, J.A.; Kingston, R.E. Mechanisms of polycomb gene silencing: Knowns and unknowns. *Nat. Rev. Mol. Cell Biol.* **2009**, *10*, 697–708.

62. Bracken, A.P.; Dietrich, N.; Pasini, D.; Hansen, K.H.; Helin, K. Genome-wide mapping of Polycomb target genes unravels their roles in cell fate transitions. G*enes Dev.* 2006, *20*, 1123–1136.

63. Lee, T.I.; Jenner, R.G.; Boyer, L.A.; Guenther, M.G.; Levine, S.S.; Kumar, R.M.; Chevalier, B.; Johnstone, S.E.; Cole, M.F.; Isono, K.; *et al.* Control of developmental regulators by Polycomb in human embryonic stem cells. *Cell* **2006**, *125*, 301–313.

64. Morey, L.; Helin, K. Polycomb group protein-mediated repression of transcription. *Trends Biochem. Sci.* **2010**, *35*, 323–332.

65. Margueron, R.; Reinberg, D. The Polycomb complex PRC2 and its mark in life. *Nature* **2011**, *469*, 343–349.

66. Pasini, D.; Bracken, A.P.; Hansen, J.B.; Capillo, M.; Helin, K. The Polycomb group protein Suz12 is required for embryonic stem cell differentiation. *Mol. Cell Biol.* **2007**, *27*, 3769–3779.

67. Surface, L.E.; Thornton, S.R.; Boyer, L.A. Polycomb group proteins set the stage for early lineage commitment. *Cell Stem. Cell* **2010**, *7*, 288–298.

68. Aldiri, I.; Vetter, M.L. PRC2 during vertebrate organogenesis: A complex in transition. *Dev. Biol.* **2012**, *367*, 91–99.

69. Studach, L.L.; Menne, S.; Cairo, S.; Buendia, M.A.; Hullinger, R.L.; Lefrançois, L.; Merle, P.; Andrisani, O.M. A subset of Suz12/PRC2 target genes is activated during hepatitis B virus replication and liver carcinogenesis associated with hepatitis B virus X protein. *Hepatology* **2012**, *56*, 1240–1251.

70. Andrisani, O.M.; Studach, L.; Merle, P. Gene signatures in hepatocellular carcinoma (HCC). *Semin. Cancer Biol.* **2001**, *21*, 4–9.

71. Yamashita, T.; Ji, J.; Budhu, A.; Forgues, M.; Yang, W.; Wang, H.Y.; Jia, H.; Ye, Q.; Qin, L.X.; Wauthier, E.; *et al.* EpCAM-positive hepatocellular carcinoma cells are tumor initiating cells with stem/progenitor cell features. *Gastroenterology* **2009**, *136*, 1012–1024.

72. Khalil, A.M.; Guttman, M.; Huarte, M.; Garber, M.; Raj, A.; Rivea Morales, D.; Thomas, K.; Presser, A.; Bernstein, B.E.; van Oudenaarden, A.; *et al.* Many human large intergenic non-coding RNAs associate with chromatin-modifying complexes and affect gene expression. *Proc. Natl. Acad. Sci. USA* **2009**, *106*, 11667–116672.

73. Zhao, J.; Ohsumi, T.K.; Kung, J.T.; Ogawa, Y.; Grau, D.J.; Sarma, K.; Song, J.J.; Kingston, R.E.; Borowsky, M.; Lee J.T. Genome-wide identification of polycomb-associated RNAs by RIP-seq. *Mol. Cell* **2010**, *40*, 939–953.

74. Toffanin, S.; Hishida, Y.; Lachenmayer, A.; Villanueva, A.; Cabellos, L.; Minguez, B.; Savic, R.; Ward, S.C.; Thung, S.; Chiang, D.Y.; *et al.* MicroRNA-based classification of hepatocellular carcinoma and oncogenic role of miR-517a. *Gastroenterology* **2011**, *140*, 1618–1628.

75. Iliopoulos, D.; Lindahl-Allen, M.; Polytarchou, C.; Hirsch, H.A.; Tsichlis, P.N.; Struhl, K. Loss of miR-200 inhibition of Suz12 leads to polycomb-mediated repression required for the formation and maintenance of cancer stem cells. *Mol. Cell* **2010**, *39*, 761–772.

76. Svotelis, A.; Bianco, S.; Matore, J.; Huppé, G.; Nordell-Markovits, A.; Mes-Masson, A.M.; Gévry, N. H3K27 demethylation by JMJD3 at a poised enhancer of anti-apoptotic gene BCL2 determines ERα ligand dependency. *EMBO J.* **2011**, *30*, 3947–3961.

77. Pasini, D.; Cloos, P.A.; Walfridsson, J.; Olsson, L.; Bukowski, J.P.; Johansen, J.V.; Bak, M.; Tommerup, N.; Rappsilber, J.; Helin, K. JARID2 regulates binding of the Polycomb repressive complex 2 to target genes in ES cells. *Nature* **2010**, *464*, 306–310.

78. Anderton, J.A.; Bose, S.; Vockerodt, M.; Vrzalikova, K.; Wei, W.; Kuo, M.; Helin, K.; Christensen, J.; Rowe, M.; Murray, P.G.; *et al.* The H3K27me3 demethylase, KDM6B, is induced by Epstein-Barr virus and over-expressed in Hodgkin's Lymphoma. *Oncogene* **2011**, *30*, 2037–2043.

79. Beausoleil, S.A.; Jedrychowski, M.; Schwartz, D.; Elias, J.E.; Villén, J.; Li, J.; Cohn, M.A.; Cantley, L.C.; Gygi, S.P. Large-scale characterization of HeLa cell nuclear phosphoproteins. *Proc. Natl. Acad. Sci. USA* **2004**, *101*, 12130–12135.

80. Tsai, M.C.; Manor, O.; Wan, Y.; Mosammaparast, N.; Wang, J.K.; Lan, F.; Shi, Y.; Segal, E.; Chang, H.Y. Long noncoding RNA as modular scaffold of histone modification complexes. *Science* **2010**, *329*, 689–693.

81. Bernstein, B.E.; Mekkelsen, T.S.; Zie, X.; Kamal, M.; Huebert, D.J.; Cuff, J.; Fry, B.; Meissner, A.; Wernig, M.; Plath, K.; *et al.* A bivalent chromatin structure marks key developmental genes in embryonic stem cells. *Cell* **2006**, *125*, 315–326.

82. Brown, D.D. The role of stable complexes that repress and activate eukaryotic genes. *Philos Trans. R. Soc. Lond. B Biol. Sci.* **1984**, *307*, 297–299.

83. Petruk, S.; Sedkov, Y.; Johnston, D.M.; Hodgson, J.W.; Black, K.L.; Kovermann, S.K.; Beck, S.; Canaani, E.; Brock, H.W.; Mazo, A. TrxG and PcG proteins but not methylated histones remain associated with DNA through replication. *Cell* **2012**, *150*, 922–933.

84. Deb-Rinker, P.; Ly, D.; Jezierski, A.; Sikorska, M.; Walker, P.R. Sequential DNA methylation of the Nanog and Oct-4 upstream regions in human NT2 cells during neuronal differentiation. *J. Biol. Chem.* **2005**, *280*, 6257–6260.

85. Meissner, A.; Mikkelsen, T.S.; Gu, H.; Wernig, M.; Hanna, J.; Sivachenko, A.; Zhang, X.; Bernstein, B.E.; Nusbaum, C.; Jaffe, D.B.; *et al.* Genome-scale DNA methylation maps of pluripotent and differentiated cells. *Nature* **2008**, *454*, 766–770.

86. Mohn, F.; Weber, M.; Rebhan, M.; Roloff, T.C.; Richter, J.; Stadler, M.B.; Bibel, M.; Schübeler, D. Lineage-specific polycomb targets and de novo DNA methylation define restriction and potential of neuronal progenitors. *Mol. Cell* **2008**, *30*, 755–766.

87. Hawkins, R.D.; Hon, G.C.; Lee, L.K.; Ngo, Q.; Lister, R.; Pelizzola, M.; Edsall, L.E.; Kuan, S.; Luu, Y.; Klugman, S.; *et al.* Distinct epigenomic landscapes of pluripotent and lineage-committed human cells. *Cell. Stem Cell.* **2010**, *6*, 479–491.

88. Brunner, A.L.; Johnson, D.S.; Kim, S.W.; Valouev, A.; Reddy, T.E.; Neff, N.F.; Anton, E.; Medina, C.; Nguyen, L.; Chiao, E.; *et al.* Distinct DNA methylation patterns characterize differentiated human embryonic stem cells and developing human fetal liver. *Genome Res.* **2009**, *19*, 1044–1056.

89. Park, I.Y.; Sohn, B.H.; Yu, E.; Suh, D.J.; Chung, Y.H.; Lee, J.H.; Surzycki, S.J.; Lee, Y.I. Aberrant epigenetic modifications in hepatocarcinogenesis induced by hepatitis B virus X protein. *Gastroenterology* **2007**, *132*, 1476–1494.

90. Zheng, D.L.; Zhang, L.; Cheng, N.; Xu, X.; Deng, Q.; Teng, X.M.; Wang, K.S.; Zhang, X.; Huang, J.; Han, Z.G. Epigenetic modification induced by hepatitis B virus X protein via interaction with *de novo* DNA methyltransferase DNMT3A. *J. Hepatol.* **2009**, *50*, 377–387.

91. Jung, K.J.; Arora, P.; Pagano, J.S.; Jang, K.L. Expression of DNA methyltransferase 1 is activated by hepatitis B virus X protein via a regulatory circuit involving the p16INK4a-cyclin D1-CDK 4/6-pRb-E2F1pathway. *Cancer Res.* **2007**, *67*, 5771–5778.

92. Chen, T.; Li, E. Structure and function of eukaryotic DNA methyltransferases. *Curr. Top. Dev. Biol.* **2004**, *60*, 55–89.
93. Vivekanandan, P.; Daniel, H.D.; Kannangai, R.; Martinez-Murillo, F.; Torbenson, M. Hepatitis B virus replication induces methylation of both host and viral DNA. *J. Virol.* **2010**, *84*, 4321–4329.
94. Vivekanandan, P.; Thomas, D.; Torbenson, M. Hepatitis B viral DNA is methylated in liver tissues. *J. Viral Hepat.* **2008**, *15*, 103–107.
95. Vivekanandan, P.; Thomas, D.; Torbenson, M. Methylation regulates hepatitis B viral protein expression. *J. Infect. Dis.* **2009**, *199*, 1286–1291.
96. Akalin, A.; Garrett-Bakelman, F.E.; Kormaksson, M.; Busuttil, J.; Zhang, L.; Khrebtukova, I.; Milne, T.A.; Huang, Y.; Biswas, D.; Hess, J.L.; *et al.* Base-pair resolution DNA methylation sequencing reveals profoundly divergent epigenetic landscapes in acute myeloid leukemia. *PLoS Genet.* **2012**, *8*, e1002781.
97. Quasdorff, M.; Hösel, M.; Odenthal, M.; Zedler, U.; Bohne, F.; Gripon, P.; Dienes, H.P.; Drebber, U.; Stippel, D.; Goeser, T.; *et al.* A concerted action of HNF4alpha and HNF1alpha links hepatitis B virus replication to hepatocyte differentiation. *Cell Microbiol.* **2008**, *10*, 1478–1490.
98. Polo, J.M.; Anderssen, E.; Walsh, R.M.; Schwarz, B.A.; Nefzger, C.M.; Lim, S.M.; Borkent, M.; Apostolou, E.; Alaei, S.; Cloutier, J.; *et al.* A molecular roadmap of reprogramming somatic cells into iPS cells. *Cell* **2012**, *151*, 1617–1632.

10

The Role of Chromatin in Adenoviral Vector Function

Carmen M. Wong [1,2], Emily R. McFall [1,2], Joseph K. Burns [1,2] and Robin J. Parks [1,2,3,*]

[1] Regenerative Medicine Program, Ottawa Hospital Research Institute, Ottawa, Ontario, K1H 8L6, Canada; E-Mails: cawong@ohri.ca (C.M.W.); emcfall@ohri.ca (E.R.M.); josburns@ohri.ca (J.K.B.)

[2] Department of Biochemistry, Microbiology and Immunology, University of Ottawa, Ottawa, Ontario K1H 8M5, Canada

[3] Department of Medicine, University of Ottawa, Ottawa, Ontario K1H 8M5, Canada

* Author to whom correspondence should be addressed; E-Mail: rparks@ohri.ca;

Abstract: Vectors based on adenovirus (Ad) are one of the most commonly utilized platforms for gene delivery to cells in molecular biology studies and in gene therapy applications. Ad is also the most popular vector system in human clinical gene therapy trials, largely due to its advantageous characteristics such as high cloning capacity (up to 36 kb), ability to infect a wide variety of cell types and tissues, and relative safety due to it remaining episomal in transduced cells. The latest generation of Ad vectors, helper-dependent Ad (hdAd), which are devoid of all viral protein coding sequences, can mediate high-level expression of a transgene for years in a variety of species ranging from rodents to non-human primates. Given the importance of histones and chromatin in modulating gene expression within the host cell, it is not surprising that Ad, a nuclear virus, also utilizes these proteins to protect the genome and modulate virus- or vector-encoded genes. In this review, we will discuss our current understanding of the contribution of chromatin to Ad vector function.

Keywords: adenovirus; chromatin; histones; DNA replication; transcription

---

1. Introduction

The biology of human adenovirus (Ad) has been studied in great detail for over 60 years, making Ad one of the best characterized human DNA viruses. These studies, while giving us a great deal of information about DNA replication, control of gene expression, and tumorigenesis, also laid the foundations for the later development of Ads as gene transfer vectors. The first suggestion that Ad could be used as a vector system for expression of foreign genes came in the late 1970s with the identification of spontaneous recombinants between Ad and SV40 which expressed T antigen fused to an Ad structural protein [1,2]. Use of this vector allowed for the purification of large quantities of a T antigen-related protein that retained biological activity and set the stage for further development of Ad as a gene delivery vehicle. A crucial development occurred when cell lines that could complement viruses deleted of the essential early region 1 (E1) were created [3]. This cell line allowed for the development of Ad-based vectors that could not replicate in most cell lines or tissues, but could provide high level expression of an exogenous transgene. Ad vectors now come in a variety of "generations" that differ in their degree of attenuation, from loss of one gene to deletion of all viral protein coding sequences. These vectors can serve a variety of functions ranging from short-term, high-level expression of a transgene in tissue culture to long-term therapeutic gene expression in animal models of human disease.

One common feature of all Ad vectors is that they remain episomal in the transduced cell and, in some animal models, the vector can persist and express a transgene for several years. This finding suggests that the vector may be able to "hide" in the nucleus through adopting a structure similar to the genomic DNA. Thus, the chromatinized viral DNA is likely impacted and influenced by all of the same factors as the native cellular DNA, such as epigenetic regulation. Indeed, recent studies have shown this to be the case, as Ad-based vector DNA associates with histones and is wrapped in nucleosomes within the host cell nucleus. This chromatinized structure strongly influences the level and duration of expression from a vector-encoded transgene. This review will discuss our current understanding of Ad vector chromatinization. For a more detailed review of the dynamic changes in nucleoprotein structure during wildtype Ad (AdWT) infection, please see [4].

2. Ad Vector Design

Although there are many different generations of Ad vectors which differ in the extent to which the genome is attenuated (reviewed by [5]), the vast majority of studies involving Ad vectors use the simple E1-deleted, first-generation Ad vector (Figure 1). Most first-generation vectors are also deleted of the E3 region, which is not required for virus replication in culture, and its removal increases the cloning capacity for foreign DNA to ~8 kb [6]. Since E1 is absolutely required for virus replication, these vectors do not replicate to any appreciable degree in most cell lines, but can be easily propagated in E1-complementing cell lines such as 293 cells [3]. However, it is important to note that the E1-deleted Ad vectors can undergo limited replication in a number of tissue culture cell lines if they are delivered at a high multiplicity of infection (MOI) [7]. Moreover, first generation Ad delivery to animals and humans is typically accompanied by the induction of very strong innate and adaptive immune responses [8,9]. These immunogenic responses are at least in part due to leaky expression of viral genes retained in the E1-deleted vectors [10], which ultimately limits the duration of transgene expression to a few days or weeks. First generation Ad vectors are usually ideal for short-term expression in tissue culture or animals, but not ideal for applications requiring long-term (months to years) expression. Second generation Ad vectors have further deletions in the E2 or E4 coding sequences. E2 encodes proteins involved in Ad DNA replication [11], so its removal will prevent replication and reduce the expression of late genes [12]. E4 encodes several proteins involved in a variety of functions that impact on both viral and cellular gene expression and signal transduction [11]; thus, removal of some or all of E4 should significantly attenuate the vector. Deletions of E2 and E4 have been shown in some studies to have beneficial effects in reducing the expression of viral proteins and vector-directed immune responses, thereby extending transgene expression [5]. However, second generation vectors are no longer in common use due to limited evidence of enhanced efficacy over first generation vectors.

Deletion of all viral protein coding sequences results in third-generation Ad vectors, also known as fully-deleted, gutted, or helper-dependent Ad (hdAd) vectors (Figure 1). This latter term arose from the fact that these vectors must be propagated in the presence of a second virus that provides all of the replication and packaging functions *in trans* for growth of the hdAd vector [13]. The hdAd vector needs only the *cis* activating elements required for virus DNA replication (the inverted terminal repeats [ITR], ~100 bp located at both ends) and the packaging sequence (~150 bp, located immediately adjacent to the left ITR). Selection against packaging of the helper virus genome is important to ensure efficient hdAd propagation. Selective packaging can be accomplished using loxP or FRT sites flanking the helper virus DNA packaging element and 293-based cell lines expressing the Cre or FLP recombinase, respectively [13–17]. Such helper viruses can replicate and produce all viral proteins necessary for replication and packaging of the hdAd, but cannot package their own genomes due to loss of the packaging element in the Cre- or FLP-expressing cells. These methods result in relatively pure stocks of hdAd. In numerous studies, we and others showed that hdAd have many desirable characteristics for gene therapy applications, including long term therapeutic gene expression (>2 years) in mice [18–20], rats [21], dogs [22] and baboons [23], and reduced toxicity relative to traditional Ad vectors [24,25]. For a more comprehensive review of hdAd vector function, please see [5,26–28].

Figure 1. Schematic of the adenovirus genome and adenovirus-based vectors. Top panel: A simplified map of the adenovirus (Ad) serotype 5 genome showing the early genes (E1–E4) and the region from which the major late transcript is produced (the L1-L5 transcripts produced from alternative splicing of the major late transcript are not shown). The relative position of pIX, VA RNA I and II and IVa2 are indicated. Also shown are the viral inverted terminal repeats (ITR) located at each end of the genome, the viral packaging element (Ψ) located adjacent to the left ITR, and the position of the major late promoter (MLP). Please note that these features are not drawn to scale. Middle panel: General structure of an early region 1 (E1)-deleted Ad vector. Most E1-deleted vectors are also deleted of the E3 region, which is not required for replication in tissue culture and increases the cloning capacity to approximately 8 kb of foreign DNA. The gene of interest (GOI) is usually introduced to replace the E1 region and is placed under control by a heterologous promoter (dark arrow). Bottom panel: General structure of a helper-dependent Ad vector. hdAd are devoid of all protein coding sequences, and need contain only the viral inverted terminal repeats and packaging element. hdAd also frequently contain non-coding stuffer DNA (shown in gray) to ensure optimal genome size.

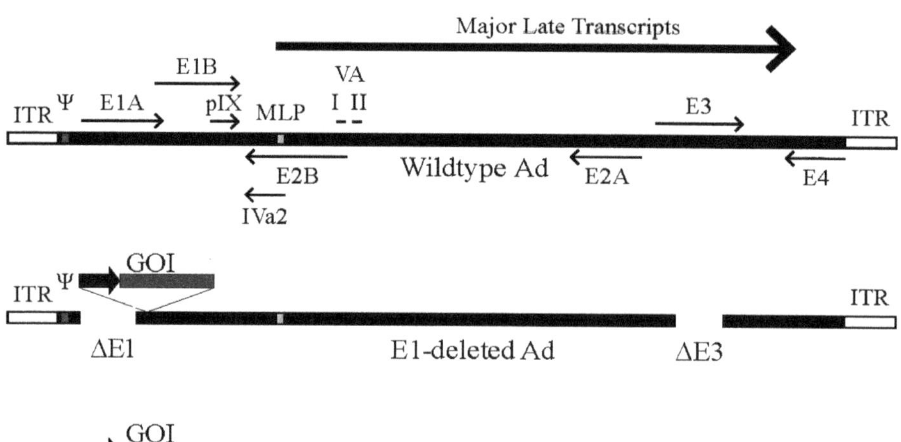

3. Ad Virion Structure

Although these Ad vectors lack some (or all) viral coding sequences, the overall virion structure appears identical to AdWT [29,30]. The Ad virion has an icosohedral, non-enveloped capsid structure (~70 to 100 nm in diameter) surrounding a nucleoprotein core containing a linear double-stranded genome that for wildtype Ads is ~30–40 kb. The Ad capsid is composed of 8 polypeptides, named in order of decreasing size [31–34]. Hexon (a trimer of protein II) assemble into a sheet-like structure called the "group-of-nine", which forms the 20 facets of the icosahedon. Protein III clusters into groups of five (known as pentons) at the vertices of the icosahedron, from which extend trimers of protein IV, known as fibre. These three polypeptides are the major capsid proteins. This general structure is supported by five minor capsid proteins (IIIa, IVa2, VI, VIII, and IX). Within the viral capsid, the viral DNA associates with three basic proteins, VII, V and Mu (μ), which function to neutralize the charge on the DNA, permitting tight packing of the DNA within the virion. Protein VII is similar to cellular protamines, and is the main protein responsible for wrapping and condensing the viral DNA [35]. A shell of protein V is postulated to coat the protein VII-DNA complex [36,37]. Pre-Mu is thought to aid in wrapping and condensing the viral DNA [38]. It is believed that cleavage of pre-Mu by the Ad-encoded protease may function to relax the viral DNA nucleoprotein structure before it enters the nucleus [39]. Since the tightly packed DNA structure is refractory to viral transcription [40,41], the nucleoprotein structure of the Ad DNA must be remodeled to achieve efficient gene expression.

Even though the viral DNA does not directly interact with the outer capsid proteins, it still contributes to the physical stability of the virion, as packaging of subgenomic sized DNA results in decreased Ad virion stability [30,42]. There seems to be a direct relationship: the smaller the genome, the less stable the virion. This observation has significant consequences for the design of Ad-based vectors. In the case of hdAd, which lacks all viral protein coding sequences, the viral genome must be replaced with alternative DNA simply to provide the necessary structural stability to support the mature capsid structure. For hdAd, reducing the genome size to less than ~27 kb causes the DNA to multimerize or rearrange to increase the genome size to between 27 and 36 kb [43]. Thus, if the transgene is large enough (e.g., a genomic loci), it may be sufficient to provide the needed support; however, a small transgene cassette may require the use of a non-coding "stuffer" element to bring the overall genome to an appropriate size. However, the nature of the stuffer DNA can significantly influence the function of the hdAd vector due to different epigenetic modifications, as discussed below [44,45].

4. Ad Infection of a Cell

The most commonly used Ad vectors are based on human Ad serotypes 2 or 5, and many of the details of the infection process have been worked out in great detail. Initially, the Ad fibre protein binds to the Coxsackie-Adenovirus receptor (CAR—a common receptor for Ad5 and Coxsackie B virus) [46,47]. Ad5 can also enter cells using heparin sulfate proteoglycans as an alternative receptor, either through direct binding to the Ad fibre shaft [48], or bridged through interaction of Ad with blood factors such as factor IX, factor X or complement component C4-binding protein [49–51]. Binding is followed by interaction between Ad penton and $\alpha_v\beta_3$ or $\alpha_v\beta_5$ integrins [52]. Ad is internalized by receptor-mediated endocytosis and escapes from the early endosome [53,54]. The virion is then transported through the cytoplasm to the nucleus along the microtubule network [53], and the capsid is slowly disassembled *en route* [55]. Upon reaching the nuclear pore, the Ad DNA complexed with protein VII is released into the nucleus [55–57], while the rest of the capsid proteins are ultimately degraded. For a more comprehensive discussion of viral entry, please see [58].

5. Ad Vector DNA Remains Primarily Episomal within the Infected Cell Nucleus

All vector systems have at least some ability to integrate into the genome of the host cell. Obviously, retrovirus- and lentivirus-based vectors integrate at very high frequencies in the target cell genome, making them ideal for studies involving rapidly dividing cell types (e.g., stem cells), but this does raise the risk of insertional activation or inactivation of cellular genes [59–61]. For Ad, the spontaneous integration rate is very low. In tissue culture studies, infection of several different cell lines with E1-deleted or hdAd vectors containing a selectable marker led to an integration frequency of 10^{-4} to 10^{-5} per cell (using an initial MOI of 10), and integration appeared to be due to non-homologous recombination [62,63]. A similar frequency was observed for hdAd in mouse hepatocytes *in vivo* [64], suggesting the vast majority of expression from hdAd in animals is due to expression from episomal vectors. Furthermore, in infected mouse hepatocytes *in vivo*, the vectors do not replicate with the cellular DNA and remain monomeric [65]. Traditional wisdom has held that in dividing tissues, non-integrated Ad DNA would be "lost" from the nucleus of transduced cells during cell division, as the virus has no known means of segregating with the host chromosomes. However, *in vivo* studies in which hdAd-transduced mouse hepatocytes were induced to divide through partial hepatectomy showed that Ad has a surprising ability to be retained in daughter cell nuclei after division, suggesting the virus may physically associate with chromosomes in the nucleus through an uncharacterized mechanism [66,67].

6. Early Events within the Infected Cell Nucleus

Much of what we know about the early stages of Ad DNA remodeling comes from studies of AdWT infection, though we assume that many of these events are similar for Ad vectors. Even though many Ad capsid proteins translocate to the periphery of the nucleus, only the VII-DNA complex enters the nucleus through the nuclear pore with the help of histone H1 (H1) [56,68]. This role of H1 appears independent of any known function in eventually condensing the viral DNA in the nucleus. Studies involving UV cross-linking of radiolabeled proteins to the AdWT DNA suggest that protein VII remains stably associated with the Ad DNA throughout the early phase of infection, from at least 2 until 13 hours post infection (hpi) [69]. Several immunofluoresence-based studies using antibody directed to protein VII have shown that protein VII-containing foci can be detected in the nucleus of both AdWT- and Ad vector-infected cells, which represent protein VII-wrapped genomes [70–73]. For AdWT, these foci remain visible for at least 8–10 hpi, but disappear around 12–16 hpi [71]. Treatment of cells with alpha-amanitin, an inhibitor of transcription, prevented loss of VII foci at late times (16 hpi), suggesting that late transcription could be involved in release of VII [70,71]. However, using a similar immunofluorescence-based approach, Karen and Hearing [72] showed that the number of protein VII foci in the nucleus steadily declined from 2 to 14 hpi. DNA replication was not required for loss of the protein VII foci, however blocking viral transcription either pharmacologically (alpha-amanitin) or through use of an E1A-deficient virus blocked the transition, once again suggesting that active viral transcription was required for release of VII from the Ad genome.

Similarly conflicting results regarding the duration and level of association of protein VII with the viral genome have been shown using ChIP-based studies. While some studies have shown that protein VII is stably associated with the Ad DNA during early stages of infection [70,74], other studies showed a gradual decrease in VII association with the viral DNA over time [75–77]. During this same time period, there was a gradual increase in the association with histone H3 (and the other core histones) over most promoter and coding regions, although the binding levels of the histones was less than cellular chromatin [74]. Similar results were observed by Haruki *et al.* [75] who demonstrated the uneven distribution of VII along the Ad genome, with relatively low occupancy at the E1A promoter and relatively high occupancy at the major late promoter (MLP) at 6 hpi. The MLP only becomes active after viral DNA replication has initiated (~8–12 hpi), suggesting protein VII association may be more prolonged for regions of the Ad genome that are activated late in the virus lifecycle. Since it is very likely that the histones were binding directly to the DNA, these observations suggest that at least a portion of protein VII must be removed or remodeled to make space for binding of the histones to the viral DNA. Indeed, protein VII and H3 could be found bound to the same DNA molecules in re-ChIP experiments [74]. Protein VII may actually play a role in regulating early viral transcription, as pre-wrapping plasmids in small quantities of purified protein VII led to higher levels of reporter gene expression compared to naked plasmid in transient transfection assays [74].

In vitro studies have shown that the protein VII-condensed DNA structure does not allow for efficient transcription [40,41], suggesting that the complex must be remodeled before efficient gene expression can occur. Again based on *in vitro* studies, three proteins have been identified that can remodel the VII-wrapped Ad genome: template activating factor Iβ (TAF-Iβ) (also known as SET [40]), TAF-II (NAP-1 [78]) and TAF-III (B23/nucleophosmin [79]). Of the three proteins, TAF-1β is the best characterized with respect to Ad DNA remodeling [70,75,80]. TAF-1β binds the VII-wrapped DNA complex, which "opens" the viral DNA to allow access to nucleases and, presumably, transcriptional activators [41]. Whether remodeling by TAF-1β involves simple translocation or actual disassociation of VII from the DNA has yet to be determined. The observation that TAF-1β knockdown in cells has only a minor effect on Ad early gene expression suggests that accessory proteins may also be required for efficient transcription from the Ad template or that redundant mechanisms exist for remodeling [74].

Whether active transcription of the Ad DNA is required to mediate VII disassociation is also a subject of debate. Although some studies showed that VII appeared to remain associated with the viral DNA for longer periods of time when transcription elongation was inhibited [71,72], other studies did not see a difference [74,76]. It has been suggested that protein VII can recruit E1A to the viral DNA, and that E1A-mediated activation of transcription may lead to removal of protein VII [71,81]. Consistent with this, infection with an E1A-deficient virus prevented loss of the protein VII foci [71]. Again based on immunofluorescence analysis, release of protein VII could be achieved in the absence of E1A or other viral proteins, if the vector contained a strong heterologous promoter, such as the CMV promoter which is not reliant on E1A for expression [71]. Since only part of the AdWT genome is actively transcribed during early times of infection, it may be that protein VII is released from transcribed regions, but remains associated with the "late" regions until these regions are subsequently transcribed. This suggestion may also be consistent with the immunofluorescence-based studies, as this technique cannot easily distinguish between full- and partial-occupancy of VII on the viral DNA.

7. Ad Vector DNA Associates with Cellular Histones in the Infected Cell Nucleus

Recent studies have established that Ad and its derivative vectors (E1-deleted, replication defective Ad or hdAd) associate with cellular histones early during infection [45,74,76,77]. Histones are detected on the Ad DNA within one hour of infection, and protein VII and histones can be found associated simultaneously with the same viral DNA fragment within the cell [74]. In general, deposition of cellular histones can occur through either a replication-coupled or replication-independent mechanism, and the specific histone variants and chaperones involved vary for each mechanism [82]. Histone H3.1, which is expressed strictly during S-phase, is deposited on newly synthesized cellular DNA in a replication-coupled mechanism by the Chromatin Assembly Factor I (CAF-1) complex [83]. Conversely, the replacement histone variant H3.3, which differs from H3.1 by only 5 amino acids and is expressed throughout the cell cycle, is deposited through a replication-independent mechanism [82]. The histone chaperone involved in the deposition of H3.3 varies depending on the region of the chromosome. Within actively transcribed genes, the chaperone HIRA mediates H3.3 deposition, whereas on telomeres and pericentric DNA repeats, the H3.3 chaperone DAXX assists in the deposition [84–86]. Recent studies have suggested that the rapid deposition of H3.3 mediated by HIRA may be an evolved mechanism to protect "naked" DNA from damage [87].

In ChIP-based studies, hdAd, E1-deleted Ad [76] and wtAd [77] DNA associates with H3.3 as early as four hours post-infection, which suggests a replication-independent mechanism is responsible for the assembly of chromatin on Ad DNA. Recent work by Komatsu *et al.* [77] showing that knocking down of CAF-1 does not affect histone deposition on the Ad genome supports this idea [77]. Knockdown of HIRA reduced association of the hdAd DNA with H3, and also reduced Ad-mediated transgene expression [76], suggesting that assembly into chromatin is required for optimal gene expression. Given that H3.3 is also deposited on incoming Herpes Simplex Virus-1 DNA [88], the cell may utilize a common mechanism for processing incoming DNA originating from nuclear viruses.

AdWT DNA associates with all core histones (H2A-H2B and H3-H4) as early as one hour post-infection [74,77]. Ad vector DNA is also found associated with all these nucleosomal proteins, and the DNA displays a classic nucleosomal laddering pattern upon micrococcal nuclease digestion [76], suggesting that the Ad DNA is wrapped into physiologically-spaced nucleosomes in the infected cell nucleus. Taken together, these studies suggest that assembly of Ad vector DNA into chromatin through deposition of histones and remodeling into nucleosomes are accomplished through a replication-independent mechanism, and this event is important in establishing optimal transgene expression.

8. Epigenetic Regulation of Ad Vectors

Assembly of hdAd DNA into chromatin is necessary for efficient expression of vector-encoded genes, and this event very likely contributes to their significant stability and efficacy *in vitro* and *in vivo* [27,65]. One of the advantages of hdAd is their large cloning capacity, which permits the use of large upstream regulator sequences, or even whole genomic loci, to permit tissue-specific gene expression [18,89,90]. Chromatin plays an important role in gene regulation [91,92], and proper placement of nucleosomes relative to the transcription start site of a gene is crucial for promoter fidelity [93,94]. The ability to incorporate large regulatory regions into hdAd coupled with its swift assembly into physiologically-spaced nucleosomes likely contributes to the maintenance of a faithful expression profile from these control elements when contained in hdAd.

As noted above, hdAd vector DNA must be designed to an optimal size in order to ensure physical stability of the capsid and genetic stability of the genome [30,42,43]. Thus, for small transgenes, additional non-coding "stuffer" DNA must be included in the vector in order to obtain an optimal size. However, the nature of this stuffer DNA can have a significant effect on function of the vector. A hdAd containing 22 kb of eukaryotic stuffer DNA expressed its transgene ~10-fold higher *in vitro* and *in vivo* compared to a vector with an identical expression cassette but containing stuffer DNA derived from prokaryotic DNA [44]. Neither of these vectors was subjected to CpG methylation and both vectors associated with histones to a similar degree. No evidence of heterochromatic methylation marks (*i.e.*, H3K9me2, H3K27me3) were observed, however hdAd-prok chromatin was markedly under-acetylated (a mark of transcriptionally inactive chromatin) [45]. This effect could be blocked through the use of a DNA insulator element or administration of trichostatin A (a histone deacetylase inhibitor), suggesting that a repressive chromatin structure assembled on the prokaryotic stuffer DNA and spread to the transgene. Cellular proteins Sp100 and DAXX were implicated in mediating this event [45], which is perhaps not surprising given that AdWT has evolved a specific mechanism to antagonize DAXX activity [95–97]. Indeed, a recent study has suggested that protein VI from the incoming virion may function to attenuate the action of DAXX, thus facilitating initiation of early gene expression [98].

A recent study has shown that virus-mediated activation of innate immune signaling can culminate in epigenetic down-regulation of expression from Ad vectors. Infection of MyD88$^{-/-}$ mouse embryonic fibroblasts with a hdAd vector resulted in a higher level of transgene expression and was associated with an increased ratio of acetylated-H3K9 to methylated-H3K9 (*i.e.*, a tendency towards "active" chromatin configuration), compared to hdAd-infected wildtype mouse embryonic fibroblasts [99]. This observation suggests that engagement of toll-like receptors (such as TLR9 [100]) by Ad vector infection, and subsequent activation of MyD88-mediated signaling cascades, can lead to epigenetic silencing of the vector DNA. Thus, this study uncovered an innate pathway designed to epigenetically regulate expression of genes located on invading DNA.

Ad-encoded proteins can also actively modulate the activity of certain cellular chromatin modifying complexes. For example, the early region 4 open reading frame 4 (E4orf4) protein was shown to bind

AcfI and modulate the activity of the ACF chromatin remodeling complex [101]. E4orf4 appears to recruit protein phosphatase 2A (PP2A) to the ACF complex (and thus to chromatin), where PP2A may dephosphorylate uncharacterized substrates and alter local chromatin structure. It is thought that this interaction may contribute to E4orf4-induced caspase-independent, non-classical apoptosis at late times of AdWT infection [101–103]. Since first-generation Ad vectors retain the E4 region, it is therefore possible that expression of E4orf4 may in part contribute to acute or chronic toxicity noted for E1-deleted vectors [5].

9. Conclusions and Future Perspectives

Ad vectors are one of the most commonly used systems to deliver genes to mammalian cells. In the nucleus, the viral DNA must conform to the rules of the host environment, and many studies have shown that histones and proper chromatin configuration are as important to Ad as it is to the host DNA. Histones deposited on the Ad DNA can adopt an "active" euchromatic state or an "inactive" heterochromatic state. In the case of more advanced generations of Ad vectors, such as the hdAd, designing the vector such that it resembles a segment of the chromosome (e.g., using genomic loci-based expression constructs or large, non-coding stuffer elements derived from the human genome) allows these vectors to retain high-level expression for many years in mice, rats, dogs and non-human primates. Improving our understanding of the mechanism of assembly of Ad DNA into chromatin, and the cellular proteins involved in modulating this nucleoprotein structure, will undoubtedly improve our ability to design the next generation of Ad vector exhibiting true tissue-specific transgene regulation, optimal safety, and expression. Similarly, uncovering aspects of Ad vector design that permit the vector to remain undetected in the host cell nucleus should improve the function and persistence of the vector DNA within the transduced cell. For AdWT, there are a few obvious areas that require further study, such as whether protein VII is truly maintained and/or required on certain regions of the Ad genome during the early phase of viral replication, and how its association is affected by active transcription. Since the wildtype virus must transition from association with protein VII to histones and back to protein VII for packaging of the DNA into progeny virions, the cellular protein(s) that facilitate these events have yet to be determined. Finally, studying how viruses and vectors have adapted to function with the context of a mammalian nucleus will undoubtedly provide novel insight into how chromatin structure impacts host cell DNA function.

Acknowledgements

We thank David J. Picketts (Ottawa Hospital Research Institute) for critical evaluation of the manuscript and helpful discussion. Research in the Parks laboratory is supported by grants from the Canadian Institutes of Health Research, National Sciences and Engineering Research Council, and the Cancer Research Society (Canada). ERM was supported by Ontario Graduate Scholarship and JKB was supported by Queen Elizabeth II Graduate Scholarships in Science and Technology from the Ontario Government.

References

1. Hassell, J.A.; Lukanidin, E.; Fey, G.; Sambrook, J. The structure and expression of two defective adenovirus 2/simian virus 40 hybrids. *J. Mol. Biol.* **1978**, *120*, 209–247.
2. Tjian, R. The binding site on SV40 DNA for a T antigen-related protein. *Cell* **1978**, *13*, 165–179.
3. Graham, F.L.; Smiley, J.; Russell, W.C.; Nairn, R. Characteristics of a human cell line transformed by DNA from human adenovirus type 5. *J. Gen. Virol.* **1977**, *36*, 59–74.
4. Giberson, A.N.; Davidson, A.R.; Parks, R.J. Chromatin structure of adenovirus DNA throughout infection. *Nucleic Acids Res.* **2012**, *40*, 2369–2376.
5. Amalfitano, A.; Parks, R.J. Separating fact from fiction: Assessing the potential of modified adenovirus vectors for use in human gene therapy. *Curr. Gene Ther.* **2002**, *2*, 111–133.
6. Bett, A.J.; Prevec, L.; Graham, F.L. Packaging capacity and stability of human adenovirus type 5 vectors. *J. Virol.* **1993**, *67*, 5911–5921.
7. Nelson, J.E.; Kay, M.A. Persistence of recombinant adenovirus *in vivo* is not dependent on vector DNA replication. *J. Virol.* **1997**, *71*, 8902–8907.
8. Ahi, Y.S.; Bangari, D.S.; Mittal, S.K. Adenoviral vector immunity: Its implications and circumvention strategies. *Curr. Gene Ther.* **2011**, *11*, 307–320.
9. Thaci, B.; Ulasov, I.V.; Wainwright, D.A.; Lesniak, M.S. The challenge for gene therapy: Innate immune response to adenoviruses. *Oncotarget* **2011**, *2*, 113–121.
10. Yang, Y.; Nunes, F.A.; Berencsi, K.; Furth, E.E.; Gonczol, E.; Wilson, J.M. Cellular immunity to viral antigens limits E1-deleted adenoviruses for gene therapy. *Proc. Natl. Acad. Sci. USA* **1994**, *91*, 4407–4411.
11. Berk, A.J. Adenoviridae: The viruses and their replication. In *Fields Virology*, 5th ed.; Knipe, D.M.; Howley, P.M., Eds.; Lippincott Williams & Wilkins: Philadelphia, PA, USA, 2007; pp. 2355–2394.
12. Thomas, G.P.; Mathews, M.B. DNA replication and the early to late transition in adenovirus infection. *Cell* **1980**, *22*, 523–533.
13. Parks, R.J.; Chen, L.; Anton, M.; Sankar, U.; Rudnicki, M.A.; Graham, F.L. A helper-dependent adenovirus vector system: Removal of helper virus by Cre-mediated excision of the viral packaging signal. *Proc. Natl. Acad. Sci. USA* **1996**, *93*, 13565–13570.
14. Hardy, S.; Kitamura, M.; Harris-Stansil, T.; Dai, Y.; Phipps, M.L. Construction of adenovirus vectors through Cre-lox recombination. *J. Virol.* **1997**, *71*, 1842–1849.
15. Umana, P.; Gerdes, C.A.; Stone, D.; Davis, J.R.; Ward, D.; Castro, M.G.; Lowenstein, P.R. Efficient FLPe recombinase enables scalable production of helper- dependent adenoviral vectors with negligible helper-virus contamination. *Nat. Biotechnol.* **2001**, *19*, 582–585.
16. Ng, P.; Beauchamp, C.; Evelegh, C.; Parks, R.; Graham, F.L. Development of a FLP/frt system for generating helper-dependent adenoviral vectors. *Mol. Ther.* **2001**, *3*, 809–815.
17. Palmer, D.; Ng, P. Improved system for helper-dependent adenoviral vector production. *Mol. Ther.* **2003**, *8*, 846–852.
18. Schiedner, G.; Morral, N.; Parks, R.J.; Wu, Y.; Koopmans, S.C.; Langston, C.; Graham, F.L.; Beaudet, A.L.; Kochanek, S. Genomic DNA transfer with a high-capacity adenovirus vector results in improved *in vivo* gene expression and decreased toxicity. *Nat. Genet.* **1998** *18*, 180–183.

19. Kim, I.H.; Jozkowicz, A.; Piedra, P.A.; Oka, K.; Chan, L. Lifetime correction of genetic deficiency in mice with a single injection of helper-dependent adenoviral vector. *Proc. Natl. Acad. Sci. USA* **2001**, *98*, 13282–13287.
20. Oka, K.; Pastore, L.; Kim, I.H.; Merched, A.; Nomura, S.; Lee, H.J.; Merched-Sauvage, M.; Arden-Riley, C.; Lee, B.; Finegold, M.; *et al.* Long-term stable correction of low-density lipoprotein receptor- deficient mice with a helper-dependent adenoviral vector expressing the very low-density lipoprotein receptor. *Circulation* **2001**, *103*, 1274–1281.
21. Toietta, G.; Mane, V.P.; Norona, W.S.; Finegold, M.J.; Ng, P.; McDonagh, A.F.; Beaudet, A.L.; Lee, B. Lifelong elimination of hyperbilirubinemia in the Gunn rat with a single injection of helper-dependent adenoviral vector. *Proc. Natl. Acad. Sci. USA* **2005**, *102*, 3930–3935.
22. Brunetti-Pierri, N.; Nichols, T.C.; McCorquodale, S.; Merricks, E.; Palmer, D.J.; Beaudet, A.L.; Ng, P. Sustained phenotypic correction of canine hemophilia B after systemic administration of helper-dependent adenoviral vector. *Hum. Gene Ther.* **2005**, *16*, 811–820.
23. Morral, N.; O'Neal, W.; Rice, K.; Leland, M.; Kaplan, J.; Piedra, P.A.; Zhou, H.; Parks, R.J.; Velji, R.; Aguilar-Cordova, E.; *et al.* Administration of helper-dependent adenoviral vectors and sequential delivery of different vector serotype for long-term liver-directed gene transfer in baboons. *Proc. Natl. Acad. Sci. USA* **1999**, *96*, 12816–12821.
24. Morral, N.; Parks, R.J.; Zhou, H.; Langston, C.; Schiedner, G.; Quinones, J.; Graham, F.L.; Kochanek, S.; Beaudet, A.L. High doses of a helper-dependent adenoviral vector yield supraphysiological levels of alpha1-antitrypsin with negligible toxicity. *Hum. Gene Ther.* **1998**, *9*, 2709–2716.
25. Muruve, D.A.; Cotter, M.J.; Zaiss, A.K.; White, L.R.; Liu, Q.; Chan, T.; Clark, S.A.; Ross, P.J.; Meulenbroek, R.A.; Maelandsmo, G.M.; *et al.* Helper-dependent adenovirus vectors elicit intact innate but attenuated adaptive host immune responses *in vivo*. *J. Virol.* **2004**, *78*, 5966–5972.
26. Parks, R.J. Improvements in adenoviral vector technology: Overcoming barriers for gene therapy. *Clin. Genet.* **2000**, *58*, 1–11.
27. Palmer, D.J.; Ng, P. Helper-dependent adenoviral vectors for gene therapy. *Hum. Gene Ther.* **2005**, *16*, 1–16.
28. Brunetti-Pierri, N.; Ng, P. Progress and prospects: Gene therapy for genetic diseases with helper-dependent adenoviral vectors. *Gene Ther.* **2008**, *15*, 553–560.
29. Parks, R.J.; Evelegh, C.M.; Graham, F.L. Use of helper-dependent adenoviral vectors of alternative serotypes permits repeat vector administration. *Gene Ther.* **1999**, *6*, 1565–1573.
30. Smith, A.C.; Poulin, K.L.; Parks, R.J. DNA genome size affects the stability of the adenovirus virion. *J. Virol.* **2009**, *83*, 2025–2028.
31. Christensen, J.B.; Byrd, S.A.; Walker, A.K.; Strahler, J.R.; Andrews, P.C.; Imperiale, M.J. Presence of the adenovirus IVa2 protein at a single vertex of the mature virion. *J. Virol.* **2008**, *82*, 9086–9093.
32. Liu, H.; Jin, L.; Koh, S.B.; Atanasov, I.; Schein, S.; Wu, L.; Zhou, Z.H. Atomic structure of human adenovirus by cryo-EM reveals interactions among protein networks. *Science* **2010**, *329*, 1038–1043.

33. Reddy, V.S.; Natchiar, S.K.; Stewart, P.L.; Nemerow, G.R. Crystal structure of human adenovirus at 3.5 A resolution. *Science* **2010**, *329*, 1071–1075.
34. Russell, W.C. Adenoviruses: Update on structure and function. *J. Gen. Virol.* **2009**, *90*, 1–20.
35. Mirza, M.A.; Weber, J. Structure of adenovirus chromatin. *Biochim. Biophys. Acta* **1982**, *696*, 76–86.
36. Everitt, E.; Sundquist, B.; Pettersson, U.; Philipson, L. Structural proteins of adenoviruses. X. Isolation and topography of low molecular weight antigens from the virion of adenovirus type 2. *Virology* **1973**, *52*, 130–147.
37. Brown, D.T.; Westphal, M.; Burlingham, B.T.; Winterhoff, U.; Doerfler, W. Structure and composition of the adenovirus type 2 core. *J. Virol.* **1975**, *16*, 366–387.
38. Anderson, C.W.; Young, M.E.; Flint, S.J. Characterization of the adenovirus 2 virion protein, mu. *Virology* **1989**, *172*, 506–512.
39. Perez-Berna, A.J.; Marabini, R.; Scheres, S.H.; Menendez-Conejero, R.; Dmitriev, I.P.; Curiel, D.T.; Mangel, W.F.; Flint, S.J.; San Martin, C. Structure and uncoating of immature adenovirus. *J. Mol. Biol.* **2009**, *392*, 547–557.
40. Matsumoto, K.; Nagata, K.; Ui, M.; Hanaoka, F. Template activating factor I, a novel host factor required to stimulate the adenovirus core DNA replication. *J. Biol. Chem.* **1993**, *268*, 10582–10587.
41. Okuwaki, M.; Nagata, K. Template activating factor-I remodels the chromatin structure and stimulates transcription from the chromatin template. *J. Biol. Chem.* **1998**, *273*, 34511–34518.
42. Kennedy, M.A.; Parks, R.J. Adenovirus virion stability and the viral genome: Size matters. *Mol. Ther.* **2009**, *17*, 1664–1666.
43. Parks, R.J.; Graham, F.L. A helper-dependent system for adenovirus vector production helps define a lower limit for efficient DNA packaging. *J. Virol.* **1997**, *71*, 3293–3298.
44. Parks, R.J.; Bramson, J.L.; Wan, Y.; Addison, C.L.; Graham, F.L. Effects of stuffer DNA on transgene expression from helper-dependent adenovirus vectors. *J. Virol.* **1999**, *73*, 8027–8034.
45. Ross, P.J.; Kennedy, M.A.; Parks, R.J. Host cell detection of noncoding stuffer DNA contained in helper-dependent adenovirus vectors leads to epigenetic repression of transgene expression. *J. Virol.* **2009**, *83*, 8409–8417.
46. Bergelson, J.M.; Cunningham, J.A.; Droguett, G.; Kurt-Jones, E.A.; Krithivas, A.; Hong, J.S.; Horwitz, M.S.; Crowell, R.L.; Finberg, R.W. Isolation of a common receptor for Coxsackie B viruses and adenoviruses 2 and 5. *Science* **1997**, *275*, 1320–1323.
47. Tomko, R.P.; Xu, R.; Philipson, L. HCAR and MCAR: The human and mouse cellular receptors for subgroup C adenoviruses and group B coxsackieviruses. *Proc. Natl. Acad. Sci. USA* **1997**, *94*, 3352–3356.
48. Smith, T.A.; Idamakanti, N.; Rollence, M.L.; Marshall-Neff, J.; Kim, J.; Mulgrew, K.; Nemerow, G.R.; Kaleko, M.; Stevenson, S.C. Adenovirus serotype 5 fiber shaft influences *in vivo* gene transfer in mice. *Hum. Gene Ther.* **2003**, *14*, 777–787.
49. Shayakhmetov, D.M.; Gaggar, A.; Ni, S.; Li, Z.Y.; Lieber, A. Adenovirus binding to blood factors results in liver cell infection and hepatotoxicity. *J. Virol.* **2005**, *79*, 7478–7491.

50. Waddington, S.N.; McVey, J.H.; Bhella, D.; Parker, A.L.; Barker, K.; Atoda, H.; Pink, R.; Buckley, S.M.K.; Greig, J.A.; Denby, L.; *et al.* Adenovirus serotype 5 hexon mediates liver gene transfer. *Cell* **2008**, *132*, 397–409.
51. Kalyuzhniy, O.; Di Paolo, N.C.; Silvestry, M.; Hofherr, S.E.; Barry, M.A.; Stewart, P.L.; Shayakhmetov, D.M. Adenovirus serotype 5 hexon is critical for virus infection of hepatocytes *in vivo*. *Proc. Natl. Acad. Sci. USA* **2008**, *105*, 5483–5488.
52. Wickham, T.J.; Mathias, P.; Cheresh, D.A.; Nemerow, G.R. Integrins alpha v beta 3 and alpha v beta 5 promote adenovirus internalization but not virus attachment. *Cell* **1993**, *73*, 309–319.
53. Leopold, P.L.; Ferris, B.; Grinberg, I.; Worgall, S.; Hackett, N.R.; Crystal, R.G. Fluorescent virions: Dynamic tracking of the pathway of adenoviral gene transfer vectors in living cells. *Hum. Gene Ther.* **1998**, *9*, 367–378.
54. Wiethoff, C.M.; Wodrich, H.; Gerace, L.; Nemerow, G.R. Adenovirus protein VI mediates membrane disruption following capsid disassembly. *J. Virol.* **2005**, *79*, 1992–2000.
55. Greber, U.F.; Willetts, M.; Webster, P.; Helenius, A. Stepwise dismantling of adenovirus 2 during entry into cells. *Cell* **1993**, *75*, 477–486.
56. Chatterjee, P.K.; Vayda, M.E.; Flint, S.J. Identification of proteins and protein domains that contact DNA within adenovirus nucleoprotein cores by ultraviolet light crosslinking of oligonucleotides 32P-labelled *in vivo*. *J. Mol. Biol.* **1986**, *188*, 23–37.
57. Strunze, S.; Engelke, M.F.; Wang, I.H.; Puntener, D.; Boucke, K.; Schleich, S.; Way, M.; Schoenenberger, P.; Burckhardt, C.J.; Greber, U.F. Kinesin-1-mediated capsid disassembly and disruption of the nuclear pore complex promote virus infection. *Cell Host Microbe* **2011**, *10*, 210–223.
58. Greber, U.F.; Puntener, D. DNA-tumor virus entry—From plasma membrane to the nucleus. *Semin. Cell Dev. Biol.* **2009**, *20*, 631–642.
59. Gabriel, R.; Schmidt, M.; von Kalle, C. Integration of retroviral vectors. *Curr. Opin. Immunol.* **2012**, *24*, 592–597.
60. Hacein-Bey-Abina, S.; von Kalle, C.; Schmidt, M.; Le Deist, F.; Wulffraat, N.; McIntyre, E.; Radford, I.; Villeval, J.L.; Fraser, C.C.; Cavazzana-Calvo, M.; *et al.* A serious adverse event after successful gene therapy for X-linked severe combined immunodeficiency. *N. Engl. J. Med.* **2003**, *348*, 255–256.
61. Hacein-Bey-Abina, S.; Von Kalle, C.; Schmidt, M.; McCormack, M.P.; Wulffraat, N.; Leboulch, P.; Lim, A.; Osborne, C.S.; Pawliuk, R.; Morillon, E.; *et al.* LMO2-associated clonal T cell proliferation in two patients after gene therapy for SCID-X1. *Science* **2003**, *302*, 415–419.
62. Harui, A.; Suzuki, S.; Kochanek, S.; Mitani, K. Frequency and stability of chromosomal integration of adenovirus vectors. *J. Virol.* **1999**, *73*, 6141–6146.
63. Hillgenberg, M.; Tonnies, H.; Strauss, M. Chromosomal integration pattern of a helper-dependent minimal adenovirus vector with a selectable marker inserted into a 27.4-kilobase genomic stuffer. *J. Virol.* **2001**, *75*, 9896–9908.
64. Stephen, S.L.; Montini, E.; Sivanandam, V.G.; Al-Dhalimy, M.; Kestler, H.A.; Finegold, M.; Grompe, M.; Kochanek, S. Chromosomal integration of adenoviral vector DNA *in vivo*. *J. Virol.* **2010**, *84*, 9987–9994.

65. Jager, L.; Ehrhardt, A. Persistence of high-capacity adenoviral vectors as replication-defective monomeric genomes *in vitro* and in murine liver. *Hum. Gene Ther.* **2009**, *20*, 883–896.
66. Ehrhardt, A.; Xu, H.; Kay, M.A. Episomal persistence of recombinant adenoviral vector genomes during the cell cycle *in vivo*. *J. Virol.* **2003**, *77*, 7689–7695.
67. Rauschhuber, C.; Noske, N.; Ehrhardt, A. New insights into stability of recombinant adenovirus vector genomes in mammalian cells. *Eur. J. Cell Biol.* **2012**, *91*, 2–9.
68. Trotman, L.C.; Mosberger, N.; Fornerod, M.; Stidwill, R.P.; Greber, U.F. Import of adenovirus DNA involves the nuclear pore complex receptor CAN/Nup214 and histone H1. *Nat. Cell Biol.* **2001**, *3*, 1092–1100.
69. Chatterjee, P.K.; Vayda, M.E.; Flint, S.J. Adenoviral protein VII packages intracellular viral DNA throughout the early phase of infection. *EMBO J.* **1986**, *5*, 1633–1644.
70. Xue, Y.; Johnson, J.S.; Ornelles, D.A.; Lieberman, J.; Engel, D.A. Adenovirus protein VII functions throughout early phase and interacts with cellular proteins SET and pp32. *J. Virol.* **2005**, *79*, 2474–2483.
71. Chen, J.; Morral, N.; Engel, D.A. Transcription releases protein VII from adenovirus chromatin. *Virology* **2007**, *369*, 411–422.
72. Karen, K.A.; Hearing, P. Adenovirus core protein VII protects the viral genome from a DNA damage response at early times after infection. *J. Virol.* **2011**, *85*, 4135–4142.
73. Walkiewicz, M.P.; Morral, N.; Engel, D.A. Accurate single-day titration of adenovirus vectors based on equivalence of protein VII nuclear dots and infectious particles. *J. Virol. Methods* **2009**, *159*, 251–258.
74. Komatsu, T.; Haruki, H.; Nagata, K. Cellular and viral chromatin proteins are positive factors in the regulation of adenovirus gene expression. *Nucleic Acids Res.* **2011**, *39*, 889–901.
75. Haruki, H.; Gyurcsik, B.; Okuwaki, M.; Nagata, K. Ternary complex formation between DNA-adenovirus core protein VII and TAF-Ibeta/SET, an acidic molecular chaperone. *FEBS Lett.* **2003**, *555*, 521–527.
76. Ross, P.J.; Kennedy, M.A.; Christou, C.; Risco Quiroz, M.; Poulin, K.L.; Parks, R.J. Assembly of helper-dependent adenovirus DNA into chromatin promotes efficient gene expression. *J. Virol.* **2011**, *85*, 3950–3958.
77. Komatsu, T.; Nagata, K. Replication-uncoupled histone deposition during adenovirus DNA replication. *J. Virol.* **2012**, *86*, 6701–6711.
78. Kawase, H.; Okuwaki, M.; Miyaji, M.; Ohba, R.; Handa, H.; Ishimi, Y.; Fujii-Nakata, T.; Kikuchi, A.; Nagata, K. NAP-I is a functional homologue of TAF-I that is required for replication and transcription of the adenovirus genome in a chromatin-like structure. *Gene. Cell.* **1996**, *1*, 1045–1056.
79. Okuwaki, M.; Iwamatsu, A.; Tsujimoto, M.; Nagata, K. Identification of nucleophosmin/B23, an acidic nucleolar protein, as a stimulatory factor for *in vitro* replication of adenovirus DNA complexed with viral basic core proteins. *J. Mol. Biol.* **2001**, *311*, 41–55.
80. Gyurcsik, B.; Haruki, H.; Takahashi, T.; Mihara, H.; Nagata, K. Binding modes of the precursor of adenovirus major core protein VII to DNA and template activating factor I: Implication for the mechanism of remodeling of the adenovirus chromatin. *Biochemistry* **2006**, *45*, 303–313.

81. Johnson, J.S.; Osheim, Y.N.; Xue, Y.; Emanuel, M.R.; Lewis, P.W.; Bankovich, A.; Beyer, A.L.; Engel, D.A. Adenovirus protein VII condenses DNA, represses transcription, and associates with transcriptional activator E1A. *J. Virol.* **2004**, *78*, 6459–6468.
82. Tagami, H.; Ray-Gallet, D.; Almouzni, G.; Nakatani, Y. Histone H3.1 and H3.3 complexes mediate nucleosome assembly pathways dependent or independent of DNA synthesis. *Cell* **2004**, *116*, 51–61.
83. Smith, S.; Stillman, B. Purification and characterization of CAF-I, a human cell factor required for chromatin assembly during DNA replication *in vitro*. *Cell* **1989**, *58*, 15–25.
84. Drane, P.; Ouararhni, K.; Depaux, A.; Shuaib, M.; Hamiche, A. The death-associated protein DAXX is a novel histone chaperone involved in the replication-independent deposition of H3.3. *Genes Dev.* **2010**, *24*, 1253–1265.
85. Lewis, P.W.; Elsaesser, S.J.; Noh, K.M.; Stadler, S.C.; Allis, C.D. Daxx is an H3.3-specific histone chaperone and cooperates with ATRX in replication-independent chromatin assembly at telomeres. *Proc. Natl. Acad. Sci. USA* **2010**, *107*, 14075–14080.
86. Goldberg, A.D.; Banaszynski, L.A.; Noh, K.M.; Lewis, P.W.; Elsaesser, S.J.; Stadler, S.; Dewell, S.; Law, M.; Guo, X.; Li, X.; *et al.* Distinct factors control histone variant H3.3 localization at specific genomic regions. *Cell* **2010**, *140*, 678–691.
87. Schneiderman, J.I.; Orsi, G.A.; Hughes, K.T.; Loppin, B.; Ahmad, K. Nucleosome-depleted chromatin gaps recruit assembly factors for the H3.3 histone variant. *Proc. Natl. Acad. Sci. USA* **2012**, *109*, 19721–19726.
88. Placek, B.J.; Huang, J.; Kent, J.R.; Dorsey, J.; Rice, L.; Fraser, N.W.; Berger, S.L. The histone variant H3.3 regulates gene expression during lytic infection with herpes simplex virus type 1. *J. Virol.* **2009**, *83*, 1416–1421.
89. Pastore, L.; Morral, N.; Zhou, H.; Garcia, R.; Parks, R.J.; Kochanek, S.; Graham, F.L.; Lee, B.; Beaudet, A.L. Use of a liver-specific promoter reduces immune response to the transgene in adenoviral vectors. *Hum. Gene Ther.* **1999**, *10*, 1773–1781.
90. Schiedner, G.; Hertel, S.; Johnston, M.; Biermann, V.; Dries, V.; Kochanek, S. Variables affecting *in vivo* performance of high-capacity adenovirus vectors. *J. Virol.* **2002**, *76*, 1600–1609.
91. Jenuwein, T.; Allis, C.D. Translating the histone code. *Science* **2001**, *293*, 1074–1080.
92. Smith, C.L.; Hager, G.L. Transcriptional regulation of mammalian genes *in vivo*. A tale of two templates. *J. Biol. Chem.* **1997**, *272*, 27493–27496.
93. Jiang, C.; Pugh, B.F. Nucleosome positioning and gene regulation: Advances through genomics. *Nat. Rev. Genet.* **2009**, *10*, 161–172.
94. Lomvardas, S.; Thanos, D. Modifying gene expression programs by altering core promoter chromatin architecture. *Cell* **2002**, *110*, 261–271.
95. Schreiner, S.; Wimmer, P.; Sirma, H.; Everett, R.D.; Blanchette, P.; Groitl, P.; Dobner, T. Proteasome-dependent degradation of Daxx by the viral E1B-55K protein in human adenovirus-infected cells. *J. Virol.* **2010**, *84*, 7029–7038.
96. Ullman, A.J.; Hearing, P. Cellular proteins PML and Daxx mediate an innate antiviral defense antagonized by the adenovirus E4 ORF3 protein. *J. Virol.* **2008**, *82*, 7325–7335.

97. Schreiner, S.; Burck, C.; Glass, M.; Groitl, P.; Wimmer, P.; Kinkley, S.; Mund, A.; Everett, R.D.; Dobner, T. Control of human adenovirus type 5 gene expression by cellular Daxx/ATRX chromatin-associated complexes. *Nucleic Acids Res.* **2013**, *41*, 3532–3550.
98. Schreiner, S.; Martinez, R.; Groitl, P.; Rayne, F.; Vaillant, R.; Wimmer, P.; Bossis, G.; Sternsdorf, T.; Marcinowski, L.; Ruzsics, Z.; *et al.* Transcriptional activation of the adenoviral genome is mediated by capsid protein VI. *PLoS Path.* **2012**, *8*, e1002549.
99. Suzuki, M.; Cerullo, V.; Bertin, T.K.; Cela, R.; Clarke, C.; Guenther, M.; Brunetti-Pierri, N.; Lee, B. MyD88-dependent silencing of transgene expression during the innate and adaptive immune response to helper-dependent adenovirus. *Hum. Gene Ther.* **2010**, *21*, 325–336.
100. Cerullo, V.; Seiler, M.P.; Mane, V.; Brunetti-Pierri, N.; Clarke, C.; Bertin, T.K.; Rodgers, J.R.; Lee, B. Toll-like receptor 9 triggers an innate immune response to helper-dependent adenoviral vectors. *Mol. Ther.* **2007**, *15*, 378–385.
101. Brestovitsky, A.; Sharf, R.; Mittelman, K.; Kleinberger, T. The adenovirus E4orf4 protein targets PP2A to the ACF chromatin-remodeling factor and induces cell death through regulation of SNF2h-containing complexes. *Nucleic Acids Res.* **2011**, *39*, 6414–6427.
102. Lavoie, J.N.; Nguyen, M.; Marcellus, R.C.; Branton, P.E.; Shore, G.C. E4orf4, a novel adenovirus death factor that induces p53-independent apoptosis by a pathway that is not inhibited by zVAD-fmk. *J. Cell Biol.* **1998**, *140*, 637–645.
103. Marcellus, R.C.; Lavoie, J.N.; Boivin, D.; Shore, G.C.; Ketner, G.; Branton, P.E. The early region 4 orf4 protein of human adenovirus type 5 induces p53- independent cell death by apoptosis. *J. Virol.* **1998**, *72*, 7144–7153.

11

Current Understanding of the Role of the Brd4 Protein in the Papillomavirus Lifecycle

Alison A. McBride * and Moon Kyoo Jang

Laboratory of Viral Diseases, National Institute of Allergy and Infectious Diseases, National Institutes of Health, Bethesda, MD 20892, USA; E-Mail: jangmk@niaid.nih.gov

* Author to whom correspondence should be addressed; E-Mail: amcbride@nih.gov;

Abstract: The Brd4 protein is an epigenetic reader that is central to regulation of cellular transcription and mitotic bookmarking. The transcription and replication proteins of many viruses interact with Brd4. We describe the multiple roles of Brd4 in the papillomavirus lifecycle.

Keywords: Brd4; BET protein; HPV; papillomavirus; transcription; chromatin; replication; tethering; partitioning; bromodomain

1. Introduction

Papillomaviruses (PVs) are an ancient group of viruses that have coevolved along with their hosts for millions of years. Each viral type infects only a particular host species and is trophic for a specific anatomical niche in the stratified epithelium of the skin or mucosa of the host. Papillomavirus infection is persistent and results in clinical outcomes, such as asymptomatic infection, verrucae, plantar and filiform warts and condylomata acuminata. A subset of oncogenic HPVs is associated with carcinomas of the oropharyngeal and anogenital tracts [1–3]. Despite the diversity of pathogenesis associated with papillomavirus infection, all papillomaviruses have similar small dsDNA genomes of approximately 8 kbp (see Figure 1), and each encodes only six to eight genes. Papillomaviruses rely on hijacking and manipulating host factors to maintain their lifestyle.

Figure 1. HPV18 genome. The circular dsDNA genome of HPV18 (7,857 bp) is shown. Viral open reading frames are depicted as red arrows. The URR (upstream regulatory region) is expanded to show transcription and replication regulatory elements. Binding sites for the E2 protein (cyan circles) and the E1 binding site (blue rectangle) are shown. The early promoter and replication origin (ori) are indicated.

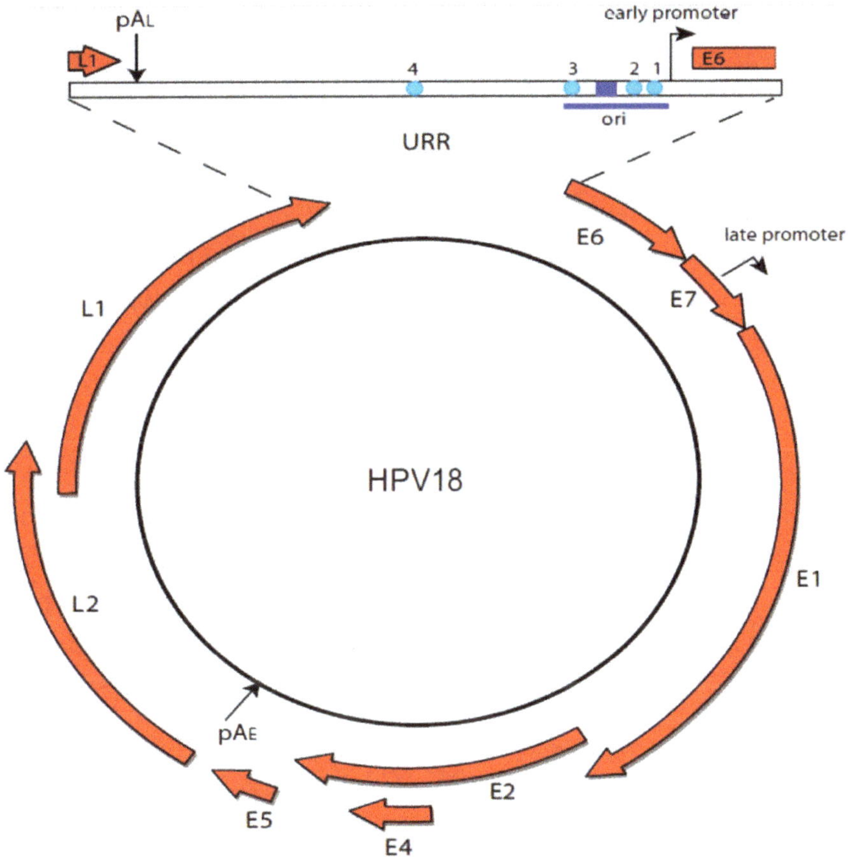

One key, cellular regulatory protein hijacked by all papillomaviruses (and other viral families) is a cellular chromatin binding protein, Brd4. Brd4 is an essential cellular protein that binds and marks chromatin to regulate several transcriptional processes. In this review, we will summarize the current knowledge pertaining to the role of Brd4 in papillomavirus infections.

2. Papillomaviruses

2.1. The Papillomavirus Lifecycle

The stratified epithelium of the skin or mucosa consists of several layers of keratinocytes in various stages of differentiation, overlying the basal layer of proliferative cells. Papillomaviruses gain access to cells in the basal layer through a microabrasion. They infect these keratinocytes, induce their proliferation by expression of the viral E7 protein and establish a persistent infection therein. The viral genome is maintained as a low copy, extrachromosomal element in the nucleus of these cells, and only low levels of viral gene products are produced. When the infected cells divide, some of the daughter cells begin the process of stratification and differentiation and progress towards the surface of the epithelium. The papillomavirus lifecycle is finely tuned to this process of differentiation; viral transcription and replication switches from early to late modes as the cell differentiates. Vegetative viral DNA replication is initiated in the mid-layers of differentiated cells, and capsid synthesis is confined to the most differentiated layers of cells.

2.2. Viral Transcription

Papillomavirus genomes can be divided into three regions (see Figure 1). The upstream regulatory region (URR) contains transcriptional enhancers and promoters and the origin of replication. The early region encodes the E (early) proteins that are expressed at early and intermediate stages of infection. Last is the late region that contains the L (late) genes. In the most undifferentiated cells, viral RNAs are transcribed from the early promoter, terminate at the early polyadenylation site (pAE) and encode the E6, E7, E1, E2, E4 and E5 proteins (reviewed in [4]). As the cells progress through differentiation, the late promoter is activated, resulting in an intermediate class of transcripts that use the late promoter and the early polyadenylation signal. These transcripts encode high levels of the E4, E1 and E2, the latter two being required for high level vegetative viral DNA replication in the mid-layers of the epithelium. Exclusively late transcripts are expressed at an even later stage of differentiation; they use both the late promoter and late polyadenylation signal (pAL) and encode the L1 and L2 capsid proteins. Complex patterns of viral mRNA species are generated by the use of alternative splicing and viral gene expression is highly regulated by differential splicing and polyadenylation (reviewed in [4]).

The E2 protein is the primary regulator of early viral transcription [5]. E2 consists of a conserved amino terminal "transactivation" domain linked to a C-terminal DNA binding/dimerization domain by a poorly conserved linker (see Figure 2) [6]. E2 specifically binds to a consensus sequence of ACCGNNNNCGGT, several copies of which are located in the viral URR [7] (see Figure 1). E2 can activate transcription from certain viral promoters [5,8–10], but the early viral promoter in the well-studied, oncogenic alpha-PVs is primarily repressed by E2 [11–13]. Early studies showed that E2 could repress the early promoter by sterically hindering the association of TBP and Sp1 with promoter elements adjacent to E2 binding sites 1 and 2 [14–16]. Subsequent studies have shown that much of this E2-mediated repression is mediated through interaction with factors that modulate cellular chromatin processes [17–20]. Disruption of E2-mediated repression (often due to HPV integration) results in increased expression of the E6 and E7 oncogenes [11,12,21]. In fact, reintroduction of the E2 protein into cervical cancer-derived lines (such as HeLa) leads to rapid senescence, as viability of these cells is completely dependent on E6 and E7 expression [22–24].

Shorter forms of the E2 protein that are lacking the transactivation domain also repress HPV transcription, in part by competing for binding to E2 binding motifs [25,26]. One of the best characterized is the E8^E2 protein (encoded from a spliced transcript), which also represses through the recruitment of chromatin-associated repressive factors [27]. As described in detail below, E2 interacts with the Brd4 protein, and this association is pivotal to transcriptional regulation of HPVs.

Figure 2. Structure of the papillomavirus E2 protein. The two domains of the E2 protein are shown. The transactivation domain structure is of HPV16 E2 bound to the Brd4 C-terminal motif (CTM). The Brd4 C-terminal peptide (residues 1343–1362) is shown in magenta. This structure is from the pdb file, 2NNU. The DNA binding domain is of the HPV18 DNA binding domain bound to DNA (shown in light purple) from the pdb file 1JJ4.

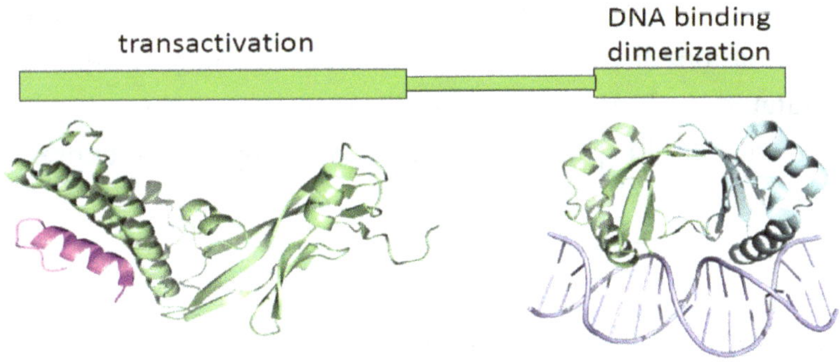

2.3. Disruption of E2 Function by HPV Integration

In the majority of HPV associated cancers, the HPV genome is integrated into the host genome (reviewed in [28]). The viral genome is most often integrated in such a way as to disrupt the E2 gene and, thus, alleviate transcriptional repression of the early viral promoter [22–24,29]. In turn, this causes dysregulation of the E6 and E7 oncogenes and promotes malignant progression [30].

2.4. Viral Replication

Papillomavirus replication requires the E1 protein, the E2 protein and the origin of replication [31–33]. E1 is the primary replication protein, an ATP-dependent helicase that binds specifically to the origin and unwinds it in a bidirectional manner to permit access by the cellular replication machinery (reviewed in [34]). E2 functions to load the E1 helicase onto the origin [35]. As depicted in Figure 1, the minimal origin consists of the E1 binding site flanked by E2 binding sites and overlaps elements regulating the early promoter.

There are three modes of viral replication in the viral lifecycle. The first is a limited amplification that occurs when the virus particle infects a basal keratinocyte. The virus must undergo a few rounds of unlicensed DNA replication to establish the genome as a low copy, nuclear, extrachromosomal element. This phase requires E1, E2 and the minimal replication origin. The second phase of replication maintains the viral genome at a low copy number during division of the proliferating basal cells. This also requires E1, E2 and the minimal origin of replication, but there is an additional requirement for additional E2 binding sites in *cis* to the origin, thus implicating the E2 protein in maintenance replication [36]. Subsequent studies showed that the role of E2 was to tether the viral genomes to the host chromatin [37–39]. The interaction of E2 with Brd4 is crucial for the tethering function of many papillomaviruses and will be discussed in detail below. Further investigation showed that the E1 protein was not always necessary for maintenance replication and, presumably, in this situation viral replication, is initiated by cellular factors, while the genome is retained by the E2 protein [40,41].

The third phase of replication is vegetative amplification, when progeny virions are produced in large numbers in differentiated cells. This requires the E1 and E2 proteins, and their expression is upregulated in differentiated cells [42,43]. There is evidence that the mode of replication changes in differentiated cells [44], and incorporation of Rad51 into replication foci indicates that the virus may replicate using a recombination directed replication mechanism [45,46]. Furthermore, the cellular ataxia telangiectasia mutated (ATM) DNA damage response pathway is required for vegetative replication in differentiated cells [47]. Nuclear foci formed by either expression of the E1 and E2 proteins [48–51] or the replicating viral genome [46,47] recruit multiple cellular proteins required for the cellular DNA damage response and repair pathways.

2.5. Differences in Transcription and Replication among Papillomaviruses

To date, there are over 240 named papillomavirus genomes that have been classified into 37 different genera [52]. The best studied are human viruses from the alpha and beta genera that infect primarily the mucosa and skin, respectively. The human mu virus, HPV1, and the ungulate delta virus, BPV1, are also well characterized. While each of these viruses has a similar organization of genes to that of HPV18 (an alpha-PV) shown in Figure 1, the number and position of the E2 binding sites can vary considerably. BPV1 has 11 E2 binding sites in the URR and six elsewhere in the genome [53], while most human alpha viruses have only the four E2 sites shown in Figure 1. In BPV1, E2 is primarily an activator of transcription [5], while E2 predominantly represses the major early promoter of alpha-PVs.

All viruses require the minimal replication origin and the E1 and E2 proteins to initiate replication, but the requirements for maintenance replication are more complex. E2 binding sites are essential for initiation of replication and for transcriptional regulation making it very difficult to separate and elucidate the role of individual sites in maintenance replication of the viral genome. Maintenance replication is best understood for BPV1, where it has been shown that at least eight E2 binding sites are required for persistent replication [36]. In the alpha-PV HPV31, only three of the four E2 binding sites are required for maintenance replication of the viral genome [54]. In agreement with this finding, using a novel complementation assay, we find that a region encompassing the 3’ half of the URR of HPV18 (containing E2 binding sites 1–3) is sufficient for long-term maintenance in the presence of the E1 and E2 proteins [55].

3. The Brd4 Protein

3.1. Brd4 Structure and Function

Brd4 was first described as an unusual chromatin binding factor that remained bound to chromosomes throughout mitosis [56]. It is a member the BET (bromodomain and extra-terminal domain) family of chromatin binding proteins and, therefore, its name was changed from MCAP (mitotic chromosome-associated protein) to bromodomain containing protein 4 (Brd4) [57]. Brd4 is an essential protein [58] that is ubiquitous in proliferating cells. The tandem bromodomains of Brd4 interact with acetylated tails of H3 and H4 histones [59], and Brd4 has been shown to be a mitotic bookmark that marks genes, which are expressed shortly after mitotic exit [60,61]. Brd4 decompacts chromatin and recruits transcriptional initiation and elongation factors to rapidly activate early G1 genes post-mitosis, as well as later in interphase [62]. Brd4 recruits the transcriptional elongation factor, p-TEFb, to promoters to enhance phosphorylation of the C-terminal tail (CTD) of RNA polymerase II promoters to stimulate transcription [63,64]. Brd4 further promotes transcription by directly phosphorylating the RNA polymerase II CTD [65]. This fundamental role of Brd4 in transcriptional regulation places it at the center of many diverse biological activities.

The Brd4 gene encodes two proteins; the short form of Brd4 contains the two bromodomains and the extra-terminal (ET) region (important for many protein-protein interactions), while the longer form of Brd4 has an additional, long unique C-terminal region (see Figure 3). The structures of both bromodomains and the ET domains have been solved [66,67]. The bromodomains bind to specific acetylated lysines on H3 and H4, but BD2 (bromodomain 2) can also interact with acetylated residues in other proteins, such as cyclin T1 (the p-TEFb subunit) and the relA subunit of NFκB [67–69].

The extra-terminal domain consists of three alpha-helices, and it seems to be a site of protein-protein interaction [70]. It binds proteins involved in transcriptional regulation, such as NSD3 (also known as WHSC1L1), a histone methyl transferase, JMJD6, a histone demethylase, and CHD4, a component of the NuRD (nuclear remodeling and deacetylase) repressor complex. Thus, Brd4 has the potential to assemble multifaceted positive and negative regulatory complexes on promoters [71].

The function of the C-terminal region is not well-characterized, except for the last 100 amino acids, which is important for interacting with the papillomavirus E2 protein [72] and with p-TEFb [73] (see Figure 3). Thus, p-TEFb interacts with two independent regions of the Brd4 protein [68].

p53 has also recently been shown to be a binding partner of Brd4, and analysis of this interaction revealed a conformational switch in Brd4 structure and protein-protein interactions modulated by CK2 phosphorylation [74]. A region between the second bromodomain and the ET domain contains two interaction regions, BID (basic residue enriched interaction domain) and NPS (N-terminal cluster of phosphorylation sites), that modulate this switch. When unphosphorylated, the NPS region interacts with the PDID (phosphorylation dependent interaction domain) that encompasses bromodomain 2, thus preventing Brd4 from binding to acetylated histones (see Figure 3). p53 binds to the BID region when Brd4 is unphosphorylated. Upon phosphorylation of NPS, p53 is released from binding to BID, and both p53 and BID now associate with phosphorylated NPS, thus exposing the bromodomain 2 in PDID and activating the complex [74].

Figure 3. Structure and function of the Brd4 protein. (**a**) Domains of the Brd4 protein. The domains shown are BD1 (bromodomain I: residues 58–169); BD2 (bromodomain 2: residues 349–461); NPS (N-terminal cluster of phosphorylation sites: residues 484–503); BID (basic residue enriched interaction domain: residues 524–579); ET (extra-terminal domain: residues 600–678); PDID (phosphorylation dependent interaction domain: residues 287–530); SEED (Ser/Glu/Asp-rich region: residues 695–720); CTM (C-terminal motif: residues 1325–1362); CTD (dominant negative domain of Brd4: residues 1047–1362) and PID (pTEF binding region: residues 1209–1362) [73]. (**b**) Viral and cellular interacting partners of Brd4. See text for references.

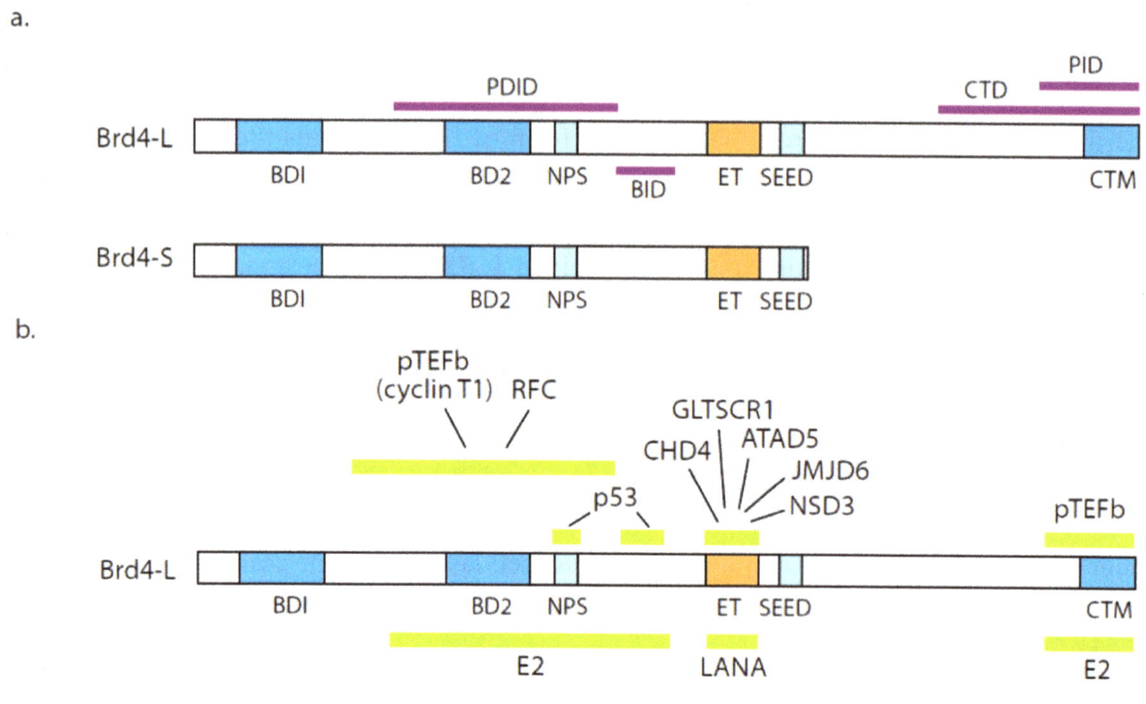

3.2. Association of Brd4 with Disease

The first association of Brd4 with human disease was the discovery that the aggressive NUT midline carcinoma (NMC) was due to a translocation (t(15;19)(q13;p13)), resulting in the fusion of Brd4 with NUT (nuclear protein in testes) [75]. The NUT protein recruits the histone acetyl transferase, p300, resulting in a feed-forward loop of histone acetylation and Brd4-NUT recruitment, which gives rise to hyperacetylated, but inactive, chromosomal foci [76]. Sequestration of Brd4 and p-TEFb to these foci promotes proliferation of Brd4-NUT cells. This can be reversed and differentiation restored, by siRNA to Brd4, by histone deacetylase inhibitors that promote global acetylation and by BET protein-specific histone mimics [77–79].

Brd4 is also a modifier of breast cancer metastasis [80] and a promising target for several cancers, because of its fundamental role in transcriptional processes. Targeted inhibition of BET bromodomain binding is potentially therapeutic for glioblastoma, lung adenocarcinoma, ALL (acute lymphoblastic leukemia) and MLL (mixed-lineage leukemia) [81–84,85].

4. Brd4 and Papillomaviruses

Brd4 was discovered to be a major interactor of the papillomavirus E2 protein by proteomic analyses [20,72], yeast two hybrid screening [86]. It was also investigated as an E2 target, because the analogous tethering protein in KSHV (LANA) interacts with the BET family member, Brd2 [87–89]. The E2 protein had previously been shown to bind and tether viral genomes to host mitotic chromosomes [37–39,90], and the Brd4 protein colocalized completely with these chromatin bound speckles of E2 [72,87,89,91]. The E2 protein is a multifunctional protein involved in papillomavirus transcription, maintenance and partitioning of extrachromosomal viral genomes and initiation of viral DNA replication. Many subsequent studies have dissected the role of Brd4 in each of these processes.

4.1. Interaction between Papillomavirus E2 and Brd4 Proteins

The Brd4 protein binds primarily to the transactivation domain of the E2 proteins (see Figure 2) [72]. The transactivation domain contacts a peptide at the extreme C-terminus of the Brd4 protein [91], and a C-terminal domain of Brd4 (CTD; residues 1047–1362) has proven useful as a dominant-negative inhibitor of the E2-Brd4 interaction [72]. The region of the E2 transactivation domain that makes contact with the Brd4 CTD is highly conserved; yet, there is a wide range of binding affinities between Brd4 and E2 proteins from different papillomaviruses [92]. The C-terminal DNA binding domain of E2 does not seem necessary for Brd4 binding, but the dimerization function of this domain greatly increases E2-Brd4 binding both *in vivo* and *in vitro*. There are hints that there may be additional contacts between E2 and Brd4: HPV11 E2 binds to the Brd4 CTD, but also to a region encompassing bromodomain 2 (BD2). The DNA binding domain of the KSHV LANA protein (a tethering protein analogous to E2 and with a DNA binding domain of similar structure) interacts with the ET domain of Brd4 [93,94]. It is likely that the interaction between Brd4 and the E2 protein will be multifactorial.

4.2. Brd4 Modulates the Stability of the E2 Proteins

Several groups have noted that the E2 protein is stabilized by interaction with Brd4 [95,96] or with the Brd4 CTD [97]. This interaction prevents proteasomal degradation of E2 by the E3 ligase cullin-3 [97] and may enhance many E2 functions, such as transcriptional regulation and stable tethering of genomes on host chromatin.

4.3. The Role of Brd4 in Viral Transcription

The E2 protein can both activate or repress viral transcription, depending on whether it binds to sites that are distal or proximal to promoter elements [5,8–10]. Binding of E2 to promoter proximal sites represses the early viral promoter in the oncogenic alpha-PVs [11–13]. A number of mutational analyses identified residues in the transactivation domain of E2 that were important for E2-mediated transcriptional activation or replication [98–103]. Prominent were two highly conserved residues (R37 and I73) that when mutated, abrogated E2-mediated transactivation, but not replication. Subsequently, it was shown that these residues were located on two adjacent alpha helices on the same face of the E2 transactivation domain [104], and later, these residues were shown to make direct contact with a C-terminal peptide (residues 1343–1362) of Brd4 [91]. In addition to binding to the Brd4 C-terminus, HPV11 E2 also interacts with Brd4 residues 280–580, which encompasses the BD2 bromodomain.

It became clear that Brd4 was essential for the transcriptional activation function of E2. A dominant negative C-terminal peptide encompassing the Brd4 CTD interfered with the E2-Brd4 interaction and inhibited transactivation by many papillomavirus E2 proteins [92,105,106]. Initially, the role of Brd4 in transcriptional repression was controversial, but it has now been proven that Brd4 is also involved in E2-mediated transcriptional repression [18–20]. However, in some cases, the dominant negative Brd4 CTD interferes with E2-mediated transactivation, but not repression, implying that there are additional or alternative modes of interaction between the Brd4 and E2 proteins [18]. Another factor that contributes to repression of the HPV early promoter is the histone acetyl transferase complex, NuA4/TIP60 [18,107]. TIP60 preferentially acetylates K14 of histone H3 and K5, K8, K12 and K16 of histone H4 [108], which are all targets of the Brd4 bromodomains [66]. Notably, the HPV E6 protein destabilizes TIP60, thereby alleviating repression of its own promoter [107].

One of the key functions of Brd4 is to recruit p-TEFb to promoters to stimulate elongation of RNA polymerase II transcription. The C-terminal region of Brd4 interacts with both E2 and p-TEFb, suggesting that these complexes are mutually exclusive. Brd4 recruitment of P-TEFb to the early promoter is required for viral transcription, and E2 disrupts this interaction [109]. In this study (unlike [18]), the dominant negative BRD4 CTD was able to inhibit E2-mediated repression.

Most HPV repression studies have analyzed viral transcription in cervical carcinoma-derived cell lines that harbor integrated HPV genomes. However, E2 may preferentially repress integrated genomes compared to episomally replicating genomes, and so, further studies are needed to define the role of Brd4 in HPV transcription [110].

4.4. The Role of Brd4 in Viral Genome Replication

Most studies have indicated that the E2-Brd4 interaction is important for transcriptional regulation and tethering of viral genomes to host chromatin. Mutated E2 proteins that are unable to bind Brd4 are able to efficiently support transient replication of an origin containing plasmid [87,98,99,105,106,111–113]. Ilves *et al.* demonstrated that the dominant negative Brd4 CTD could inhibit the replication of BPV1 genomes or origins in rodent cells, but not in human C-33A cells [113]. Furthermore, this inhibition was not dependent on the interaction of Brd4 with E2 (at least through the R37 and I73 residues) and was not specific for papillomavirus replication [113].

Wang *et al.* find that Brd4 is recruited to foci formed by HPV16 E1 and E2 in a replication origin-dependent fashion in C-33A cells [114]. An E2 protein mutated in both Brd4 interacting residues (R37 and I73) is defective in replication, thus leading the authors to propose that Brd4 is required for replication. However, as previously found by others, E2 proteins with a single substitution in I73 are not defective in replication, despite an inability to bind to Brd4 [87,99,105,106,111–113]. Because downregulation of Brd4 has detrimental effects on cell growth and proliferation (making it difficult to interpret HPV replication experiments), Wang *et al.* demonstrated that Brd4 could stimulate HPV replication *in vitro* [114].

Somewhat similarly, we find that Brd4 is recruited to replication foci formed by the E1-E2 proteins in keratinocytes [49], in a process that is completely dependent on E1, E2 and Brd4. However, we find that Brd4 is displaced to the periphery of these foci in the presence of an actively replicating origin or genome, and Brd4 is no longer required for their formation [115]. Brd4 is also found in a satellite pattern around late replication foci that contain amplified genomes in differentiated keratinocytes [115], but it does not seem to be essential for viral DNA amplification [116]. The HPV replication foci induce a cellular DNA damage response and recruit repair proteins [46–50], and it is tempting to speculate that Brd4 is involved in these processes. The replication factor, RF/C, is found in Brd4 [117] and E2-Brd4 protein complexes [20,118]. Furthermore, the alternative RFC1 subunit, ATAD5, which is involved in the DNA damage response, interacts with the ET domain of Brd4 [71], suggesting that it might play a role in HPV replication. Clearly, more studies are required to elucidate the exact role of Brd4 in the papillomavirus replication process, but there are several hints that Brd4 might be involved in viral and cellular DNA replication and repair processes.

4.5. The Role of Brd4 in Viral Genome Maintenance and Partitioning

The E1 and E2 proteins support transient replication, but long-term persistence of viral-derived DNA requires additional E2 binding sites in *cis* to the replication origin [36]. The first clue to the role of E2 in viral DNA persistence was the observation that both viral DNA and the BPV1 E2 protein are localized in punctate foci on the host mitotic chromosomes [37]. This led to the model (as shown in Figure 4) that E2 associates with host chromosomes through the transactivation domain [39], while the DNA binding domain binds to E2 sites in the viral genomes and tethers them to the host chromosomes to promote retention and partitioning [119]. This tethering mechanism ensures that the low copy viral genome is retained in the nucleus and is partitioned to daughter cells.

At least for BPV1, the cellular target that mediates mitotic tethering is the Brd4 protein [72,87,89]. Brd4 is usually observed as a diffuse cloud (if at all) around the condensed mitotic chromosomes [59], but in the presence of E2, both proteins colocalize in punctate foci [89]. Brd4 has a high on-off rate and can be easily extracted from chromatin [59], but E2 dramatically stabilizes the interaction of Brd4 with chromatin forming a stable anchor in interphase and mitosis [89]. As described above, two highly conserved residues in the transactivation domain of E2 (R37 and I73) mediate the interaction with Brd4, and mutations in these residues abrogate the interaction of E2 with Brd4 and mitotic chromatin [87]. The DNA binding domain of E2 is not required for the interaction with Brd4, but it is required to link the viral genomes to chromatin [119]. The dimerization function of the E2 C-terminal domain greatly increases the affinity of Brd4 for chromatin both *in vivo* and *in vitro*, most likely by promoting the assembly of higher order E2-Brd4 complexes [120]. Expression of the dominant negative Brd4 CTD resulted in inhibition of E2 mitotic chromosome binding and loss of BPV1 genomes from BPV1 transformed cells [89,113,121]. Moreover, BPV1 E2-mediated plasmid maintenance could be reconstituted in *Saccharomyces cerevisiae* by exogenously expressed Brd4 [122].

Figure 4. Model of E2-mediated tethering of the viral genome to host chromatin. The Brd4 protein interacts with acetylated lysine residues on histone tails protruding from the host nucleosomes (shown in purple). The papillomavirus E2 protein interacts with the C-terminal region of Brd4 through the E2 transactivation domain. The DNA binding-dimerization domain of E2 links the viral genome to the chromatin complex.

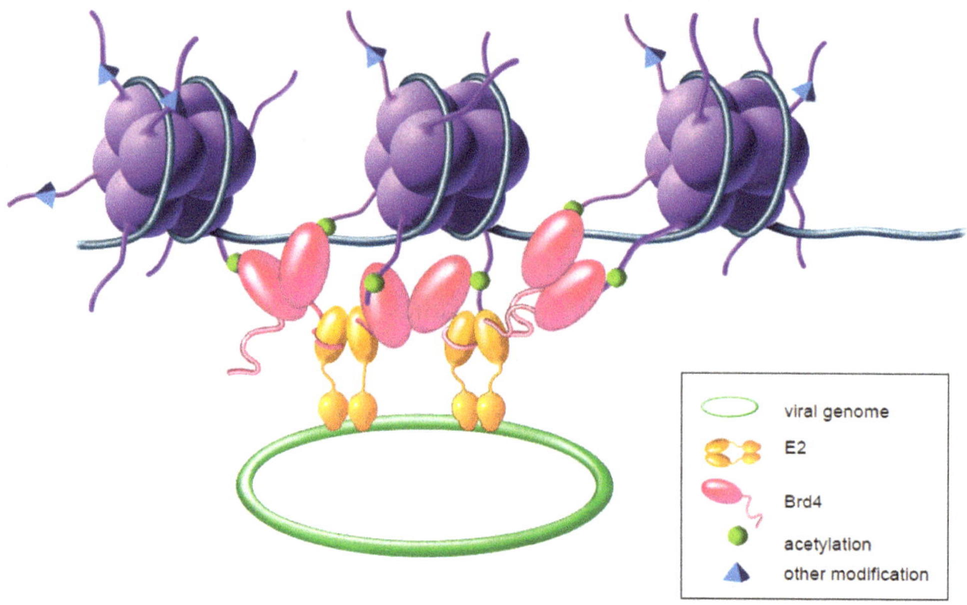

Although the E2 proteins from all papillomaviruses interact with the C-terminal region of Brd4 (through the R37 and I73 residues in E2), there are differences in the strength of binding [92,118]. Furthermore, not all E2 proteins are as readily observed bound to mitotic chromosomes as BPV1 E2 [92,123]. A careful analysis of the E2 proteins from numerous different papillomaviruses showed that there were three different phenotypes of mitotic chromosome binding that segregated perfectly according to the phylogeny of papillomaviruses [123]. These groups were comprised of the alpha-papillomaviruses, a large genus that encompasses mainly human viruses that infect the oral and genital mucosa; the beta and gamma papillomaviruses, another large group containing mainly human viruses that infect the cutaneous epithelium in an asymptomatic manner and a diverse group of viruses from the delta (BPV1), mu (HPV1), kappa (OcPV1 and SfPV1) and other genera. The E2 proteins from this latter group bind tightly to Brd4, stabilize its association with interphase chromatin and colocalize with Brd4 on the arms of mitotic chromosomes in punctate dots [92,123].

In contrast, the beta-PV E2 proteins bind strongly to pericentromeric regions of mitotic chromosomes that overlap the loci for the ribosomal RNA genes [123,124]. The determinants of the E2 protein required for this perichromosomal binding are quite different from those required for the E2 Brd4 chromosomal foci. The primary requirements are the E2 DNA binding domain and a short peptide from the hinge region that facilitates interaction with chromatin [125]. Phosphorylation of this peptide by PKA (protein kinase A) stabilizes the E2 protein and promotes chromosomal binding [126] in a manner analogous to that of the KSHV LANA tethering protein [127]. However, the beta E2 proteins do have high affinity for Brd4, and if the chromosomal binding peptide in the hinge is mutated, E2-directed foci of Brd4 can be observed on mitotic chromosomes [128]. The significance of these two binding modes has yet to be determined, as beta-PV genomes do not readily replicate in cell culture.

For alpha-PVs, the mechanism of E2-mediated viral genome tethering and E2-Brd4 chromosomal binding is still elusive. Alpha-PV E2 proteins bind to Brd4 relatively weakly, they do not stabilize the association of Brd4 with host chromatin and cannot be easily detected on mitotic chromosomes, except in late telophase [123,129]. When cells are pre-extracted before fixation, the alpha-PV E2 proteins bind to the peri-centromeric regions of host chromosomes in a Brd4-independent manner similar to that of the beta-PVs [123]. Difficulties in detecting alpha-PV E2-Brd4 mitotic foci have led to the proposal of other targets, such as the mitotic spindle [130], a mitotic kinesin-like protein, MKlp2 [131], ChlR1 (an ATP-dependent DNA helicase important for sister chromatid cohesion) [132] and TopBP1 [129]. Furthermore, HPV31 genomes that encode a Brd4 binding defective E2 protein (an I73L mutation) can still maintain extrachromosomal viral genomes and undergo amplification in differentiated keratinocytes [54,105]. Recent findings indicate that Brd4 colocalizes with nuclear foci formed by the alpha-PV E1 and E2 proteins [114,115], and we find that the alpha-PV E1-E2 protein complex binds to the same regions of host chromatin as the stable HPV1 E2-Brd4 complex in C-33A cells [133].

Therefore, many questions remain, and it seems that the interaction of E2 and Brd4 with host chromatin is complex. The tethering mechanism is likely to be coupled with transcriptional and replication processes. Silla *et al.* have shown that simple attachment of genomes to chromatin is not sufficient [134]; chromatin attachment and transactivation functions must cooperate to ensure proper plasmid segregation. A genome-wide ChIP-on-chip analysis showed that BPV1 E2 and Brd4 were bound to transcriptionally active regions of chromatin, perhaps to ensure that the viral genome localized to transcriptionally active regions of the nucleus [135]. Brd4 is recruited to HPV replication centers containing alpha-PV proteins that do not tightly associate with Brd4 [114,115]. Thus, transcription, replication and genome partitioning are most likely intertwined processes.

4.6. Association of Brd4 with Other Viruses

Papillomaviruses are not the only viruses that have discovered the versatility and usefulness of BET proteins [136]. The EBNA and LANA tethering proteins of the gamma herpes viruses, EBV and KSHV, interact with Brd2 and Brd4 for transcriptional regulation [88,93,137,138]. Polyoma viruses also recruit Brd4 to viral replication centers [139]. Brd4 represses HIV expression by competing with the HIV TAT transactivator for recruitment of p-TEFb to the HIV promoter [73]. Inhibition of Brd4 with BET inhibitors reactivates latent HIV with great therapeutic potential [140–143].

5. Conclusions

Viruses have always alerted us to the key players in cellular processes. Papillomaviruses, in particular, have small genomes with limited coding capacity and rely almost completely on using and manipulating cellular factors for viral processes. Brd4 is clearly a central player in HPV biology, and a complete understanding of its role in essential viral processes will provide deeper insight into its role in host biology.

Acknowledgments

We are grateful to Koenraad van Doorslaer and Wesley Stepp for critical reading of the manuscript. This work was funded by the Intramural Research Program of the NIAID, NIH.

References

1. Bouvard, V.; Baan, R.; Straif, K.; Grosse, Y.; Secretan, B.; El, G.F.; Benbrahim-Tallaa, L.; Guha, N.; Freeman, C.; Galichet, L.; *et al.* A review of human carcinogens—Part B: Biological agents. *Lancet Oncol.* **2009**, *10*, 321–322.
2. Walboomers, J.M.; Jacobs, M.V.; Manos, M.M.; Bosch, F.X.; Kummer, J.A.; Shah, K.V.; Snijders, P.J.; Peto, J.; Meijer, C.J.; Muñoz, N. Human papillomavirus is a necessary cause of invasive cervical cancer worldwide. *J. Pathol.* **1999**, *189*, 12–19.
3. Gillison, M.L.; Lowy, D.R. A causal role for human papillomavirus in head and neck cancer. *Lancet* **2004**, *363*, 1488–1489.
4. Johansson, C.; Schwartz, S. Regulation of human papillomavirus gene expression by splicing and polyadenylation. *Nat. Rev. Microbiol.* **2013**, *11*, 239–251.
5. Spalholz, B.A.; Yang, Y.C.; Howley, P.M. Transactivation of a bovine papilloma virus transcriptional regulatory element by the E2 gene product. *Cell* **1985**, *42*, 183–191.
6. McBride, A.A.; Byrne, J.C.; Howley, P.M. E2 polypeptides encoded by bovine papillomavirus type 1 form dimers through the common carboxyl-terminal domain: Transactivation is mediated by the conserved amino-terminal domain. *Proc. Natl. Acad. Sci. USA* **1989**, *86*, 510–514.
7. Androphy, E.J.; Lowy, D.R.; Schiller, J.T. Bovine papillomavirus E2 trans-activating gene product binds to specific sites in papillomavirus DNA. *Nature* **1987**, *325*, 70–73.
8. Cripe, T.P.; Haugen, T.H.; Turk, J.P.; Tabatabai, F.; Schmid, P.G., 3rd.; Dürst, M.; Gissmann, L.; Roman, A.; Turek, L.P. Transcriptional regulation of the human papillomavirus- 16 E6-E7 promoter by a keratinocyte-dependent enhancer, and by viral E2 trans-activator and repressor gene products: Implications for cervical carcinogenesis. *EMBO J.* **1987**, *6*, 3745–3753.
9. Chin, M.T.; Hirochika, R.; Hirochika, H.; Broker, T.R.; Chow, L.T. Regulation of human papillomavirus type 11 enhancer and E6 promoter by activating and repressing proteins from the E2 open reading frame: Functional and biochemical studies. *J. Virol.* **1988**, *62*, 2994–3002.
10. Steger, G.; Corbach, S. Dose-dependent regulation of the early promoter of human papillomavirus type 18 by the viral E2 protein. *J. Virol.* **1997**, *71*, 50–58.

11. Thierry, F.; Yaniv, M. The BPV1-E2 trans-acting protein can be either an activator or a repressor of the HPV18 regulatory region. *EMBO J.* **1987**, *6*, 3391–3397.
12. Bernard, B.A.; Bailly, C.; Lenoir, M.C.; Darmon, M.; Thierry, F.; Yaniv, M. The human papillomavirus type 18 (HPV18) E2 gene product is a repressor of the HPV18 regulatory region in human keratinocytes. *J. Virol.* **1989**, *63*, 4317–4324.
13. Romanczuk, H.; Thierry, F.; Howley, P.M. Mutational analysis of cis elements involved in E2 modulation of human papillomavirus type 16 P 97 and type 18 P 105 promoters. *J. Virol.* **1990**, *64*, 2849–2859.
14. Tan, S.H.; Gloss, B.; Bernard, H.U. During negative regulation of the human papillomavirus-16 E6 promoter, the viral E2 protein can displace Sp1 from a proximal promoter element. *Nucleic Acids Res.* **1992**, *20*, 251–256.
15. Dong, G.; Broker, T.R.; Chow, L.T. Human papillomavirus type 11 E2 proteins repress the homologous E6 promoter by interfering with the binding of host transcription factors to adjacent elements. *J. Virol.* **1994**, *68*, 1115–1127.
16. Tan, S.H.; Leong, L.E.; Walker, P.A.; Bernard, H.U. The human papillomavirus type 16 E2 transcription factor binds with low cooperativity to two flanking sites and represses the E6 promoter through displacement of Sp1 and TFIID. *J. Virol.* **1994**, *68*, 6411–6420.
17. Nishimura, A.; Ono, T.; Ishimoto, A.; Dowhanick, J.J.; Frizzell, M.A.; Howley, P.M.; Sakai, H. Mechanisms of human papillomavirus E2-mediated repression of viral oncogene expression and cervical cancer cell growth inhibition. *J. Virol.* **2000**, *74*, 3752–3760.
18. Smith, J.A.; White, E.A.; Sowa, M.E.; Powell, M.L.; Ottinger, M.; Harper, J.W.; Howley, P.M. Genome-wide siRNA screen identifies SMCX, EP400, and Brd4 as E2-dependent regulators of human papillomavirus oncogene expression. *Proc. Natl. Acad. Sci. USA* **2010**, *107*, 3752–3757.
19. Schweiger, M.R.; Ottinger, M.; You, J.; Howley, P.M. Brd4 independent transcriptional repression function of the papillomavirus E2 proteins. *J. Virol.* **2007**, *81*, 9612–9622.
20. Wu, S.Y.; Lee, A.Y.; Hou, S.Y.; Kemper, J.K.; Erdjument-Bromage, H.; Tempst, P.; Chiang, C.M. Brd4 links chromatin targeting to HPV transcriptional silencing. *Genes Dev.* **2006**, *20*, 2383–2396.
21. Thierry, F.; Howley, P.M. Functional analysis of E2-mediated repression of the HPV18 P105 promoter. *New Biol.* **1991**, *3*, 90–100.
22. Hwang, E.S.; Riese, D.J.D.; Settleman, J.; Nilson, L.A.; Honig, J.; Flynn, S.; DiMaio, D. Inhibition of cervical carcinoma cell line proliferation by the introduction of a bovine papillomavirus regulatory gene. *J. Virol.* **1993**, *67*, 3720–3729.
23. Dowhanick, J.J.; McBride, A.A.; Howley, P.M. Suppression of cellular proliferation by the papillomavirus E2 protein. *J. Virol.* **1995**, *69*, 7791–7799.
24. Desaintes, C.; Demeret, C.; Goyat, S.; Yaniv, M.; Thierry, F. Expression of the papillomavirus E2 protein in HeLa cells leads to apoptosis. *EMBO J.* **1997**, *16*, 504–514.
25. Stubenrauch, F.; Zobel, T.; Iftner, T. The E8 domain confers a novel long-distance transcriptional repression activity on the E8E2C protein of high-risk human papillomavirus type 31. *J. Virol.* **2001**, *75*, 4139–4149.

26. Chiang, C.M.; Broker, T.R.; Chow, L.T. An E1M^E2C fusion protein encoded by human papillomavirus type 11 is a sequence-specific transcription repressor. *J. Virol.* **1991**, *65*, 3317–3329.
27. Powell, M.L.; Smith, J.A.; Sowa, M.E.; Harper, J.W.; Iftner, T.; Stubenrauch, F.; Howley, P.M. NCoR1 mediates papillomavirus E8;E2C transcriptional repression. *J. Virol.* **2010**, *84*, 4451–4460.
28. Pett, M.; Coleman, N. Integration of high-risk human papillomavirus: A key event in cervical carcinogenesis? *J. Pathol.* **2007**, *212*, 356–367.
29. Francis, D.A.; Schmid, S.I.; Howley, P.M. Repression of the integrated papillomavirus E6/E7 promoter is required for growth suppression of cervical cancer cells. *J. Virol.* **2000**, *74*, 2679–2686.
30. Jeon, S.; Allen-Hoffmann, B.L.; Lambert, P.F. Integration of human papillomavirus type 16 into the human genome correlates with a selective growth advantage of cells. *J. Virol.* **1995**, *69*, 2989–2997.
31. Mohr, I.J.; Clark, R.; Sun, S.; Androphy, E.J.; MacPherson, P.; Botchan, M.R. Targeting the E1 replication protein to the papillomavirus origin of replication by complex formation with the E2 transactivator. *Science* **1990**, *250*, 1694–1699.
32. Ustav, M.; Stenlund, A. Transient replication of BPV-1 requires two viral polypeptides encoded by the E1 and E2 open reading frames. *EMBO J.* **1991**, *10*, 449–457.
33. Ustav, M.; Ustav, E.; Szymanski, P.; Stenlund, A. Identification of the origin of replication of bovine papillomavirus and characterization of the viral origin recognition factor E1. *EMBO J.* **1991**, *10*, 4321–4329.
34. McBride, A.A. Replication and partitioning of papillomavirus genomes. *Adv. Virus Res.* **2008**, *72*, 155–205.
35. Sanders, C.M.; Stenlund, A. Recruitment and loading of the E1 initiator protein: An ATP-dependent process catalysed by a transcription factor. *EMBO J.* **1998**, *17*, 7044–7055.
36. Piirsoo, M.; Ustav, E.; Mandel, T.; Stenlund, A.; Ustav, M. Cis and trans requirements for stable episomal maintenance of the BPV-1 replicator. *EMBO J.* **1996**, *15*, 1–11.
37. Skiadopoulos, M.H.; McBride, A.A. Bovine papillomavirus type 1 genomes and the E2 transactivator protein are closely associated with mitotic chromatin. *J. Virol.* **1998**, *72*, 2079–2088.
38. Ilves, I.; Kivi, S.; Ustav, M. Long-term episomal maintenance of bovine papillomavirus type 1 plasmids is determined by attachment to host chromosomes, which is mediated by the viral E2 protein and its binding sites. *J. Virol.* **1999**, *73*, 4404–4412.
39. Bastien, N.; McBride, A.A. Interaction of the papillomavirus E2 protein with mitotic chromosomes. *Virology* **2000**, *270*, 124–134.
40. Kim, K.; Lambert, P.F. E1 protein of bovine papillomavirus 1 is not required for the maintenance of viral plasmid DNA replication. *Virology* **2002**, *293*, 10–14.
41. Egawa, N.; Nakahara, T.; Ohno, S.; Narisawa-Saito, M.; Yugawa, T.; Fujita, M.; Yamato, K.; Natori, Y.; Kiyono, T. The E1 protein of human papillomavirus type 16 is dispensable for maintenance replication of the viral genome. *J. Virol.* **2012**, *86*, 3276–3283.
42. Xue, Y.; Bellanger, S.; Zhang, W.; Lim, D.; Low, J.; Lunny, D.; Thierry, F. HPV16 E2 is an immediate early marker of viral infection, preceding E7 expression in precursor structures of cervical carcinoma. *Canc. Res.* **2010** *70*, 5316–5325.

43. Penrose, K.J.; McBride, A.A. Proteasome-mediated degradation of the papillomavirus E2-TA protein is regulated by phosphorylation and can modulate viral genome copy number. *J. Virol.* **2000**, *74*, 6031–6038.
44. Flores, E.R.; Lambert, P.F. Evidence for a switch in the mode of human papillomavirus type 16 DNA replication during the viral life cycle. *J. Virol.* **1997**, *71*, 7167–7179.
45. Sakakibara, N.; Chen, D.; McBride, A.A. Papillomaviruses use Recombination Dependent Replication to Vegetatively Amplify their Genomes in Differentiated Cells. *PLoS Pathog.* **2013**, in press.
46. Gillespie, K.A.; Mehta, K.P.; Laimins, L.A.; Moody, C.A. Human papillomaviruses recruit cellular DNA repair and homologous recombination factors to viral replication centers. *J. Virol* **2012**, *86*, 9520–9526.
47. Moody, C.A.; Laimins, L.A. Human papillomaviruses activate the ATM DNA damage pathway for viral genome amplification upon differentiation. *PLoS Pathog.* **2009**, *5*, e1000605.
48. Fradet-Turcotte, A.; Bergeron-Labrecque, F.; Moody, C.A.; Lehoux, M.; Laimins, L.A.; Archambault, J. Nuclear accumulation of the papillomavirus E1 helicase blocks S-phase progression and triggers an ATM-dependent DNA damage response. *J. Virol.* **2011**, *85*, 8996–9012.
49. Sakakibara, N.; Mitra, R.; McBride, A.A. The papillomavirus E1 helicase activates a cellular DNA damage response in viral replication foci. *J. Virol.* **2011**, *85*, 8981–8995.
50. Reinson, T.; Toots, M.; Kadaja, M.; Pipitch, R.; Allik, M.; Ustav, E.; Ustav, M. Engagement of the ATR-dependent DNA damage response at the human papillomavirus 18 replication centers during the initial amplification. *J. Virol.* **2013**, *87*, 951–964.
51. Swindle, C.S.; Zou, N.; Van Tine, B.A.; Shaw, G.M.; Engler, J.A.; Chow, L.T. Human papillomavirus DNA replication compartments in a transient DNA replication system. *J. Virol.* **1999**, *73*, 1001–1009.
52. Van Doorslaer, K.; Tan, Q.; Xirasagar, S.; Bandaru, S.; Gopalan, V.; Mohamoud, Y.; Huyen, Y.; McBride, A.A. The Papillomavirus Episteme: A central resource for papillomavirus sequence data and analysis. *Nucleic Acids Res.* **2013**, *41*, D571–D578.
53. Li, R.; Knight, J.; Bream, G.; Stenlund, A.; Botchan, M. Specific recognition nucleotides and their DNA context determine the affinity of E2 protein for 17 binding sites in the BPV-1 genome. *Genes Dev.* **1989**, *3*, 510–526.
54. Stubenrauch, F.; Lim, H.B.; Laimins, L.A. Differential requirements for conserved E2 binding sites in the life cycle of oncogenic human papillomavirus type 31. *J. Virol.* **1998**, *72*, 1071–1077.
55. Van Doorslaer, K.; Khan, J.; Chapman, S.; McBride, A.A. Three E2 binding sites are sufficient for stable episomal maintenance of HPV18. National Institutes of Health, Bethesda, MD, USA. To be submitted for publication, 2013.
56. Dey, A.; Ellenberg, J.; Farina, A.; Coleman, A.E.; Maruyama, T.; Sciortino, S.; Lippincott-Schwartz, J.; Ozato, K. A bromodomain protein, MCAP, associates with mitotic chromosomes and affects G(2)-to-M transition. *Mol. Cell Biol.* **2000**, *20*, 6537–6549.
57. Florence, B.; Faller, D.V. You bet-cha: A novel family of transcriptional regulators. *Front. Biosci.* **2001**, *6*, D1008–D1018.

58. Houzelstein, D.; Bullock, S.L.; Lynch, D.E.; Grigorieva, E.F.; Wilson, V.A.; Beddington, R.S. Growth and early postimplantation defects in mice deficient for the bromodomain-containing protein Brd4. *Mol. Cell Biol.* **2002**, *22*, 3794–3802.
59. Dey, A.; Chitsaz, F.; Abbasi, A.; Misteli, T.; Ozato, K. The double bromodomain protein Brd4 binds to acetylated chromatin during interphase and mitosis. *Proc. Natl. Acad. Sci. USA* **2003**, *100*, 8758–8763.
60. Dey, A.; Nishiyama, A.; Karpova, T.; McNally, J.; Ozato, K. Brd4 marks select genes on mitotic chromatin and directs postmitotic transcription. *Mol. Biol. Cell* **2009**, *20*, 4899–4909.
61. Mochizuki, K.; Nishiyama, A.; Jang, M.K.; Dey, A.; Ghosh, A.; Tamura, T.; Natsume, H.; Yao, H.J.; Ozato, K. The bromodomain protein Brd4 stimulates G(1) gene transcription and promotes progression to S phase. *J. Biol. Chem.* **2008**, *283*, 9040–9048.
62. Zhao, R.; Nakamura, T.; Fu, Y.; Lazar, Z.; Spector, D.L. Gene bookmarking accelerates the kinetics of post-mitotic transcriptional re-activation. *Nat. Cell Biol.* **2011**, *13*, 1295–1304.
63. Jang, M.K.; Mochizuki, K.; Zhou, M.; Jeong, H.S.; Brady, J.N.; Ozato, K. The bromodomain protein Brd4 is a positive regulatory component of P-TEFb and stimulates RNA polymerase II-dependent transcription. *Mol. Cell* **2005**, *19*, 523–534.
64. Yang, Z.; Yik, J.H.; Chen, R.; He, N.; Jang, M.K.; Ozato, K.; Zhou, Q. Recruitment of P-TEFb for stimulation of transcriptional elongation by the bromodomain protein Brd4. *Mol. Cell* **2005**, *19*, 535–545.
65. Devaiah, B.N.; Singer, D.S. Two faces of brd4: Mitotic bookmark and transcriptional lynchpin. *Transcription* **2013**, *4*, 13–17.
66. Filippakopoulos, P.; Picaud, S.; Mangos, M.; Keates, T.; Lambert, J.P.; Barsyte-Lovejoy, D.; Felletar, I.; Volkmer, R.; Muller, S.; Pawson, T.; *et al.* Histone recognition and large-scale structural analysis of the human bromodomain family. *Cell* **2012**, *149*, 214–231.
67. Vollmuth, F.; Blankenfeldt, W.; Geyer, M. Structures of the dual bromodomains of the P-TEFb-activating protein Brd4 at atomic resolution. *J. Biol. Chem.* **2009**, *284*, 36547–36556.
68. Schröder, S.; Cho, S.; Zeng, L.; Zhang, Q.; Kaehlcke, K.; Mak, L.; Lau, J.; Bisgrove, D.; Schnölzer, M.; Verdin, E. Two-pronged binding with bromodomain-containing protein 4 liberates positive transcription elongation factor b from inactive ribonucleoprotein complexes. *J. Biol. Chem.* **2012**, *287*, 1090–1099.
69. Huang, B.; Yang, X.D.; Zhou, M.M.; Ozato, K.; Chen, L.F. Brd4 coactivates transcriptional activation of NF-kappaB via specific binding to acetylated RelA. *Mol. Cell Biol.* **2009**, *29*, 1375–1387.
70. Lin, Y.J.; Umehara, T.; Inoue, M.; Saito, K.; Kigawa, T.; Jang, M.K.; Ozato, K.; Yokoyama, S.; Padmanabhan, B.; Guntert, P. Solution structure of the extraterminal domain of the bromodomain-containing protein BRD4. *Protein Sci.* **2008**, *17*, 2174–2179.
71. Rahman, S.; Sowa, M.E.; Ottinger, M.; Smith, J.A.; Shi, Y.; Harper, J.W.; Howley, P.M. The Brd4 extraterminal domain confers transcription activation independent of pTEFb by recruiting multiple proteins, including NSD3. *Mol. Cell Biol.* **2011**, *31*, 2641–2652.

72. You, J.; Croyle, J.L.; Nishimura, A.; Ozato, K.; Howley, P.M. Interaction of the bovine papillomavirus E2 protein with Brd4 tethers the viral DNA to host mitotic chromosomes. *Cell* **2004**, *117*, 349–360.
73. Bisgrove, D.A.; Mahmoudi, T.; Henklein, P.; Verdin, E. Conserved P-TEFb-interacting domain of BRD4 inhibits HIV transcription. *Proc. Natl. Acad. Sci. USA* **2007**, *104*, 13690–13695.
74. Wu, S.Y.; Lee, A.Y.; Lai, H.T.; Zhang, H.; Chiang, C.M. Phospho switch triggers brd4 chromatin binding and activator recruitment for gene-specific targeting. *Mol. Cell* **2013**, *49*, 843–857.
75. French, C.A.; Miyoshi, I.; Aster, J.C.; Kubonishi, I.; Kroll, T.G.; Dal Cin, P.; Vargas, S.O.; Perez-Atayde, A.R.; Fletcher, J.A. BRD4 bromodomain gene rearrangement in aggressive carcinoma with translocation t(15;19). *Am. J. Pathol.* **2001**, *159*, 1987–1992.
76. Reynoird, N.; Schwartz, B.E.; Delvecchio, M.; Sadoul, K.; Meyers, D.; Mukherjee, C.; Caron, C.; Kimura, H.; Rousseaux, S.; Cole, P.A.; *et al.* Oncogenesis by sequestration of CBP/p300 in transcriptionally inactive hyperacetylated chromatin domains. *EMBO J.* **2010**, *29*, 2943–2952.
77. Filippakopoulos, P.; Qi, J.; Picaud, S.; Shen, Y.; Smith, W.B.; Fedorov, O.; Morse, E.M.; Keates, T.; Hickman, T.T.; Felletar, I.; *et al.* Selective inhibition of BET bromodomains. *Nature* **2010**, *468*, 1067–1073.
78. Schwartz, B.E.; Hofer, M.D.; Lemieux, M.E.; Bauer, D.E.; Cameron, M.J.; West, N.H.; Agoston, E.S.; Reynoird, N.; Khochbin, S.; Ince, T.A.; *et al.* Differentiation of NUT midline carcinoma by epigenomic reprogramming. *Canc. Res.* **2011**, *71*, 2686–2696.
79. Yan, J.; Diaz, J.; Jiao, J.; Wang, R.; You, J. Perturbation of BRD4 protein function by BRD4-NUT protein abrogates cellular differentiation in NUT midline carcinoma. *J. Biol. Chem.* **2011**, *286*, 27663–27675.
80. Crawford, N.P.S.; Alsarraj, J.; Lukes, L.; Walker, R.C.; Officewala, J.S.; Yang, H.H.; Lee, M.P.; Ozato, K.; Hunter, K.W. Bromodomain 4 activation predicts breast cancer survival. *Proc. Natl. Acad. Sci. USA* **2008**, *105*, 6380–6385.
81. Lockwood, W.W.; Zejnullahu, K.; Bradner, J.E.; Varmus, H. Sensitivity of human lung adenocarcinoma cell lines to targeted inhibition of BET epigenetic signaling proteins. *Proc. Natl. Acad. Sci. USA* **2012**, *109*, 19408–19413.
82. Ott, C.J.; Kopp, N.; Bird, L.; Paranal, R.M.; Qi, J.; Bowman, T.; Rodig, S.J.; Kung, A.L.; Bradner, J.E.; Weinstock, D.M. BET bromodomain inhibition targets both c-Myc and IL7R in high-risk acute lymphoblastic leukemia. *Blood* **2012**, *120*, 2843–2852.
83. Dawson, M.A.; Prinjha, R.K.; Dittmann, A.; Giotopoulos, G.; Bantscheff, M.; Chan, W.I.; Robson, S.C.; Chung, C.W.; Hopf, C.; Savitski, M.M.; *et al.* Inhibition of BET recruitment to chromatin as an effective treatment for MLL-fusion leukaemia. *Nature* **2011**, *478*, 529–533.
84. Delmore, J.E.; Issa, G.C.; Lemieux, M.E.; Rahl, P.B.; Shi, J.; Jacobs, H.M.; Kastritis, E.; Gilpatrick, T.; Paranal, R.M.; Qi, J.; *et al.* BET bromodomain inhibition as a therapeutic strategy to target c-Myc. *Cell* **2011**, *146*, 904–917.
85. Mertz, J.A.; Conery, A.R.; Bryant, B.M.; Sandy, P.; Balasubramanian, S.; Mele, D.A.; Bergeron, L.; Sims, R.J., 3rd. Targeting MYC dependence in cancer by inhibiting BET bromodomains. *Proc. Natl. Acad. Sci. USA* **2011**, *108*, 16669–16674.

86. Olejnik-Schmidt, A.K.; Schmidt, M.T.; Kedzia, W.; Gozdzicka-Jozefiak, A. Search for cellular partners of human papillomavirus type 16 E2 protein. *Arch. Virol.* **2008**, *153*, 983–990.
87. Baxter, M.K.; McPhillips, M.G.; Ozato, K.; McBride, A.A. The mitotic chromosome binding activity of the papillomavirus E2 protein correlates with interaction with the cellular chromosomal protein, Brd4. *J. Virol.* **2005**, *79*, 4806–4818.
88. Platt, G.M.; Simpson, G.R.; Mittnacht, S.; Schulz, T.F. Latent nuclear antigen of Kaposi's sarcoma-associated herpesvirus interacts with RING3, a homolog of the Drosophila female sterile homeotic (fsh) gene. *J. Virol.* **1999**, *73*, 9789–9795.
89. McPhillips, M.G.; Ozato, K.; McBride, A.A. Interaction of bovine papillomavirus E2 protein with Brd4 stabilizes its association with chromatin. *J. Virol.* **2005**, *79*, 8920–8932.
90. Lehman, C.W.; Botchan, M.R. Segregation of viral plasmids depends on tethering to chromosomes and is regulated by phosphorylation. *Proc. Natl. Acad. Sci. USA* **1998**, *95*, 4338–4343.
91. Abbate, E.A.; Voitenleitner, C.; Botchan, M.R. Structure of the papillomavirus DNA-tethering complex E2:Brd4 and a peptide that ablates HPV chromosomal association. *Mol. Cell* **2006**, *24*, 877–889.
92. McPhillips, M.G.; Oliveira, J.G.; Spindler, J.E.; Mitra, R.; McBride, A.A. Brd4 is required for e2-mediated transcriptional activation but not genome partitioning of all papillomaviruses. *J. Virol.* **2006**, *80*, 9530–9543.
93. Ottinger, M.; Christalla, T.; Nathan, K.; Brinkmann, M.M.; Viejo-Borbolla, A.; Schulz, T.F. The Kaposi's Sarcoma-Associated Herpesvirus LANA-1 interacts with the short variant of BRD4 and releases cells from a BRD4- and BRD2/RING3-induced G1 cell cycle arrest. *J. Virol.* **2006**, *80*, 10772–10786.
94. You, J.; Srinivasan, V.; Denis, G.V.; Harrington, W.J., Jr.; Ballestas, M.E.; Kaye, K.M.; Howley, P.M. Kaposi's sarcoma-associated herpesvirus latency-associated nuclear antigen interacts with bromodomain protein Brd4 on host mitotic chromosomes. *J. Virol.* **2006**, *80*, 8909–8919.
95. Lee, A.Y.; Chiang, C.M. Chromatin adaptor Brd4 modulates E2 transcription activity and protein stability. *J. Biol. Chem.* **2009**, *284*, 2778–2786.
96. Gagnon, D.; Joubert, S.; Senechal, H.; Fradet-Turcotte, A.; Torre, S.; Archambault, J. Proteasomal degradation of the papillomavirus E2 protein is inhibited by overexpression of bromodomain-containing protein 4. *J. Virol.* **2009**, *83*, 4127–4139.
97. Zheng, G.; Schweiger, M.R.; Martinez-Noel, G.; Zheng, L.; Smith, J.A.; Harper, J.W.; Howley, P.M. Brd4 regulation of papillomavirus protein E2 stability. *J. Virol.* **2009**, *83*, 8683–8692.
98. Winokur, P.L.; McBride, A.A. Separation of the transcriptional activation and replication functions of the bovine papillomavirus-1 E2 protein. *EMBO J.* **1992**, *11*, 4111–4118.
99. Sakai, H.; Yasugi, T.; Benson, J.D.; Dowhanick, J.J.; Howley, P.M. Targeted mutagenesis of the human papillomavirus type 16 E2 transactivation domain reveals separable transcriptional activation and DNA replication functions. *J. Virol.* **1996**, *70*, 1602–1611.
100. Abroi, A.; Kurg, R.; Ustav, M. Transcriptional and replicational activation functions in the BPV1 E2 protein are encoded by different structural determinants. *J. Virol.* **1996**, *70*, 6169–6179.

101. Breiding, D.E.; Grossel, M.J.; Androphy, E.J. Genetic analysis of the bovine papillomavirus E2 transcriptional activation domain. *Virology* **1996**, *221*, 34–43.
102. Ferguson, M.F.; Botchan, M.R. Genetic analysis of the activation domain of bovine papillomavirus protein E2:its role in transcription and replication. *J. Virol.* **1996**, *70*, 4193–4199.
103. Cooper, C.S.; Upmeyer, S.N.; Winokur, P.L. Identification of single amino acids in the human papillomavirus 11 E2 protein critical for the transactivation or replication functions. *Virology* **1998**, *241*, 312–322.
104. Antson, A.A.; Burns, J.E.; Moroz, O.V.; Scott, D.J.; Sanders, C.M.; Bronstein, I.B.; Dodson, G.G.; Wilson, K.S.; Maitland, N.J. Structure of the intact transactivation domain of the human papillomavirus E2 protein. *Nature* **2000**, *403*, 805–809.
105. Senechal, H.; Poirier, G.G.; Coulombe, B.; Laimins, L.A.; Archambault, J. Amino acid substitutions that specifically impair the transcriptional activity of papillomavirus E2 affect binding to the long isoform of Brd4. *Virology* **2007**, *358*, 10–17.
106. Schweiger, M.R.; You, J.; Howley, P.M. Bromodomain protein 4 mediates the papillomavirus e2 transcriptional activation function. *J. Virol.* **2006**, *80*, 4276–4285.
107. Jha, S.; Vande, P.S.; Banerjee, N.S.; Dutta, A.B.; Chow, L.T.; Dutta, A. Destabilization of TIP60 by human papillomavirus E6 results in attenuation of TIP60-dependent transcriptional regulation and apoptotic pathway. *Mol. Cell* **2010**, *38*, 700–711.
108. Kimura, A.; Horikoshi, M. Tip60 acetylates six lysines of a specific class in core histones *in vitro*. *Gene. Cell.* **1998**, *3*, 789–800.
109. Yan, J.; Li, Q.; Lievens, S.; Tavernier, J.; You, J. Abrogation of the Brd4-positive transcription elongation factor B complex by papillomavirus E2 protein contributes to viral oncogene repression. *J. Virol.* **2010**, *84*, 76–87.
110. Bechtold, V.; Beard, P.; Raj, K. Human papillomavirus type 16 E2 protein has no effect on transcription from episomal viral DNA. *J. Virol.* **2003**, *77*, 2021–2028.
111. Baxter, M.K.; McBride, A.A. An acidic amphipathic helix in the Bovine Papillomavirus E2 protein is critical for DNA replication and interaction with the E1 protein. *Virology* **2005**, *332*, 78–88.
112. Brokaw, J.L.; Blanco, M.; McBride, A.A. Amino acids critical for the functions of the bovine papillomavirus type 1 E2 transactivator. *J. Virol.* **1996**, *70*, 23–29.
113. Ilves, I.; Maemets, K.; Silla, T.; Janikson, K.; Ustav, M. Brd4 is involved in multiple processes of the bovine papillomavirus type 1 life cycle. *J. Virol.* **2006**, *80*, 3660–3665.
114. Wang, X.; Helfer, C.M.; Pancholi, N.; Bradner, J.E.; You, J. Recruitment of brd4 to the human papillomavirus type 16 DNA replication complex is essential for replication of viral DNA. *J. Virol.* **2013**, *87*, 3871–3884.
115. Sakakibara, N.; Chen, D.; Jang, M.K.; McBride, A.A. The Brd4 Chromatin Adaptor Protein is displaced from nuclear foci as the HPV E2 protein switches from Transcriptional to Replicational Modes. National Institutes of Health, Bethesda, MD, USA. Submitted for publication, 2013.
116. Stubenrauch, F.; Colbert, A.M.; Laimins, L.A. Transactivation by the E2 protein of oncogenic human papillomavirus type 31 is not essential for early and late viral functions. *J. Virol.* **1998**, *72*, 8115–8123.

117. Maruyama, T.; Farina, A.; Dey, A.; Cheong, J.; Bermudez, V.P.; Tamura, T.; Sciortino, S.; Shuman, J.; Hurwitz, J.; Ozato, K. A Mammalian bromodomain protein, Brd4, interacts with replication factor C and inhibits progression to S phase. *Mol. Cell Biol.* **2002**, *22*, 6509–6520.
118. Jang, M.K.; McBride, A.A. National Institutes of Health, Bethesda, MD, USA. Unpublished work, 2013.
119. Abroi, A.; Ilves, I.; Kivi, S.; Ustav, M. Analysis of chromatin attachment and partitioning functions of bovine papillomavirus type 1 E2 protein. *J. Virol.* **2004**, *78*, 2100–2113.
120. Cardenas-Mora, J.; Spindler, J.E.; Jang, M.K.; McBride, A.A. Dimerization of the papillomavirus E2 protein is required for efficient mitotic chromosome association and Brd4 binding. *J. Virol.* **2008**, *82*, 7298–7305.
121. You, J.; Schweiger, M.R.; Howley, P.M. Inhibition of E2 binding to Brd4 enhances viral genome loss and phenotypic reversion of bovine papillomavirus-transformed cells. *J. Virol.* **2005**, *79*, 14956–14961.
122. Brannon, A.R.; Maresca, J.A.; Boeke, J.D.; Basrai, M.A.; McBride, A.A. Reconstitution of papillomavirus E2-mediated plasmid maintenance in Saccharomyces cerevisiae by the Brd4 bromodomain protein. *Proc. Natl. Acad. Sci. USA* **2005**, *102*, 2998–3003.
123. Oliveira, J.G.; Colf, L.A.; McBride, A.A. Variations in the association of papillomavirus E2 proteins with mitotic chromosomes. *Proc. Natl. Acad. Sci. USA* **2006**, *103*, 1047–1052.
124. Poddar, A.; Reed, S.C.; McPhillips, M.G.; Spindler, J.E.; McBride, A.A. The human papillomavirus type 8 E2 tethering protein targets the ribosomal DNA loci of host mitotic chromosomes. *J. Virol.* **2009**, *83*, 640–650.
125. Sekhar, V.; Reed, S.C.; McBride, A.A. Interaction of the betapapillomavirus E2 tethering protein with mitotic chromosomes. *J. Virol.* **2010**, *84*, 543–557.
126. Sekhar, V.; McBride, A.A. Phosphorylation regulates binding of the human papillomavirus type 8 E2 protein to host chromosomes. *J. Virol.* **2012**, *86*, 10047–10058.
127. Woodard, C.; Shamay, M.; Liao, G.; Zhu, J.; Ng, A.N.; Li, R.; Newman, R.; Rho, H.S.; Hu, J.; Wan, J.; *et al.* Phosphorylation of the chromatin binding domain of KSHV LANA. *PLoS Pathog.* **2012**, *8*, e1002972.
128. McBride, A.A.; van Doorslaer, K. National Institutes of Health, Bethesda, MD, USA. Unpublished work, 2013.
129. Donaldson, M.M.; Boner, W.; Morgan, I.M. TopBP1 regulates human papillomavirus type 16 E2 interaction with chromatin. *J. Virol.* **2007**, *81*, 4338–4342.
130. Dao, L.D.; Duffy, A.; van Tine, B.A.; Wu, S.Y.; Chiang, C.M.; Broker, T.R.; Chow, L.T. Dynamic localization of the human papillomavirus type 11 origin binding protein E2 through mitosis while in association with the spindle apparatus. *J. Virol.* **2006**, *80*, 4792–4800.
131. Yu, T.; Peng, Y.C.; Androphy, E.J. Mitotic kinesin-like protein 2 binds and colocalizes with papillomavirus E2 during mitosis. *J. Virol.* **2007**, *81*, 1736–1745.
132. Parish, J.L.; Bean, A.M.; Park, R.B.; Androphy, E.J. ChlR1 is required for loading papillomavirus E2 onto mitotic chromosomes and viral genome maintenance. *Mol. Cell* **2006**, *24*, 867–876.

133. Jang, M.K.; Sakakibara, N.; McBride, A.A. Papillomavirus Genomes associate with the Cellular Protein Brd4 to replicate at Fragile Sites in the Host Genome. National Institutes of Health, Bethesda, MD, USA. Submitted for publication, 2013.

134. Silla, T.; Mannik, A.; Ustav, M. Effective formation of the segregation-competent complex determines successful partitioning of the bovine papillomavirus genome during cell division. *J. Virol.* **2010**, *84*, 11175–11188.

135. Jang, M.K.; Kwon, D.; McBride, A.A. Papillomavirus E2 proteins and the host BRD4 protein associate with transcriptionally active cellular chromatin. *J. Virol.* **2009**, *83*, 2592–2600.

136. Weidner-Glunde, M.; Ottinger, M.; Schulz, T.F. WHAT do viruses BET on? *Front. Biosci.* **2010**, *15*, 537–549.

137. Lin, A.; Wang, S.; Nguyen, T.; Shire, K.; Frappier, L. The EBNA1 protein of Epstein-Barr virus functionally interacts with Brd4. *J. Virol.* **2008**, *82*, 12009–12019.

138. Viejo-Borbolla, A.; Kati, E.; Sheldon, J.A.; Nathan, K.; Mattsson, K.; Szekely, L.; Schulz, T.F. A Domain in the C-terminal region of latency-associated nuclear antigen 1 of Kaposi's sarcoma-associated Herpesvirus affects transcriptional activation and binding to nuclear heterochromatin. *J. Virol.* **2003**, *77*, 7093–7100.

139. Wang, X.; Li, J.; Schowalter, R.M.; Jiao, J.; Buck, C.B.; You, J. Bromodomain protein Brd4 plays a key role in Merkel cell polyomavirus DNA replication. *PLoS Pathog.* **2012**, *8*, e1003021.

140. Li, Z.; Guo, J.; Wu, Y.; Zhou, Q. The BET bromodomain inhibitor JQ1 activates HIV latency through antagonizing Brd4 inhibition of Tat-transactivation. *Nucleic Acids Res.* **2013**, *41*, 277–287.

141. Boehm, D.; Calvanese, V.; Dar, R.D.; Xing, S.; Schroeder, S.; Martins, L.; Aull, K.; Li, P.C.; Planelles, V.; Bradner, J.E.; *et al.* BET bromodomain-targeting compounds reactivate HIV from latency via a Tat-independent mechanism. *Cell Cycle* **2013**, *12*, 452–462.

142. Zhu, J.; Gaiha, G.D.; John, S.P.; Pertel, T.; Chin, C.R.; Gao, G.; Qu, H.; Walker, B.D.; Elledge, S.J.; Brass, A.L. Reactivation of latent HIV-1 by inhibition of BRD4. *Cell Rep.* **2012**, *2*, 807–816.

143. Banerjee, C.; Archin, N.; Michaels, D.; Belkina, A.C.; Denis, G.V.; Bradner, J.; Sebastiani, P.; Margolis, D.M.; Montano, M. BET bromodomain inhibition as a novel strategy for reactivation of HIV-1. *J. Leukoc. Biol.* **2012**, *92*, 1147–1154.

12

Interpreting the Epstein-Barr Virus (EBV) Epigenome Using High-Throughput Data

Aaron Arvey [1], Italo Tempera [2] and Paul M. Lieberman [3,*]

[1] Memorial Sloan Kettering Cancer Center, NY, NY and Howard Hughes Medical Institute; E-Mail: aarvey@cbio.mskcc.org

[2] The Fels Cancer Institute and Department of Microbiology Temple University School of Medicine, Philadelphia, PA; E-Mail: Tempera@temple.edu

[3] The Wistar Institute Philadelphia, PA 19104; E-Mail: Lieberman@wistar.org

* Author to whom correspondence should be addressed; E-Mail: Lieberman@wistar.org (F.L.);

Abstract: The Epstein-Barr virus (EBV) double-stranded DNA genome is subject to extensive epigenetic regulation. Large consortiums and individual labs have generated a vast number of genome-wide data sets on human lymphoblastoid and other cell lines latently infected with EBV. Analysis of these data sets reveals important new information on the properties of the host and viral chromosome structure organization and epigenetic modifications. We discuss the mapping of these data sets and the subsequent insights into the chromatin structure and transcription factor binding patterns on latent EBV genomes. Colocalization of multiple histone modifications and transcription factors at regulatory loci are considered in the context of the biology and regulation of EBV.

Keywords: Epstein-Barr virus; gammaherpesvirus; chromatin; histone modification; CTCF; OriP

---

1. Introduction

Epstein-Barr virus (EBV) is a human gammaherpesvirus that establishes long-term latent infection in B-lymphocytes [2,3]. The latent infection is associated with various B-cell malignancies, including Burkitt's lymphoma, Hodgkin's disease and lymphoproliferative diseases, following immunosuppression. EBV infection can efficiently immortalize naive resting B-cells and establish long-term quasi-homogenous lymphoblastoid cell lines (LCLs). In LCLs, the majority of viral genomes adopt a gene expression program, referred to as type III latency, which represents the most permissive form of latent infection [4]. In type III latency, the complete set of viral genes required for B-cell proliferation and survival are expressed, while the viral genes required for lytic replication and virion production are repressed. The viral genomes are maintained as multicopy circular mini-chromosomes that reside in the nuclear compartment. Viral gene expression is regulated by a combination of host and viral regulatory factors, and latent replication is limited to once per cell cycle in concert with host chromosomes [5]. While most cells maintain the viral genome in a type III latent state, a percentage of cells in the population can undergo spontaneous lytic replication, and the extent of this lytic replication depends on the LCL and culture conditions [6].

To appreciate the relevance of the EBV epigenome, it is first necessary to highlight some of the major properties of the EBV genome during latency. The type III latency-associated gene expression program in LCLs consists of nine protein coding genes, 21 microRNAs and several non-coding RNAs. The protein coding genes include the Epstein-Barr Nuclear Antigens (EBNAs) EBNA-LP, 1, 2, 3a, 3b and 3c, as well as the Latency Membrane Proteins, LMP1, LMP2a and LMP2b. Two small non-coding RNAs, EBER1 and EBER2, are generated by RNA polymerase III. The miRNAs are generated from two different host transcripts from the BHRF1 or BART regions of the genome [7]. The latent genome is circularized through the joining of the terminal repeats (TRs), which generates the template for the LMP2a and LMP2b transcripts. The viral episome is maintained through the interaction of the EBNA1 proteins with the viral origin of plasmid replication (OriP), which consists of a family of repeats (FR) and a dyad symmetry (DS) element. The FR is required for maintenance through a mechanism that involves tethering to metaphase chromosomes and the DS functions as an efficient origin of bidirectional DNA replication. EBNA1 also binds to the Q promoter (Qp), which functions as an alternative promoter for expressing the EBNA1 transcript only. OriP can also function as an EBNA1-dependent transcriptional enhancer of the C promoter (Cp), which controls the transcription of a large multicistronic transcript encoding the EBNA-LP, -2, -3a, -3b, -3c and -1 genes. LMP1 transcription can initiate from the TR or from regions near the TR, and its poly A site resides in the first intron of the LMP2 transcripts that are transcribed in the opposite orientation from the complementary DNA strand of LMP1. Lytic origins of DNA replication remain mostly inactive in LCLs, but contain promoters for non-coding RNAs and miRNAs that can be generated at high levels during latency. How these genetic elements are coordinately regulated may be partly revealed through analysis of the viral epigenome.

2. Assaying the EBV Epigenome

Epigenetically regulated loci in the EBV genome can be elucidated by high-throughput sequencing data in latently infected human cell lines. Large data sets generated by labs around the world are deposited in standardized databases, such as the NCBI sequence read archive (SRA) and gene expression omnibus (GEO). The raw data can be downloaded and reanalyzed with respect to EBV by aligning the reads to EBV and subtracting any reads that map to the human genome [1]. We have developed a simple open access browser for viewing ENCODE ChIP-seq data sets mapped to the EBV genome (http://ebv.wistar.upenn.edu). The data deposited to this site include raw alignments, coverage tracks and use original accessions as filenames to ensure reproducible analysis.

Due to the small size of the EBV genome relative to the human genome, the alignment can be performed orders of magnitude faster by common tools, such as bowtie and bwa [8,9]. Interestingly, the average number of reads mapping to the viral genome tend to be an order of magnitude more than what would be expected from a randomly selected equally sized portion of the human genome given the estimated episome copy number. This suggests that the viral chromatin may be more soluble and/or amenable to sonication and enzyme digestion chromatin fragmentation.

The EBV genome contains several loci that should be interpreted with caution when using sequencing data. Regions that are seemingly depleted may in fact be regions whose copy number was overestimated (and thus, over-normalized, e.g., terminal or W repeats) or has orthologous regions in the human genome and, therefore, is unmappable (e.g., the simple repeat elements in EBNA1 and EBNA2). Furthermore, an initial challenge in any large data study is segregating the data into what is robust, spurious or artifactual. In the case of ChIP, the traditional controls of sonicated genomic DNA ("input") and non-specific IgG ChIP provide information on two independent background noises. The EBV genome has no regions that appear enriched in the input controls, indicating that the genome is fairly uniform with no genomic regions being more easily sonicated than others. However, the FR repeats are enriched in several IgG ChIP controls, which suggests that FR lacks antibody specificity and is likely to be some form of "sticky" chromatin, possibly due to its potential role as a nuclear matrix attachment region [10]. Even though FR immunoprecipitates upon non-specific IgG interrogation, it is possible that this non-specific interaction occurs *in vivo*, with many proteins genuinely binding the chromatin. However, these two scenarios cannot be disambiguated using current technologies.

Since meta-analyzing genomics experiments for EBV comes with the same caveats as analyzing data for human, it is highly recommended that all experiments be first mapped to the human genome. Quality statistics should be generated from the typically millions of mapping reads and thousands of relevant human loci instead of the typically <20 sites in the viral episome. Quality metrics include cross-strand correlation, which is an effective measure for fragment length and enrichment relative to genomic background [11] and enrichment estimates via percentage reads in peaks.

Experiment reproducibility should also be examined in both the human and EBV genomes. However, even examining biological replicates across only the EBV genome can generate an estimate of reproducibility. For instance, NF-kB experiments give widely varying peak results. In this case, only the best replicates can be selected from the human aligned data. In some cases, even when an experiment is highly reproducible in human, a low number of reads mapping to the viral episome makes one or multiple replicates unreliable; however, this has mostly ceased being a problem with the advent of deeper sequencers.

One complication of analyzing the EBV epigenome through publically available data is that most LCLs are transformed using the B95.8 genome, which contains a large deletion in the Bam HI A region that encompasses the duplicated lytic origin (OriLyt right or DSr) and many BamHI A non-coding RNAs and miRNAs [7,12]. Even though the B95.8 strain is more commonly used, all recent studies, including our own, map to the complete EBV reference genome (NC_007605). Consequently, many of the data sets fail to map to the BamHI A region and lack information on the chromatin structure and transcripts generated from this region. Nevertheless, much information exists for the remaining regulatory elements of the B95.8 genome, which functions efficiently in B-cell immortalization and maintenance of latent infection.

3. Tour of the EBV Epigenome

3.1. Overview of Chromatin Structure

In latently infected cells, the EBV genome is chromatinized with density similar to that of the host genome. Nucleosome position and histone tail modifications are strong indicators of chromatin structure and gene regulation. Micrococcal nuclease I (MNase I) and DNase I mapping studies can be used to assess the overall chromatin density and structure of viral genetic loci. For EBV, the majority of the genome is occupied by nucleosomes with varying degrees of static positioning or phasing, consistent with the dynamic nature of the viral genomes in LCL populations [13].

3.2. Histone Modifications

Mapping histone modifications across the EBV genome reveals enrichment of several marks at specific genome positions (Figure 1B). Enrichment can be assessed based on background input or IgG control DNA, as well as relative to average values for all histone modification specific ChIP assays and MNase I nucleosome density mapping [14]. Using these guidelines, histone modifications, H3K4m1, H3K4m2 and H3K4m3, are similarly enriched at the EBER-OriP-Cp locus (~7,000–13,000), the BART transcript promoter region (BARTp) (~138,500) and the LMP2-LMP1 promoter locus (~165,400–169,600). These regions represent the major sites of RNA polymerase II and III loading for type III latency transcripts. This is consistent with the established role of H3K4 methylation in transcription enhancer and promoter function, as well as sites of DNA replication [15]. Acetylated histones (H3K9ac and H3K27ac) are enriched at much sharper peaks that correlate well with sites of transcription initiation at Cp (~11,537), the BARTp (~138,563), LMP1p (~169,246) and LMP2a promoter region (~165,319).

Figure 1. Chromatin overview of the Epstein-Barr virus (EBV) epigenome. ChIP-seq in lymphoblastoid cell lines (LCLs) are mapped to the wild-type HHV4 genome for CTCF, histone variant, H2A.Z, histone modifications and RNAPII. Many colocalized modifications are sites of type III latent gene transcription, such as Cp, BARTp and the LMP locus. RNAPII tracks illustrate the heterogeneous and dynamic nature of recruitment across the viral genome.

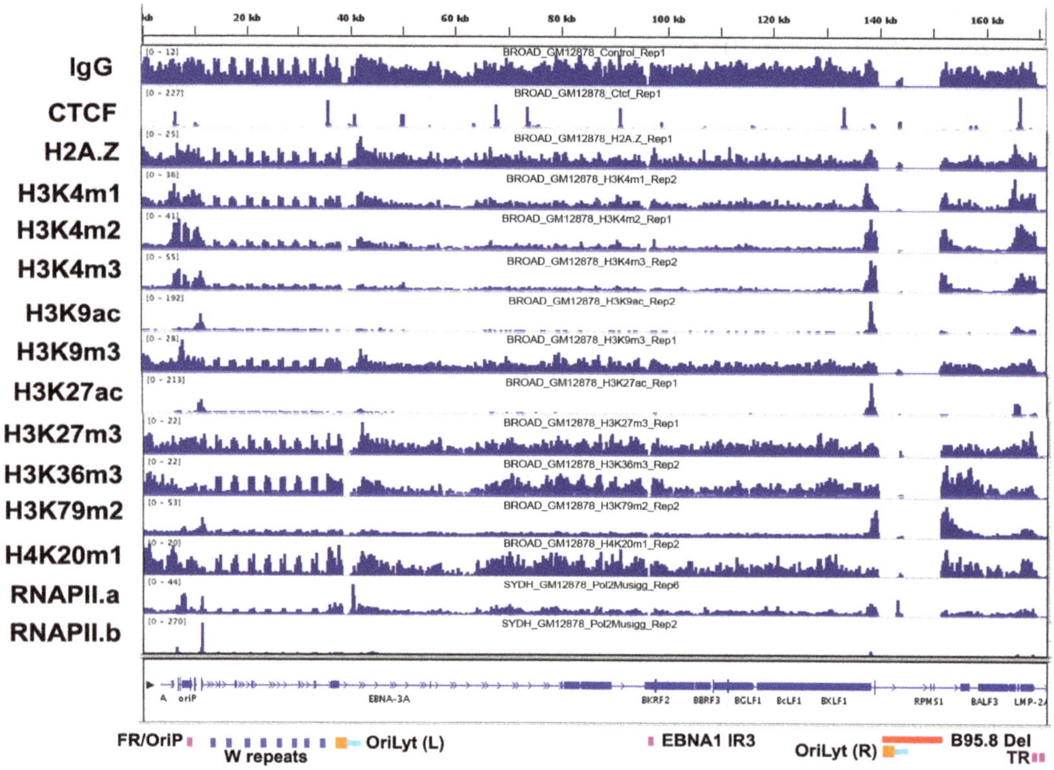

Histone modifications associated with facultative (H3K27m3) or constitutive (H3K9m3) heterochromatin appear generally low throughout the EBV genome. This may be due to the type III latency program in which most of the latent genome is transcribed. It may also be due to the partial or abortive lytic gene expression observed in some LCLs. In contrast, the latent KSHV genome has several broad peaks of H3K9m3 and bivalent K3K27m3 and H3K4m3 marks at lytic switch regulatory regions [16]. For EBV, only modestly enriched peaks for H3K27 and H3K9 trimethylation and no apparent bivalent control regions exist. The enrichment of H3K9m3 at the FR region of OriP, while very likely to be the result of sticky chromatin, since this locus also IPs with IgG, is potentially intriguing, because of colocalization with the Origin Recognition Complex (ORC), which has been implicated in H3K9 heterochromatin formation, as well as in replication origin function [17,18]. H3K27m3 is modestly elevated at the BHRF1 promoter control region (~41,852), which may regulate aspects of EBV miRNA production. H3K79m2 is found elevated at the 5' end of the Cp generated EBNA2 transcript (~11,292) and the BARTp generated BART transcripts (~139,054–155,254). H3K79m2 is conferred by the Dot1 methyltransferase, and recent studies have implicated Dot1 and

H3K79m2 in pluripotent stem cell reprogramming [19]. Additionally, Dot1 and H3K79m2 have been implicated in controlling DNA damage response during DNA replication and colocalizing with BAT3 transcription factors [20]. Each of these potential functions are worthy of further investigation at EBV regulatory elements.

3.3. CTCF and Cohesin Binding Sites

CTCF is an eleven zinc finger DNA binding protein that has been implicated in chromatin boundary function, enhancer blocking and DNA-loop formation [21,22]. CTCF ChIP-seq reveals at least 19 sites of significant enrichment in multiple replicates, each of which contains a strong CTCF binding motif. These include binding sites at ~6,559 (5' EBER-1 promoter), ~10,494 (5' of Cp), ~36,000 (5' EBNA2 ORF), ~40,792 (OriLyt between divergent promoter of BHLF1 and BHRF1), ~49,973 (5' Qp), ~67,812 (BMRF1 ORF), ~73,845 (BSLF1/BMLF1 ORF), ~91,290 (BZLF1p), 99,028 (BKRF3 ORF); 133,524 (BVRF1 ORF), 139,033 (BART intron), 143,866 (BARF1 transcript) and 166,446 (LMP2 first intron/LMP1 poly A). It is remarkable that most of these CTCF sites can be assigned to important regulatory regions of the genome. However, it is impossible to assign a single function to CTCF that explains the binding to each of these sites. Surprisingly, many CTCF binding sites are proximal to RNA polymerase regulatory elements, which is in contrast to the host genome, where the vast majority of CTCF sites are located at positions far from transcription initiation. This finding is consistent with other gammaherpesvirus studies, including those with Kaposi's sarcoma-associated herpesvirus (KSHV) multicistronic LANA-vCyclin-vFLIP transcript, that suggest CTCF regulates RNA polymerase programming [23,24]. It is also likely that some of these CTCF sites represent DNA loop junctions and inter-chromosomal linkages, as was found for the CTCF-mediated interactions between the OriP and Qp [25] or OriP and LMP1/2 region [1]. It is also worth noting that CTCF peak heights vary substantially, suggesting that some sites may be stronger or perhaps only bound to a subset of episomes.

3.4. Transcription Factor Binding Sites

EBV gene expression is regulated by mechanisms similar, if not identical, to host cell genes. Therefore, it is not surprising that many cellular transcription factors bind at multiple locations across the EBV genome (Figure 2). Transcription factor binding at known viral promoter regulatory elements is expected, and many of these interactions have been described previously. For example, PU.1 and Sp1 co-regulate Cp/Wp and LMP1 and are found colocalized at these loci and at an unanticipated site within a cluster of lytic genes (e.g., BGLF1 ORF) not expressed during latent infection. The function of PU.1/Sp1 binding at this site in latently infected LCLs is not obvious. YY1 has also been implicated in regulation of Wp and is highly enriched in at least one, possibly all, W repeats. Given the role of YY1 in polycomb-mediated chromatin regulation [26], it is tempting to speculate that the function of YY1 in these repeats is related to H3K27m3 formation and higher order chromatin organization at these internal repeats.

Figure 2. Transcription factor occupancy on the EBV epigenome. ChIP-seq tracks for various transcription factors (as indicated) were mapped from B95-8 LCLs. There is extensive colocalization at multiple loci across the genome.

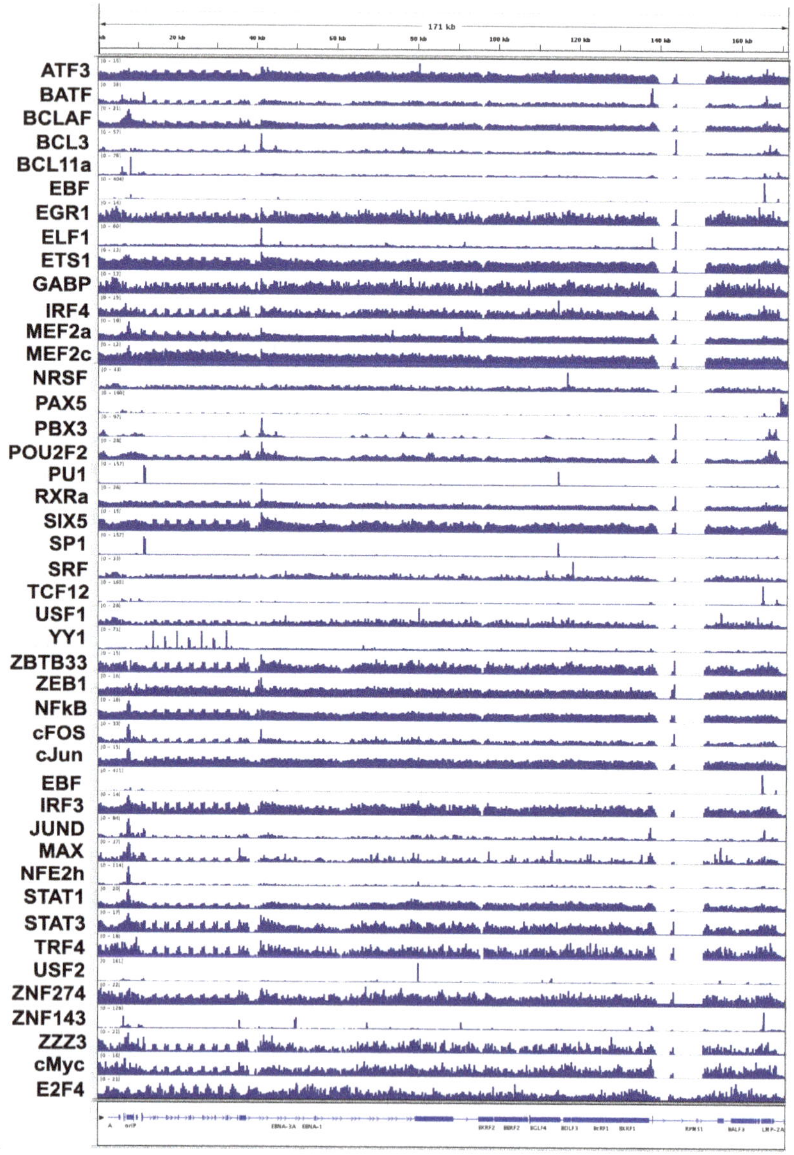

Transcription factor co-occupancy is observed at several key regulatory elements of EBV. The combination of factors at each of these sites may provide interesting new insights into signaling pathways and interactive transcription factor networks. For instance, BATF, JunD, Max and TRF4 are enriched at Cp; OriLyt-L (BHLF1/BHRF1 divergent promoter) contains binding sites for BCL3, ELF1, PBX3, POU2F2, RXRa and cFOS; and the LMP2 promoter binds TCF12, EBF, ZNF143 and JUND. Several cellular factors were found to bind to regions of the viral episome with no known regulatory functions. For example, ATF3, USF1 and USF2 show strong colocalization at ~80,655, which falls within the first internal repeat of the EBNA3A transcript. Another example is SRF and NRSF binding at 112,407, which falls near the putative promoter elements of the capsid protein

BGLF3 promoter, a lytic protein not likely to be expressed during latent infection. The colocalization of this particular subset of factors at these genetic regulatory elements suggests a partitioning of factor functions and warrants further investigation.

3.5. Co-Activator Binding Sites

Examination of non-sequence specific transcription co-activators reveals a remarkable enrichment at the OriLyt (L) or OriLyt (R) control elements (Figure 3). In particular, enrichment of GCN5, p300, BRCA1 and CHD21 occurs at the BHRF1 promoter in OriLyt, while TAFs and Pol II are enriched at the divergently transcribed BHLF1 promoter. A CTCF binding site sits between these two different regulatory elements, possibly functioning as a latent/lytic insulator. Also remarkable is that TBP was highly enriched at the EBERs, colocalizing with RNA Pol III.

Figure 3. RNA polymerases and transcriptional co-factor occupancy on the EBV genome. ChIP-seq tracks for RNA Pol III, TBP, TAFii, TAF1, RNA Pol II, GCN5, p300, SPT20, BRCA1 and CHD21 for B95-8 LCLs. EBERS oriLyt (R) and BART promoter are indicated below. B) Zoom of the OriLyt region of EBV.

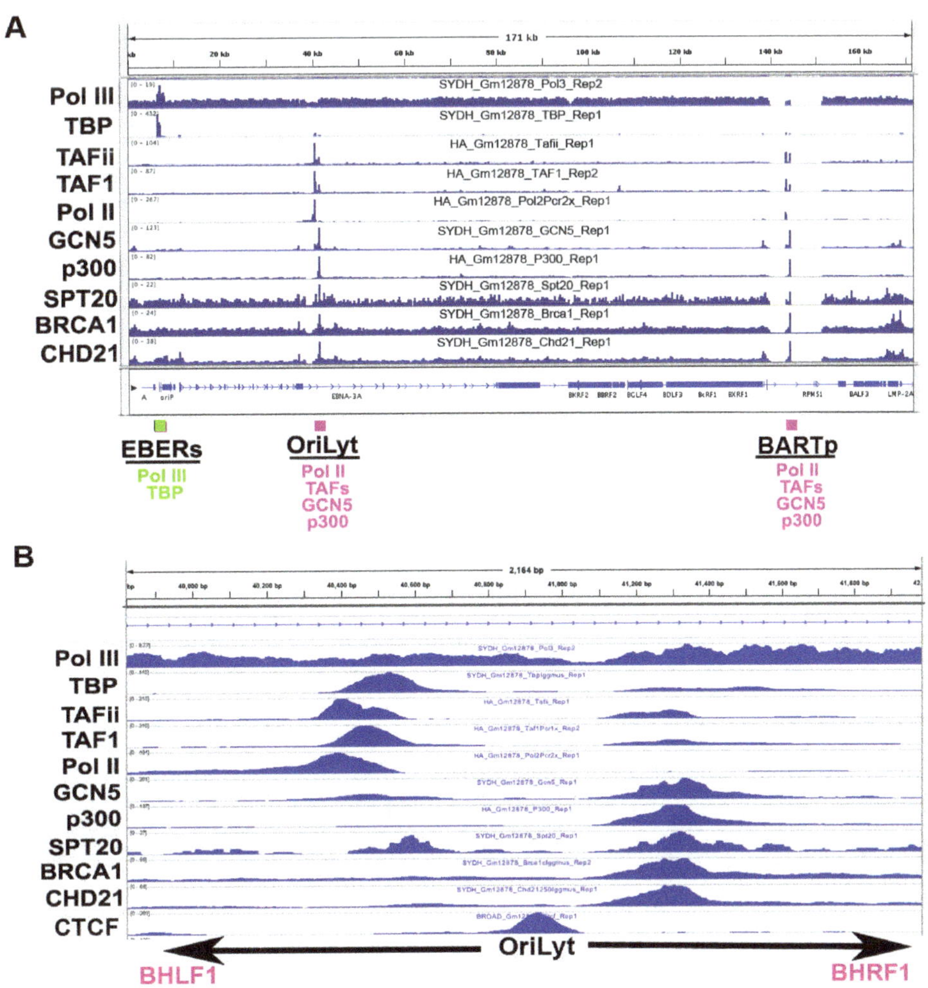

3.6. Origin of Latent Replication

The origin of latent replication (OriP) is the episomal maintenance element that can serve as an origin of DNA replication and tethers the viral genome to host metaphase chromosomes during mitosis [27,28]. As such, it is possible that some of the factors that associate with OriP may reflect close interactions of OriP with host chromosomal proteins or histone modifications. As mentioned above, OriP can function as a transcriptional enhancer for Cp and LMP1/LMP2, and recent studies have implicated CTCF and cohesins in loop formation between OriP and these promoters [1,25]. CTCF binding sites appear to bracket the entire EBER-OriP region, potentially forming a functional DNA loop for OriP enhancer mobilization and insulation of other gene activation. Examination of the epigenomic features of OriP reveals a nucleosome-free region overlapping EBNA1 binding sites at FR and DS, but a strong positioning and phasing of nucleosomes at positions flanking DS and FR (Figure 4A). Strong nucleosome position flanking DS was reported previously using conventional methods [29]. The epigenetic modification of these nucleosomes are not clear, since H3K4m3 was reported to be elevated, but has significantly higher peaks at regions 5' to FR and overlapping EBER transcripts. H2A.Z appears to be enriched at these positions, but the relative enrichment is modest.

As mentioned above, several transcription factors colocalize at OriP. Previous studies have shown that Oct2 (Pou2F2) can bind to FR, and ENCODE ChIP-seq shows strong enrichment of Pou2F2 at FR (Figure 4B). A number of other factors show ChIP-seq signal at FR (e.g., BCLAF, BCL11a, NFE2h, cFos, RNA Pol III and others); however, this region is also elevated in non-specific IgG immunoprecipitation. BCL11a showed a more discrete peak that overlapped with the Oct2 binding site, suggesting that this may reflect-specific binding. As noted above, the relative enrichment of IgG at the FR complicates interpretation of ChIP-Seq data and may reflect important physical features of OriP, including nuclear matrix attachment [10].

3.7. DNA Methylation

DNA methylation contributes to the balance of limiting gene expression and avoiding immune detection during latency, while establishing a landscape that can be overcome during lytic reactivation to express the >70 gene products involved in replication. The EBV genome packaged in virions is unmethylated and gradually becomes methylated by host factors during initial cellular infection. Genome-wide analysis of methylated CpG levels in the EBV genome has revealed that the origin of plasmid replication OriP, the Cp and the Qp promoters, and the region for the noncoding RNA EBERS lack significant levels of DNA methylation in lymphoblastoid cell lines during latency [30,31]. Interestingly, CTCF demarcates the boundaries of unmethylated high CpG frequency regions in EBV, and at least in the case of the Qp and Cp, the loss of CTCF binding alters the functionality of these regions [31,32]. Highly methylated loci inhibit the transition from the latent to lytic phase; however, the Zta transcription factor selectively activates methylated promoters of lytic genes, including genes encoding for the viral helicase, the DNA polymerase and the DNA polymerase processivity factor [33, 34].

Figure 4. Histone modifications and transcription factor occupancy at OriP. (**A**) MNase I seq analysis for MutuI (type I latent lymphoma cell line) and MutuLCL (type III latent LCL using the same viral strain as MutuI), showing nucleosome depletion at the EBNA1 binding sites in DS. (**B**) ChIP-seq for CTCF, H2A.Z, histone modifications and EBNA1 binding at OriP region. (**C**) ChIP-seq tracks for transcription factors CTCF, POU2F2, BCL11a, BCLAF, cFOS, NFE2h, RNA Pol III, TBP, ZNF143 and EBNA1 at the OriP region.

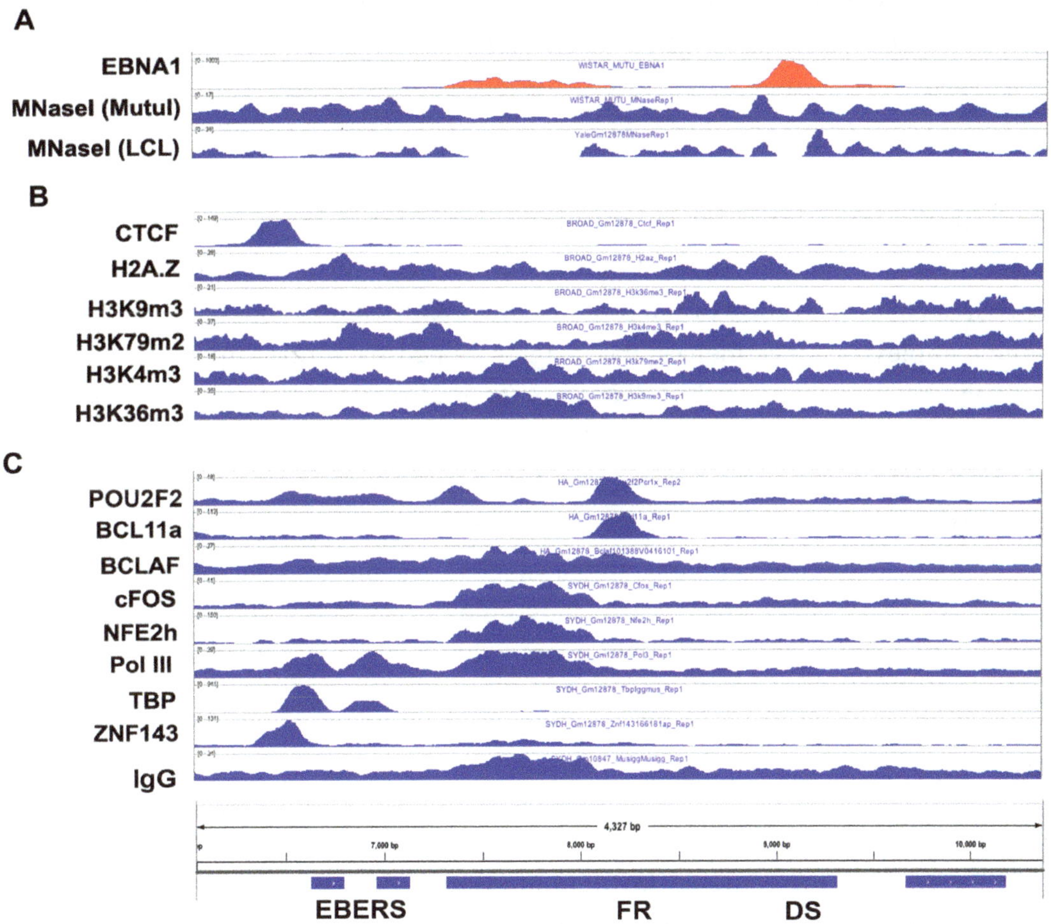

3.8. Negative Results

Through meta-analysis, it is possible to discover and observe many phenomena; however, just as notable are the phenomena that are not observed. While negative results are typically not formally reported, they can be accrued in unbiased databases of experiments mapped to the viral genome [1]. For instance, of the 68 transcriptional regulators previously examined, only 26 have had reproducible binding sites in the EBV genome. While some of the 42 TFs may bind the viral genome, possibly with lower affinity, it seems more likely that the majority of host transcriptional regulators do not physically interact with the viral episome. Furthermore, repressive histone modifications, such as H3K27me3, are largely absent from the viral genome (or at the very least, had no spatial enrichment, meaning that if H3K27me3 is present on viral nucleosomes, the modification lacks spatial regulatory specificity).

Previously identified regulatory interactions are largely confirmed in high throughput analyses. However, a small subset of experiments yielded surprising negative results. For instance, NF-kB binding at LMP1p was either weak or non-existent. Additionally, ZEB1 binding to Zp could not be confirmed. In both of these examples, it was crucial that positive controls in the viral and host genomes were provided. Importantly, the ChIP-seq methods are only semi-quantitative, and observed peaks of significant interest need to be validated by conventional ChIP and qPCR methods, which have been performed at only a small subset of these sites.

4. Conclusions

The EBV epigenome, as revealed by data mining, reflects only a small fraction of the protein interactions and histone modifications that define the viral chromosome. It is certainly not a complete nor comprehensive characterization of the proteins and modifications that regulate the EBV genome in all its dynamic complexity. Nevertheless, the insights gained from this "tip of the iceberg" glimpse of the EBV epigenome suggest that this discovery approach can reveal many new and previously unanticipated regulatory features of viral-host interactions, gene regulation and chromosome organization. Many of the observations discussed in this review need to be experimentally validated and further characterized to fully assess their functional significance. However, these observations indicate that "omics" dissection of viral and host gene regulation can generate new concepts and hypotheses and a deeper understanding of how the viral and cellular genomes persist during latent infection.

Acknowledgments

This work was supported by grants from NIH CA085678, CA093606 and DE017336 to PML and a K99AI099153 award from the National Institute of Allergy And Infectious Diseases to IT. We thank Louise Showe and Priyankara Wikramasinghe from the Wistar Institute Genomics and Bioinformatics facilities and the support of the Wistar Institute Cancer Center Core grant P30 CA10815. We also thank Chris Wawak and Joanne Edington for technical support.

References

1. Arvey, A.; Tempera, I.; Tsai, K.; Chen, H.S.; Tikhmyanova, N.; Klichinsky, M.; Leslie, C.; Lieberman, P.M. An atlas of the epstein-barr virus transcriptome and epigenome reveals host-virus regulatory interactions. *Cell. Host. Microbe.* **2012**, *12*, 233–245.

2. Kieff, E. *Epstein-Barr Virus and its replication.* 5th ed.; Wolters Kluwer Health/Lippincott Williams & Wilkins: Philadelphia, 2007; p 2 v. (xix, 3091, 86 p.).
3. Rickinson, A. B., and Kieff, E., *Epstein-Barr Virus.* 5th ed.; Wolters Kluwer Health/Lippincott Williams & Wilkins: Philadelphia, 2007; p 2 v. (xix, 3091, 86 p.).
4. Rowe, M.; Lear, A.L.; Croom-Carter, D.; Davies, A.H.; Rickinson, A.B. Three pathways of Epstein-Barr virus gene activation from EBNA1-positive latency in B lymphocytes. *J. Virol.* **1992**, *66*, 122–131.
5. Yates, J.L.; Guan, N. Epstein-Barr virus-derived plasmids replicate only once per cell cycle and are not amplified after entry into cells. *J. Virol.* **1991**, *65*, 483–488.
6. Amon, W.; Farrell, P.J. Reactivation of Epstein-Barr virus from latency. *Rev. Med. Virol.* **2005**, *15*, 149–156.
7. Cai, X.; Schafer, A.; Lu, S.; Bilello, J.P.; Desrosiers, R.C.; Edwards, R.; Raab-Traub, N.; Cullen, B.R. Epstein-Barr virus microRNAs are evolutionarily conserved and differentially expressed. *PLoS Pathog.* **2006**, *2*, e23.
8. Li, H.; Durbin, R. Fast and accurate short read alignment with Burrows-Wheeler transform. *Bioinformatics* **2009**, *25*, 1754–1760.
9. Langmead, B.; Trapnell, C.; Pop, M.; Salzberg, S.L. Ultrafast and memory-efficient alignment of short DNA sequences to the human genome. *Genome. Biol.* **2009**, *10*, R25.
10. Jankelevich, S.; Kolman, J.L.; Bodnar, J.W.; Miller, G. A nuclear matrix attachment region organizes the Epstein-Barr viral plasmid in Raji cells into a single DNA domain. *EMBO J.* **1992**, *11*, 1165–1176.
11. Kundaje, A.; Kyriazopoulou-Panagiotopoulou, S.; Libbrecht, M.; Smith, C.L.; Raha, D.; Winters, E.E.; Johnson, S.M.; Snyder, M.; Batzoglou, S.; Sidow, A. Ubiquitous heterogeneity and asymmetry of the chromatin environment at regulatory elements. *Genome. Res.* **2012**, *22*, 1735–1747.
12. Baer, R.; Bankier, A.T.; Biggin, M.D.; Deininger, P.L.; Farrell, P.J.; Gibson, T.J.; Hatfull, G.; Hudson, G.S.; Satchwell, S.C.; Seguin, C.; *et al.* DNA sequence and expression of the B95-8 Epstein-Barr virus genome. *Nature* **1984**, *310*, 207–211.
13. Dyson, P.J.; Farrell, P.J. Chromatin structure of Esptein-Barr virus. *J. Gen. Virol.* **1985**, *66*, 1931–1940.
14. Pepke, S.; Wold, B.; Mortazavi, A. Computation for ChIP-seq and RNA-seq studies. *Nat. Methods* **2009**, *6*, 22–32.
15. Shilatifard, A. Molecular implementation and physiological roles for histone H3 lysine 4 (H3K4) methylation. *Curr. Opin. Cell. Biol.* **2008**, *20*, 341–348.
16. Toth, Z.; Maglinte, D.T.; Lee, S.H.; Lee, H.R.; Wong, L.Y.; Brulois, K.F.; Lee, S.; Buckley, J.D.; Laird, P.W.; Marquez, V.E.; Jung, J.U. Epigenetic analysis of KSHV latent and lytic genomes. *PLoS Pathog.* **2010**, *6*, e1001013.
17. Prasanth, S.G.; Shen, Z.; Prasanth, K.V.; Stillman, B. Human origin recognition complex is essential for HP1 binding to chromatin and heterochromatin organization. *Proc. Natl. Acad. Sci. USA* **2010** *107*, 15093–15098.

18. Chakraborty, A.; Shen, Z.; Prasanth, S.G. "ORCanization" on heterochromatin: linking DNA replication initiation to chromatin organization. *Epigenetics* **2011**, *6*, 665–670.
19. Onder, T.T.; Kara, N.; Cherry, A.; Sinha, A.U.; Zhu, N.; Bernt, K.M.; Cahan, P.; Marcarci, B.O.; Unternaehrer, J.; Gupta, P.B.; *et al.* Chromatin-modifying enzymes as modulators of reprogramming. *Nature* **2012**, *483*, 598–602.
20. Wakeman, T.P.; Wang, Q.; Feng, J.; Wang, X.F. Bat3 facilitates H3K79 dimethylation by DOT1L and promotes DNA damage-induced 53BP1 foci at G1/G2 cell-cycle phases. *EMBO J.* **2012**, *31*, 2169–2181.
21. Phillips, J.E.; Corces, V.G. CTCF: Master weaver of the genome. *Cell* **2009**, *137*, 1194–1211.
22. Ohlsson, R.; Lobanenkov, V.; Klenova, E. Does CTCF mediate between nuclear organization and gene expression? *Bioessays* **2010**, *32*, 37-50.
23. Kang, H.; Wiedmer, A.; Yuan, Y.; Robertson, E.; Lieberman, P.M. Coordination of KSHV latent and lytic gene control by CTCF-cohesin mediated chromosome conformation. *PLoS Pathog.* **2011**, *7*, e1002140.
24. Kang, H.; Lieberman, P.M. Mechanism of Glycyrrhizic Acid Inhibition of Kaposi's Sarcoma-Associated Herpesvirus: Disruption of CTCF-Cohesin-Mediated RNA Polymerase II Pausing and Sister Chromatid Cohesion. *J. Virol.* **2011**, *85*, 11159–11169.
25. Tempera, I.; Klichinsky, M.; Lieberman, P.M. EBV latency types adopt alternative chromatin conformations. *PLoS Pathog.* **2011**, *7*, e1002180.
26. Atchison, M.; Basu, A.; Zaprazna, K.; Papasani, M. Mechanisms of Yin Yang 1 in oncogenesis: the importance of indirect effects. *Crit. Rev. Oncog.* **2012**, *16*, 143–161.
27. Wang, J.; Sugden, B. Origins of bidirectional replication of Epstein-Barr virus: Models for understanding mammalian origins of DNA synthesis. *J. Cell. Biochem.* **2005**, *94*, 247–256.
28. Lindner, S.E.; Sugden, B. The plasmid replicon of Epstein-Barr virus: mechanistic insights into efficient, licensed, extrachromosomal replication in human cells. *Plasmid.* **2007**, *58*, 1–12.
29. Zhou, J.; Chau, C.M.; Deng, Z.; Shiekhattar, R.; Spindler, M.P.; Schepers, A.; Lieberman, P.M. Cell cycle regulation of chromatin at an origin of DNA replication. *Embo J.* **2005**, *24*, 1406–1417.
30. Kalla, M.; Hammerschmidt, W. Human B cells on their route to latent infection--early but transient expression of lytic genes of Epstein-Barr virus. *Eur. J. Cell. Biol.* **2011**, *91*, 65-69.
31. Tempera, I.; Wiedmer, A.; Dheekollu, J.; Lieberman, P.M. CTCF prevents the epigenetic drift of EBV latency promoter Qp. *PLoS Pathog.* **2010**, *6*, e1001048.
32. Hughes, D.J.; Marendy, E.M.; Dickerson, C.A.; Yetming, K.D.; Sample, C.E.; Sample, J.T. Contributions of CTCF and DNA methyltransferases DNMT1 and DNMT3B to Epstein-Barr virus restricted latency. *J. Virol.* **2011**, *86*, 1034–1045.
33. Bergbauer, M.; Kalla, M.; Schmeinck, A.; Gobel, C.; Rothbauer, U.; Eck, S.; Benet-Pages, A.; Strom, T.M.; Hammerschmidt, W. CpG-methylation regulates a class of Epstein-Barr virus promoters. *PLoS Pathog.* **2010**, *6*, 1001114.
34. Ramasubramanyan, S.; Kanhere, A.; Osborn, K.; Flower, K.; Jenner, R.G.; Sinclair, A.J. Genome-Wide Analyses of Zta Binding to the Epstein-Barr Virus Genome Reveals Interactions in both Early and Late Lytic Cycles and an Epigenetic Switch Leading to an Altered Binding Profile. *J. Virol.* **2012**, *86*, 12494–12502.

Permissions

All chapters in this book were first published by MDPI; hereby published with permission under the Creative Commons Attribution License or equivalent. Every chapter published in this book has been scrutinized by our experts. Their significance has been extensively debated. The topics covered herein carry significant findings which will fuel the growth of the discipline. They may even be implemented as practical applications or may be referred to as a beginning point for another development.

The contributors of this book come from diverse backgrounds, making this book a truly international effort. This book will bring forth new frontiers with its revolutionizing research information and detailed analysis of the nascent developments around the world.

We would like to thank all the contributing authors for lending their expertise to make the book truly unique. They have played a crucial role in the development of this book. Without their invaluable contributions this book wouldn't have been possible. They have made vital efforts to compile up to date information on the varied aspects of this subject to make this book a valuable addition to the collection of many professionals and students.

This book was conceptualized with the vision of imparting up-to-date information and advanced data in this field. To ensure the same, a matchless editorial board was set up. Every individual on the board went through rigorous rounds of assessment to prove their worth. After which they invested a large part of their time researching and compiling the most relevant data for our readers.

The editorial board has been involved in producing this book since its inception. They have spent rigorous hours researching and exploring the diverse topics which have resulted in the successful publishing of this book. They have passed on their knowledge of decades through this book. To expedite this challenging task, the publisher supported the team at every step. A small team of assistant editors was also appointed to further simplify the editing procedure and attain best results for the readers.

Apart from the editorial board, the designing team has also invested a significant amount of their time in understanding the subject and creating the most relevant covers. They scrutinized every image to scout for the most suitable representation of the subject and create an appropriate cover for the book.

The publishing team has been an ardent support to the editorial, designing and production team. Their endless efforts to recruit the best for this project, has resulted in the accomplishment of this book. They are a veteran in the field of academics and their pool of knowledge is as vast as their experience in printing. Their expertise and guidance has proved useful at every step. Their uncompromising quality standards have made this book an exceptional effort. Their encouragement from time to time has been an inspiration for everyone.

The publisher and the editorial board hope that this book will prove to be a valuable piece of knowledge for researchers, students, practitioners and scholars across the globe.

List of Contributors

Luis M. Agosto
Department of Medicine, Boston University School of Medicine, Boston, MA 02118, USA

Matthew Gagne
Graduate Program in Microbiology, Boston University School of Medicine, Boston, MA 02118, USA

Andrew J. Henderson
Department of Medicine, Boston University School of Medicine, Boston, MA 02118, USA
Graduate Program in Microbiology, Boston University School of Medicine, Boston, MA 02118, USA

Timsy Uppal and Subhash C. Verma
Department of Microbiology and Immunology, School of Medicine, University of Nevada, 1664 N Virginia Street, MS 320, Reno, NV 89557, USA

Hem C. Jha and Erle S. Robertson
Department of Microbiology and the Tumor Virology Program of the Abramson Cancer Center, Perelman School of Medicine at the University of Pennsylvania, 201E Johnson Pavilion, 3610 Hamilton Walk, Philadelphia, PA 19104, USA

Amanda J. Guise, Hanna G. Budayeva, Benjamin A. Diner and Ileana M. Cristea
Department of Molecular Biology, Princeton University, Washington Road, Princeton, NJ 08544, USA

Jessica N. Groen
School of Biotechnology and Biomolecular Sciences, The University of New South Wales, Sydney, NSW 2052, Australia

Kevin V. Morris
School of Biotechnology and Biomolecular Sciences, The University of New South Wales, Sydney, NSW 2052, Australia
Department of Molecular and Experimental Medicine, The Scripps Research Institute, La Jolla, CA 92037, USA

Margaret E. McLaughlin-Drubin and Karl Munger
Division of Infectious Diseases, Brigham and Women's Hospital and Department of Medicine, Harvard Medical School, 181 Longwood Avenue, MCP 861, Boston, MA 02115, USA

Daniela Boehm Ryan J. Conrad and Melanie Ott
Gladstone Institute of Virology and Immunology, San Francisco, CA 94158, USA
Department of Medicine, University of California, San Francisco, CA 94158, USA

Zsolt Toth, Kevin Brulois and Jae U. Jung
Department of Molecular Microbiology and Immunology, Keck School of Medicine, University of Southern California, Harlyne J. Norris Cancer Research Tower, 1450 Biggy Street, Los Angeles, CA 90033, USA

Matthew Reeves and John Sinclair
Department of Medicine, University of Cambridge, Addenbrooke's Hospital, Hills Road, Cambridge, CB2 0QQ, UK

Ourania M. Andrisani
Department of Basic Medical Science and Center for Cancer Research, Purdue University West Lafayette, IN 47907, USA

Carmen M. Wong, Emily R. McFall and Joseph K. Burns
Regenerative Medicine Program, Ottawa Hospital Research Institute, Ottawa, Ontario, K1H 8L6, Canada
Department of Biochemistry, Microbiology and Immunology, University of Ottawa, Ottawa, Ontario K1H 8M5, Canada

Robin J. Parks
Regenerative Medicine Program, Ottawa Hospital Research Institute, Ottawa, Ontario, K1H 8L6, Canada
Department of Biochemistry, Microbiology and Immunology, University of Ottawa, Ottawa, Ontario K1H 8M5, Canada
Department of Medicine, University of Ottawa, Ottawa, Ontario K1H 8M5, Canada

Alison A. McBride and Moon Kyoo Jang
Laboratory of Viral Diseases, National Institute of Allergy and Infectious Diseases, National Institutes of Health, Bethesda, MD 20892, USA

Aaron Arvey
Memorial Sloan Kettering Cancer Center, NY, USA
NY and Howard Hughes Medical Institute, USA

Italo Tempera
The Fels Cancer Institute and Department of Microbiology Temple University School of Medicine, Philadelphia, PA, USA

Paul M. Lieberman
The Wistar Institute Philadelphia, PA, USA

Index

Printed in the USA
CPSIA information can be obtained
at www.ICGtesting.com
LVHW080036211023
761596LV00010BA/1787

9 781639 877874